Essential Haematology

Essential Haematology

A.V. Hoffbrand MA DM FRCP
FRCPath FRCP(Edin) DSc
Professor of Haematology, Royal Free Hospital
and School of Medicine, London

J.E. Pettit MD FRCPA FRCPath
Director and Haematologist, Medlab South,
Christchurch, New Zealand

Third Edition

**Blackwell
Science**

© 1980, 1984, 1993 by
Blackwell Science Ltd
Editorial Offices:
Osney Mead, Oxford OX2 0EL
25 John Street, London WC1N 2BL
23 Ainslie Place, Edinburgh EH3 6AJ
350 Main Street, Malden
 MA 02148 5018, USA
54 University Street, Carlton
 Victoria 3053, Australia
10, rue Casimir Delavigne
 75006 Paris, France

Other Editorial Offices:
Blackwell Wissenschafts-Verlag GmbH
Kurfürstendamm 57
10707 Berlin, Germany

Blackwell Science KK
MG Kodenmacho Building
7–10 Kodenmacho Nihombashi
Chuo-ku, Tokyo 104, Japan

First published 1980
Reprinted 1981, 1982, 1983 (twice)
Second edition 1984
Reprinted 1985
Reprinted with corrections 1985, 1988 (twice),
 1989
German edition 1986
Japenese edition 1986
Spanish edition 1987 (reprinted twice)
Indonesian edition 1987
Third edition 1993
Four Dragons edition 1993
Reprinted with corrections 1993, 1994, 1995,
 1996, 1997, 1998, 1999, 2000

DISTRIBUTORS

Marston Book Services Ltd
PO Box 269
Abingdon, Oxon OX14 4YN
(*Orders*: Tel: 01235 465500
        Fax: 01235 465555)

USA
Blackwell Science, Inc.
Commerce Place
350 Main Street
Malden, MA 02148 5018
(*Orders*: Tel: 800 759 6102
        781 388 8250
      Fax: 781 388 8255)

Canada
Login Brothers Book Company
324 Saulteaux Crescent
Winnipeg, Manitoba R3J 3T2
(*Orders*: Tel: 204 837-2987)

Australia
Blackwell Science Pty Ltd
54 University Street
Carlton, Victoria 3053
(*Orders*: Tel: 3 9347 0300
        Fax: 3 9347 5001)

A catalogue record for this title
is available from the British Library

ISBN 0-632-01954-9 (BSL)
ISBN 0-632-03083-6 (IE)

Set by Setrite Typesetters Ltd, Hong Kong
Printed and bound in Italy by Vincenzo
Bona, srl, Turin

The Blackwell Science logo is a
trade mark of Blackwell Science Ltd,
registered at the United Kingdom
Trade Marks Registry

For further information on
Blackwell Science, visit our website:
www.blackwell-science.com

Contents

Preface to Third Edition, vii

Preface to First Edition, viii

Bibliography, ix

1 Blood Cell Formation (Haemopoiesis), 1

2 Erythropoiesis and General Aspects of Anaemia, 12

3 Iron Deficiency and Other Hypochromic Anaemias, 36

4 Megaloblastic Anaemias and Other Macrocytic Anaemias, 53

5 Haemolytic Anaemias, 74

6 Genetic Defects of Haemoglobin, 94

7 Aplastic Anaemia and Bone Marrow Transplantation, 121

8 The White Cells 1: Granulocytes, Monocytes and their Benign Disorders, 141

9 The White Cells 2: Lymphocytes and their Benign Disorders, 161

10 Haematological Malignancies: General Aspects, 186

11 Acute Leukaemias, 209

12 Chronic Leukaemias and Myelodysplastic Syndromes, 232

13 Malignant Lymphomas, 251

14 Multiple Myeloma and Related Disorders, 272

15 Myeloproliferative Disorders, 286

16 Platelets, Blood Coagulation and Haemostasis, 299

17 Bleeding Disorders due to Vascular and Platelet Abnormalities, 318

18 Coagulation Disorders, 332

19 Thrombosis and Antithrombotic Therapy, 350

20 Haematological Changes in Systemic Disease, 366

21 Blood Transfusion, 392

    Appendices
 1 Recognized HLA Specificities, 416
 2 Principal Features of Known Cluster Differentiation
    Molecules, 417
 3 Normal Values, 419

    Glossary of Molecular Genetics, 420

    Index, 425

Preface to Third Edition

In the 8 years since the publication of the previous edition of *Essential Haematology* there have been great advances in molecular biology. These have had a major impact on the understanding of normal physiological processes and the basis of disease within the field of haematology. It has proved a difficult task, therefore, in writing this third edition to maintain the size and style of the previous editions. The authors appreciate that the scope of this book is now beyond that strictly required by an undergraduate course, but we feel that the extra information is necessary for an understanding of this broad and scientifically advanced subject. The sections on haemopoiesis, genetic defects of haemoglobin, antenatal diagnosis, leucocytes, leukaemias, haemostasis and blood transfusion, in particular, have been expanded to incorporate this new knowledge. Advances in therapy (such as the use of haemopoietic growth factors), broadening indications for allogeneic and autologous bone marrow transplantation, and the use of thrombolytic agents have also been incorporated. We have attempted to reflect the relative frequency of diseases more equitably by increasing the space allotted to such topics as the blood in systemic diseases, AIDS, myelodysplasia and thrombosis, as compared with rarer entities.

New figures and tables appear in all chapters, and most illustrations are now in colour. The authors and publishers are grateful to Gower Medical Publishing for use of the following figures from *Sandoz Atlas of Clinical Haematology* (Hoffbrand & Pettit, 1988): 2.14a−b, 2.15, 3.4a−c, 4.6, 4.7, 4.8, 5.4b, 6.4, 6.11, 6.21, 7.2, 8.7, 8.8f, 9.6, 9.7, 9.8, 10.4a, 10.7, 11.10, 12.10a, 13.9a−c, 13.14, 14.6d, 14.7a−b, 15.3a, 18.3, 18.4, 20.6, 20.7a, 20.10a−b, 20.12c and 21.1; and to Mosby-Wolfe for Fig. 16.6 redrawn from *Color Atlas of Clinical Hematology* (Hoffbrand & Pettit, 1994).

We are grateful to P. Amlot, M.K. Brenner, M. Contreras, J.F. Hancock, G. Hazelhurst, D.S.C. Huang, R.A. Hutton, C.A. Lee, D.L. Linch, A. Lubenko, A.B. Mehta, K.J. Pasi, H.G. Prentice, L. Secker-Walker, E.G.D. Tuddenham, D.J. Weatherall, B. Wonke, M.E. Wood and R.G. Wickremasinghe for reviewing various sections of the manuscript, Mrs Charlotte Huang and Mrs Maria Evans for typing and retyping the text, and to our publishers.

AVH, JEP

Note to the corrected reprint For this new printing of the third edition we have indicated by a red vertical line in the margin those sections of the text which we consider less 'essential' for undergraduate medical students approaching their final examination.

Preface to First Edition

The major changes that have occurred in all fields of medicine over the last decade have been accompanied by an increased understanding of the biochemical, physiological and immuno-logical processes involved in normal blood cell formation and function and the disturbances that may occur in different diseases. At the same time, the range of treatment available for patients with diseases of the blood and blood-forming organs has widened and improved substantially as understanding of the disease processes has increased and new drugs and means of support care have been introduced.

We hope the present book will enable the medical student of the 1980s to grasp the essential features of modern clinical and laboratory haematology and to achieve an understanding of how many of the manifestations of blood diseases can be explained with this new knowledge of the disease processes.

We would like to thank many colleagues and assistants who have helped with the preparation of the book. In particular, Dr H.G. Prentice cared for the patients whose haematological responses are illustrated in Figs 5.3 and 7.8 and Dr J. McLaughlin supplied Fig. 8.6. Dr S. Knowles reviewed critically the final manuscript and made many helpful suggestions. Any remaining errors are, however, our own. We also thank Mr J.B. Irwin and R.W. McPhee who drew many excellent diagrams, Mr Cedric Gilson for expert photomicrography, Mrs T. Charalambos, Mrs B. Elliot, Mrs M. Evans and Miss J. Allaway for typing the manuscript, and Mr Jony Russell of Blackwell Scientific Publications for his invaluable help and patience.

AVH, JEP

Bibliography

Alter B.P. (ed.) (1990) *Perinatal Hematology*. Methods in Haematology, Vol. 21. Churchill Livingstone, Edinburgh.

Babior B.M. & Stossel T.P. (1989) *Haematology: A Pathophysiologic Approach*. Churchill Livingstone, New York.

Bain B. (1989) *Blood Cells: A Practical Guide*. Gower Medical Publishing, London.

Bain B., Clark D.M. & Lampert I.A. (1992) *Bone Marrow Pathology*. Blackwell Scientific Publications, Oxford.

Bick R.L., Bennett J.M., Byrnes R.K., Cline M.J., Kass L., Shohet S.B. & Ward P.C.J. (1992) *Hematology. Clinical and Laboratory Practice*. C.V. Mosby, St Louis.

Brain M.C. & Carbone P.P. (eds) (1992) *Current Therapy in Hematology–Oncology*, 4th Edition. B.C. Decker, Philadelphia.

Chanarin I. (ed.) (1989) *Laboratory Haematology: An Account of Laboratory Techniques*. Churchill Livingstone, Edinburgh.

Dacie J.V. & Lewis S.M. (eds) (1991) *Practical Haematology*, 6th Edition, Churchill Livingstone, Edinburgh.

Erslev A.J. & Gabuzda F. (1985) *Pathophysiology of Blood*, 3rd Edition. W.B. Saunders, Philadelphia.

Firkin F., Chesterman N., Penington D. & Rush B. (1989) *De Gruchy's Clinical Haematology in Medical Practice*, 5th Edition. Blackwell Scientific Publications, Oxford.

Hann I.M. & Letzky E. (1991) *Fetal and Neonatal Haematology*, Baillière Tindall, London.

Hann I.M., Rankin A., Lake B.D. & Pritchard J. (1990) *Colour Atlas of Paediatric Haematology*, 2nd Edition. Oxford Medical Publications, Oxford.

Hoffbrand A.V. (ed.) (1988) *Recent Advances in Haematology*, 5. Churchill Livingstone, Edinburgh.

Hoffbrand A.V. & Brenner M.K. (1992) *Recent Advances in Haematology*, 6. Churchill Livingstone, Edinburgh.

Hoffbrand A.V. & Lewis S.M. (eds) (1989) *Postgraduate Haematology*, 3rd Edition. Heinemann Medical, Oxford.

Hoffbrand A.V. & Pettit J.E. (1988) *Sandoz Atlas of Clinical Haematology*. Gower Medical, London and Sandoz, Basel.

Hoffman R., Benz E.J., Shattil S.J., Furie B. & Cohen H.J. (1991) *Hematology: Basic Principles and Practice*. Churchill Livingstone, New York.

Jandl J.H. (1987) *Blood: Textbook of Haematology*. Churchill Livingstone, Edinburgh.

Jandl J.H. (1991) *Blood: Pathophysiology*. Blackwell Scientific Publications, Boston.

Lee G.R., Bithell T.C., Foerster J., Athens J.W. & Lukens J.N. (1992) *Wintrobe's Clinical Hematology*, 9th Edition. Lea & Febiger, Philadelphia.

Lilleyman J.S. & Hann I.M. (eds) (1992) *Paediatric Haematology*. Churchill Livingstone, Edinburgh.

Ludlam C.A. (ed.) (1990) *Clinical Haematology*. Churchill Livingstone, Edinburgh.

MacDonald G.A., Paul J. & Cruickshank B. (1989) *Atlas of Haematology*, 5th Edition. Churchill Livingstone, Edinburgh.

Miller D.R. & Baehner R.L. (eds) (1990) *Blood Diseases in Infancy and Childhood*, 6th Edition. C.V. Mosby, St Louis.

Nathan D.G. & Oski F. (1992) *Hematology of Infancy and Childhood*, 4th Edition. W.B. Saunders, Philadelphia.

Roberts B. (ed.) (1991) *Standard Haematological Practice*. Blackwell Scientific Publications, Oxford.

Stamatoyannopoulos G., Nienhuis A.W., Leder P. & Majerus P.W. (1987) *Molecular Basis of Blood Diseases*. W.B. Saunders, Philadelphia.

Thorup O.A. (1987) *Leavell and Thorup's Fundamental of Clinical Haematology*. W.B. Saunders, Philadelphia.

Weatherall D.J. (1991) *The New Genetics and Clinical Practice*, 3rd Edition. Oxford University Press, Oxford.

Williams W.J., Beutler E., Erslev A.J. & Lichtman M.A. (eds) (1990) *Haematology*, 4th Edition. MacGraw-Hill, New York.

Zucker-Frankin D., Greaves M.F. & Marmont A.M. (1988) *Atlas of Blood Cells, Functions and Pathology*, 2nd Edition. Lea & Febiger, Philadelphia.

Chapter 1
Blood Cell Formation (Haemopoiesis)

This first chapter mainly concerns general aspects of blood cell formation (haemopoiesis) and the early stages of formation of red cells (erythropoiesis), granulocytes and monocytes (myelopoiesis) and platelets (thrombopoiesis).

Site

[handwritten margin notes: haemopoiesis: 1) yolk sac 0-6 wks 2) liver, spleen — 6 wks – 2 wks After Birth 3) BM 6 mths – adulthood]

In the first few weeks of gestation the yolk sac is the main site of haemopoiesis. From 6 weeks until 6−7 months of foetal life the liver and spleen are the main organs involved and they continue to produce blood cells until about 2 weeks after birth (Table 1.1, Fig. 6.1b). The bone marrow is the most important site from 6−7 months of foetal life and, during normal childhood and adult life, the marrow is the only source of new blood cells. The developing cells are situated outside the bone marrow sinuses and mature cells are released into the sinus spaces, the marrow microcirculation and so into the general circulation.

In infancy, all the bone marrow is haemopoietic but, during childhood, there is progressive fatty replacement of marrow throughout the long bones so that, in adult life, haemopoietic marrow is confined to the central skeleton and proximal ends of the femurs and humeri (Table 1.1). Even in these haemopoietic areas, approximately 50% of the marrow consists of fat (Fig. 1.1). The remaining fatty marrow is capable of reversion to haemopoiesis and in many diseases there is also expansion of haemopoiesis down the long bones. Morever, the liver and spleen can resume their foetal haemopoietic role (so-called 'extramedullary haemopoiesis').

Haemopoietic stem and progenitor cells

[handwritten margin notes: erythroid → granulocytic monocytic pleuripotent stem cell → megakaryocytic → lymphoid]

It is now thought that a common (pluripotential) stem cell gives rise after a number of cell divisions and differentiation steps to a series of progenitor cells for three main marrow cell lines: (a) erythroid, (b) granulocytic and monocytic, and (c) megakaryocytic, as well as to a common lymphoid stem cell (Fig. 1.2). Although the appearance of the pluripotential stem cells is probably similar to that of small- or intermediate-sized lymphocytes, their presence can be shown in mice, at least, by culture

• Foetus	0−2 months — yolk sac
	2−7 months — liver, spleen
	5−9 months — bone marrow
• Infants	Bone marrow (practically all bones)
• Adults	Vertebrae, ribs, sternum, skull, sacrum and pelvis, proximal ends of femur

Table 1.1 Sites of haemopoiesis.

techniques. The existence of the separate progenitor cells, which also resemble lymphocytes, for the three cell lines has also been demonstrated by *in vitro* culture techniques. The earliest detectable myeloid precursor gives rise to granulocytes, erythrocytes, monocytes and megakaryocytes and is termed CFU_{GEMM} (CFU = colony-forming unit in agar culture medium). More mature and specialized progenitors are then formed (Fig. 1.2).

The stem cell also has the capability of self-renewal (Fig. 1.3) so that, although the marrow is a major site of new cell production, its overall cellularity remains constant in a normal healthy steady state. The precursor cells are, however, capable of responding to haemopoietic growth factors with increased production of one or other cell line when the need arises. There is considerable amplification in the system: one stem cell, for example is normally capable of producing about 10^6 mature blood cells after 20 cell divisions (Fig. 1.3).

The bone marrow is also the primary site of origin of lymphocytes in humans (Chapter 9) and there is evidence for a common precursor cell of both the myeloid and lymphoid systems.

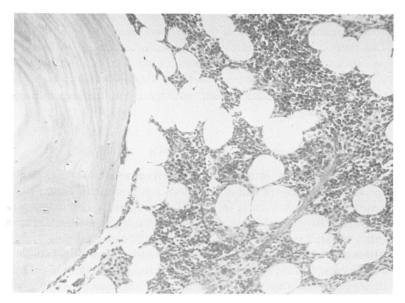

Fig. 1.1 A normal bone marrow trephine biopsy (posterior iliac crest). Haematoxylin and eosin stain; approximately 50% of the intertrabecular tissue is haemopoietic tissue and 50% is fat.

CFU – colony forming units

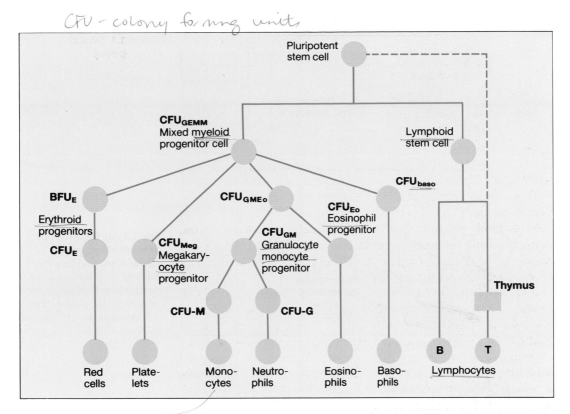

Fig. 1.2 Diagrammatic representation of the bone marrow pluripotent stem cell and the cell lines that arise from it. Various progenitor cells can now be identified by culture in semi-solid medium by the type of colony they form. BFU$_E$, burst-forming unit, erythroid; CFU, colony-forming unit; E, erythroid; Eo, eosinophil; GEMM, mixed granulocyte, erythroid, monocyte, megakaryocyte; GM, granulocyte, monocyte; Meg, megakaryocyte.

Haemopoietic stem cells also give rise to osteoclasts which are part of the monocyte–phagocyte system. The development of the mature cells — red cells, granulocytes, monocytes, megakaryocytes and lymphocytes — is further considered in other sections of this book.

Bone marrow stroma

The bone marrow forms a suitable environment for stem cell growth and development. It is composed of stromal cells and a microvascular network (Fig. 1.4). If haemopoietic stem cells are infused intravenously into a suitably prepared recipient, they circulate and seed the marrow successfully but do not thrive at other sites. This is the basis of bone marrow transplantation performed for a number of serious bone marrow and other diseases. The direction in which stem and progenitor cells

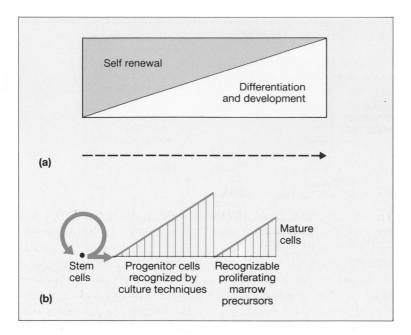

Fig. 1.3 (a) Bone marrow cells are increasingly differentiated and lose the capacity for self-renewal as they mature. (b) A single stem cell gives rise, after multiple cell divisions, to >10^6 mature cells.

differentiate depends largely on the spectrum of growth factors to which they are exposed. As the marrow cells differentiate they lose cell adhesion molecules (CAMs), changes allowing the cells to leave the marrow and enter the circulation. Stem cells also circulate and in the early foetus, the yolk sac, and in later foetal life the liver and spleen, as well as the bone marrow, provide the correct environment for stem cell survival and proliferation.

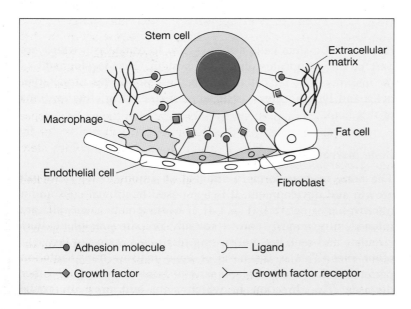

Fig. 1.4 Haemopoiesis occurs in a suitable microenvironment provided by a stromal matrix on which stem cells grow and divide. There are probably specific recognition and adhesion sites; extracellular glycoproteins and other compounds are involved in the binding (Table 1.2).

Table 1.2 The composition of the bone marrow microenvironment.

Extracellular matrix	Stromal cells
Fibronectin (binds erythroid precursors)	Macrophages
Haemonectin (binds granulocyte precursors)	Fibroblasts
Laminin	Endothelial cells
Collagen	Fat cells
Proteoglycans (acid mucopolysaccharides), e.g. chondroitin, heparan	Reticulum ('blanket') cells

Haemopoietic growth factors

The haemopoietic growth factors are glycoprotein hormones that regulate the proliferation and differentiation of haemopoietic progenitor cells and the function of mature blood cells (Table 1.3). They may act locally at the site where they are produced or circulate in plasma. They share a number of common properties (Table 1.4). T lymphocytes, monocytes (and macrophages), endothelial cells and fibroblasts (stromal cells) are the major cell sources except for erythropoietin, 90% of which is synthesized in the kidney. The biological effects of the growth factors are mediated through specific receptors on target cells. Some growth factors are found normally in plasma but others cannot be detected except when there is an inflammatory or other stimulus. Antigens or endotoxins activate T lymphocytes or macrophages to release IL-1 (interleukin-1) and tumour necrosis factor (TNF) which then stimulate other cells including endothelial cells, fibroblasts and other T cells and macrophages to produce GM-CSF (CSF = colony-stimulating factor), G-CSF, M-CSF, IL-6 and other growth factors in an interacting network (Fig. 1.5). T lymphocytes appear to be the sole source of IL-3 and IL-5. An important feature of growth factor action is that two or more factors may synergize in stimulating a particular cell to proliferate or differentiate. Moreover, the action of one growth factor on a cell may stimulate production of another growth factor or growth factor receptor. Within the marrow the growth factors, particularly those acting at the earliest stages of haemopoiesis, may act locally by cell to cell contact or by binding to the extracellular matrix to form niches to which stem and progenitor cells adhere.

IL-1 has a wide variety of biological activities mainly related to inflammation. Stem cell factor acts locally on the pluripotential stem cells and on early myeloid and lymphoid progenitors (Fig. 1.6). IL-3 and GM-CSF are multi-potential growth factors with overlapping activates, IL-3 being more active on the earliest marrow progenitors. IL-3 activity also leads to increased platelet as well as granulocyte and monocyte production. IL-1 and IL-6 enhance the effects of SCF, IL-3 and GM-CSF on survival

Act on stromal cells
IL-1 } stimulate production of GM-CSF,
TNF } G-CSF, M-CSF, IL-6

Act on pluripotential cells
SCF (stem cell factor, kit ligand, Steel factor)

Act on early multipotential cells
IL-3
IL-6
GM-CSF

Act on late cells committed to one (or two) lineages
G-CSF
M-CSF
IL-5 (Eo-CSF)
Erythropoietin
Thrombopoietin

Notes:
1 TGFβ (transforming growth factor-β) acts as a growth-inhibiting factor for a wide variety of haemopoietic and non-haemopoietic cells. Both TNF and IL-4 also have inhibitory effects for late myeloid progenitors.
2 IL-3 and GM-CSF have synergistic effects with the more restricted growth factors on later cells.
3 A number of other factors (IL-8, IL-9, IL-10, IL-11) are described but less well characterized.
4 Growth factors acting on lymphoid progenitors are described in Chapter 9.
CSF, colony-stimulating factor; Eo, eosinophil; G, granulocytes; IL, interleukin; M, monocyte; TNF, tumour necrosis factor.

Table 1.3 Haemopoietic growth factors.

1 Glycoproteins that act at very low concentrations
2 Act hierarchically
3 Usually produced by many cell types
4 Usually affect more than one lineage
5 Usually active on stem/progenitor cells and on functional end cells
6 Usually show synergistic or additive interactions with other growth factors
7 Often act on the neoplastic equivalent of a normal cell
8 Multiple actions: proliferation, differentiation, maturation, membrane integrity, functional activation, prevention of apoptosis

Table 1.4 General characteristics of myeloid and lymphoid growth factors.

and differentiation of the early haemopoietic cells. Together these factors maintain a pool of haemopoietic stem and progenitor cells on which later acting factors may act to stimulate increased production of one or other cell lineage in response to the body's needs, e.g. in infection (Fig. 1.5), haemorrhage or hypoxia.

Erythropoietin, G-CSF, M-CSF, IL-5 (an eosinophilic growth factor) and thrombopoietin act on later cells which are more

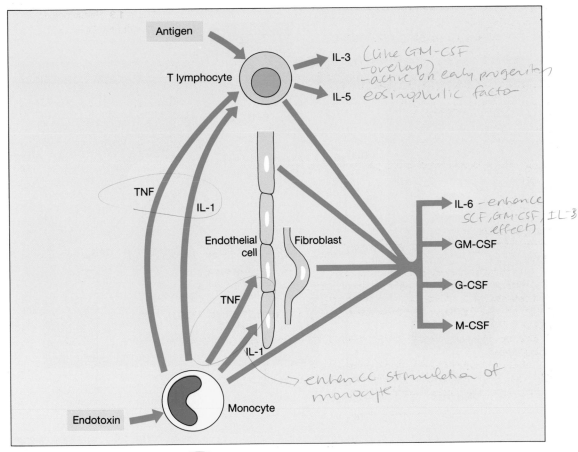

Handwritten annotations on figure:
- Near IL-3: (like GM-CSF -overlap) -active on early progenitors
- Near IL-5: eosinophilic factor
- Near IL-6: - enhance SCF, GM-CSF, IL-3 effect)
- Near Monocyte: → enhance stimulation of monocyte
- Left margin: CSF - colony stimulating factor / GM - Granulocyte monocyte

Fig. 1.5 Regulation of haemopoiesis; pathways of stimulation of leucopoiesis by endotoxin, for example from infection. It is likely that endothelial and fibroblast cells release basal quantities of GM-CSF and G-CSF in the normal resting state and that this is enhanced substantially by the monokines TNF (tumour necrosis factor) and IL-1 (interleukin-1), released in response to infection. IL-1 and TNF also stimulate T cells and antigen may stimulate T cells directly. CSF, colony-stimulating factor; G, granulocyte; M, monocyte.

committed to one cell lineage (Fig. 1.6). IL-6 also has a particular role in megakaryocyte formation. The growth factors also affect the survival and function of mature cells, e.g. GM-CSF potentiates viability and microbial killing and the production of cytokines by mature neutrophils, monocytes and eosinophils (Fig. 1.7).

A common action of the growth factors is to inhibit apoptosis (programmed cell death) of target cells. Apoptosis is a gene-directed process requiring ongoing protein synthesis in which Ca^{2+} ions activate endonucleases, the dying cells being removed by phagocytosis.

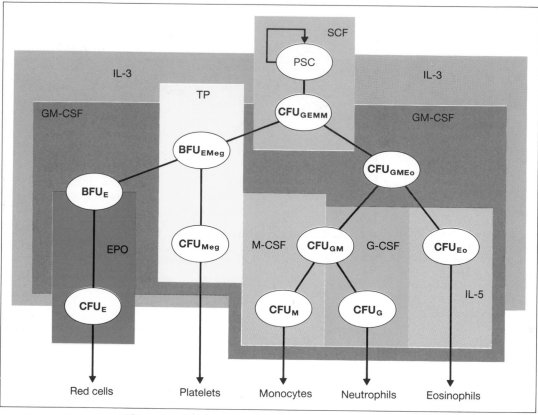

BFU – burst
forming
unit

Fig. 1.6 A simplified diagram
of the role of growth factors in
normal haemopoiesis. Multiple
growth factors act on the
earlier marrow stem and
progenitor cells. EPO,
erythropoietin; TP,
thrombopoietin; PSC,
pluripotential stem cell; SCF,
stem cell factor. For other
abbreviations see Fig. 1.2 and
Table 1.3.

Signal transduction

Several different mechanisms have been identified by which a
growth factor signal for the cell to proliferate or differentiate is
transduced through the target cell membrane to the cell nucleus
(Fig. 1.8 and 1.9). The first event, however, is the binding of the
growth factor to its receptor on the cell membrane.

Growth factor receptors

Each of the growth factors binds with high affinity to its corresponding receptor on the target cell. Most of the receptors belong
to a structurally related set of membrane glycoproteins, the
haematopoietin receptor family (Table 1.5). Binding of the growth
factor to these receptors causes alteration of the intracellular
domains of the receptor protein. Dimerization of two identical,
or the two different, receptor molecules in response to growth
factor binding appears to be necessary for signal transduction

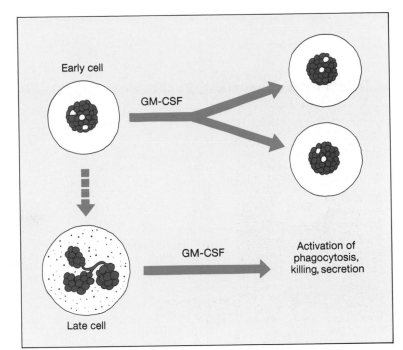

Fig. 1.7 Growth factors may stimulate proliferation of early bone marrow cells and affect the function of mature non-dividing cells, as illustrated here for GM-CSF for an early myeloid progenitor and a neutrophil.

(Fig. 1.8). This initiates a series of phosphorylation events in other proteins but the details of how this is generated is unclear since the receptor does not have a protein kinase domain.

A second smaller group of growth factor receptors have an

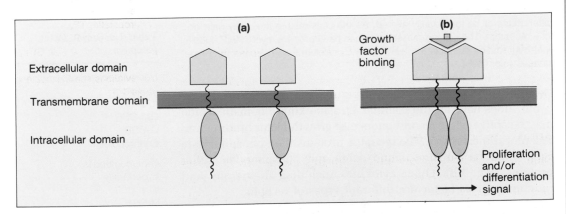

Fig. 1.8 Binding of a growth factor to its receptor may cause dimerization of the receptor and a change in its intracellular domain (e.g. phosphorylation) by which the growth signal is transduced to the cell interior.

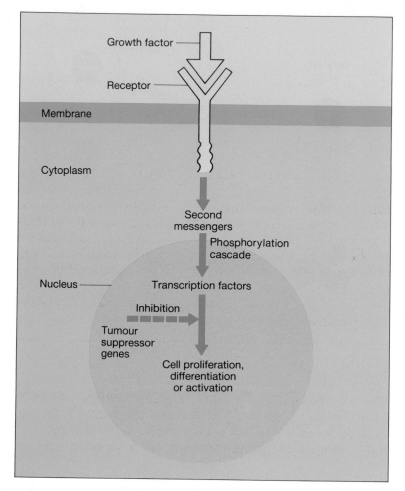

Fig. 1.9 Control of haemopoiesis by growth factors. The growth factors act on cells expressing the corresponding receptor. The cell may then proliferate or differentiate or be functionally altered. As the cells mature they may gain or lose receptors. The second messengers can be G proteins, cyclic AMP, inositol lipid degradation products, protein kinase C, calcium ions or serine/threonine kinases (e.g. *RAF*).

external immunoglobulin-like structure. For this group, the receptor does have an intracellular tyrosine kinase domain which may be activated as a consequence of growth factor binding and receptor dimerization. The receptor proteins then phosphorylate each other on tyrosine amino acids and phosphorylate other proteins (Fig. 1.8). Other cytokines including interferons and tumour necrosis factor use different types of receptor.

Second messengers and intracellular signal pathways

The number of low molecular weight compounds may be released in response to growth factor binding and receptor acti-

Table 1.5 Growth factor receptors.

Haematopoietin superfamily receptors
IL-2–6
GM-CSF
G-CSF
Erythropoietin

Immunoglobulin superfamily
IL-1
M-CSF
SCF

Others
Tumour necrosis factor (TNF), interferons

vation. These include cyclic AMP, cyclic GMP, diacylglycerol and inositol tris- and tetrakisphosphate (IP_3 and IP_4) (see Fig. 9.3), phosphatidylinositol triphosphate (PtIn 3,4,5 phosphate) and calcium ions. These compounds activate, often by phosphorylation, proteins involved in intracellular signal transduction.

The membrane and intracellular signals form complex interacting and feedback loops. The enzymes involved in signal transduction may bind together via SH (SRC homology) domains. A cascade of phosphorylation events is involved. In one pathway GRB2 binds to activated receptor, and to SOS which then activates RAS triggering phosphorylation of RAF. The products of *RAF*, a serine tyrosine kinase and mitogen activated kinases (MAPK) transmit signals for further transmission to the nucleus (Fig. 10.4a, p. 196). In the nucleus, activation of transcription factors by phosphorylation or other mechanisms is an early event before DNA synthesis is initiated. A number of proteins called cyclins bind to protein kinases in the cdcd2 family to form a complex involved in transition of cell from G_1 to S phase and from the S phase into G_2 and mitosis (see Fig. 10.4b).

Bibliography

Alison M.R. & Sarraf C.E. (1992) Apoptosis: a gene-directed programme of cell death. *Journal of the Royal College of Physicians*, **26**, 25−35.

Balkwill F.R. (1989) *Cytokines in Cancer Therapy*. Oxford University Press, Oxford.

Bybee A. & Thomas N.S.B. (1991) Cell cycle regulation. *Blood Reviews*, **5**, 177−192.

Dexter T.M., Garland J.M. & Testa N.G. (eds) (1990) *Colony-Stimulating Factors: Molecular and Cellular Biology*. Immunology Series 49. Marcel Dekker, Inc., New York.

Golde D.W. (ed.) (1989) Hematopoietic growth factors. *Hematology/Oncology Clinics of North America*, **3**, 369−557.

Green A. (ed.) (1989) *Peptide Regulatory Factors*. Edward Arnold, London.

Groopman J.E., Molina J.M. & Scadden D.T. (1989) Hematopoietic growth factors: biology and clinical applications. *New England Journal of Medicine*, **321**, 1449−1459.

Kaczmarski R.S. & Mufti G.J. (1991) The cytokine receptor superfamily. *Blood Reviews*, **5**, 193−203.

Lord B.J. & Dexter T.M. (1992) Growth factors in haemopoiesis. *Clinical Haematology*, **5** (in press).

Metcalfe D. (1989) Haematopoietic growth factors. *Lancet*, **i**, 825−827, 885−887.

Nathan D.G. (ed.) (1991) The molecular biology of hematopoiesis. *Seminars in Hematology*, **28**, 114−176.

Nicola N.A. (1989) Hemopoietic growth factors and their receptors. *Annual Review of Biochemistry*, **58**, 45−77.

Sachs L., Abraham N.G., Wideman C.J., Konwalinka G. & Levine A.S. (eds) (1990) *Molecular Biology of Haematopoiesis*. Intercept, Andover.

Witte O.N. (1990) Steel locus defines new multi-potent growth factor. *Cell*, **63**, 5−6.

Chapter 2
Erythropoiesis and General Aspects of Anaemia

As discussed in Chapter 1, the earliest stages of erythropoiesis from the pluripotent stem cell can only be detected by *in vitro* assays for the progenitor cells, CFU_{GEMM}, BFU_E and CFU_E (BFU = burst-forming unit; CFU = colony-forming unit). The earliest recognizable erythroid cell in the marrow is the pronormoblast which — on the usual Romanowsky (e.g. May−Grünwald Giemsa, Leishman or Wright) stain — is a large cell with dark-blue cytoplasm, a central nucleus with nucleoli and slightly clumped chromatin (Fig. 2.1). This gives rise to a series of progressively smaller normoblasts by a number of cell divisions. They also contain progressively more haemoglobin (which stains pink) in the cytoplasm; the cytoplasm stains paler blue as it loses its RNA and protein synthetic apparatus while the nuclear chromatin becomes more condensed (Figs 2.1, 2.2). The nucleus is finally extruded from the late normoblast within the marrow and a reticulocyte stage results which still contains some ribosomal RNA and is still able to synthesize haemoglobin (Fig. 2.3). This cell is slightly larger than a mature red cell, spends 1−2 days in the marrow and also circulates in the peripheral blood for 1−2 days before maturing, mainly in the spleen, when RNA is completely lost. A completely pink-staining, mature erythrocyte (red cell) results which is a non-nucleated biconcave disc. A single pronormoblast usually gives rise to 16 mature red cells (Fig. 2.2). Nucleated red cells (normoblasts) appear in the blood if erythropoiesis is occurring outside the marrow (extramedullary erythropoiesis) and also with some marrow diseases. Normoblasts are not present in normal human peripheral blood.

Erythropoietin

Erythropoietic activity is regulated by the hormone erythropoietin. Erythropoietin has a molecular weight of 30 400; it is heavily glycosylated (39% carbohydrate) with a polypeptide of 165 amino acids. It has a plasma half-life of 6−9 hours and distributes in the plasma volume. Normally 90% of the hormone is produced in the peritubular complex of the kidney and 10% in the liver and elsewhere. There are no preformed stores and the stimulus to erythropoietin production is the oxygen (O_2) tension in the tissues of the kidney (Fig. 2.4). When anaemia

contain more Hb in cytoplasm (more pink)

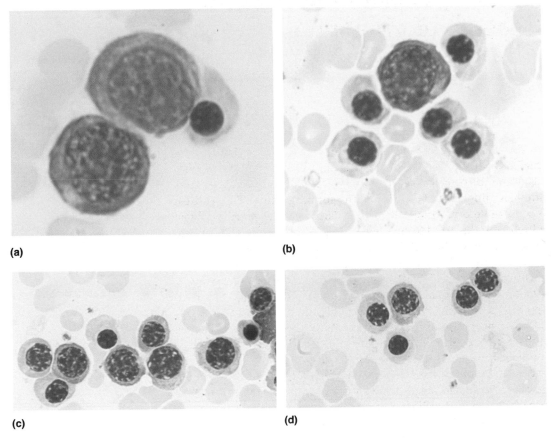

(a)

(b)

(c)

(d)

Fig. 2.1 Erythroblasts (normoblasts) at varying stages of development. The earlier cells are larger, with more basophilic cytoplasm and a more open nuclear chromatin pattern. The cytoplasm of the later cells is more eosinophilic due to haemoglobin formation.

occurs, or haemoglobin for some metabolic or structural reason is unable to give up O_2 normally or atmospheric O_2 is low or defective cardiac or pulmonary function or damage to the renal circulation affects O_2 delivery to the kidney, erythropoietin production increases and stimulates erythropoiesis by increasing the number of progenitor cells committed to erythropoiesis. Late BFU_E and CFU_E which have erythropoietin receptors are stimulated to proliferate, differentiate and produce haemoglobin. The proportion of erythroid cells in the marrow increases and, in the chronic state, there is anatomical expansion of erythropoiesis into fatty marrow and sometimes into extramedullary sites. In infants, the marrow cavity may expand into cortical bone resulting in bone deformities with frontal bossing and protrusion of the maxilla (p. 103).

On the other hand, increased O_2 supply to the tissues (due to an increased red cell mass or because haemoglobin is able to release its O_2 more readily than normal) reduces the erythropoietin drive.

Plasma erythropoietin levels can be measured although the

14

CHAPTER 2

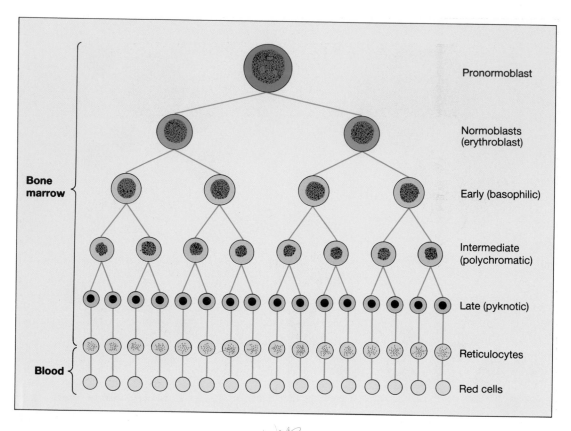

still has some ribosomal RNA

Fig. 2.2 Diagram illustrating the amplification and maturation sequence in the development of mature red cells from the pronormoblast.

	Normoblast	Reticulocyte	Mature RBC
Nuclear DNA	Yes	No	No
RNA in cytoplasm	Yes	Yes	No
In marrow	Yes	Yes	Yes
In blood	No	Yes	Yes

Fig. 2.3 Comparison of the DNA and RNA content, and marrow and peripheral blood distribution of the erythroblast (normoblast), reticulocyte and mature red cell (RBC).

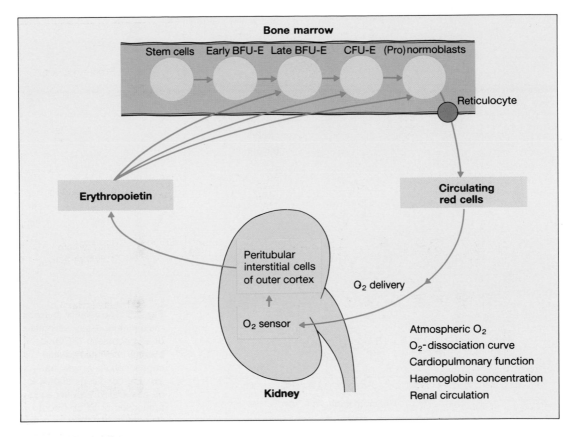

Fig. 2.4 The production of erythropoietin by the kidney in response to its oxygen (O_2) supplies. Erythropoietin stimulates erythropoiesis and so increases O_2 delivery. (From Erslev & Gabuzda, 1985.)

techniques are difficult. They may be of clinical value if a tumour-secreting erythropoietin is considered to be a cause of polycythaemia. They are low in severe renal disease despite anaemia (Fig. 2.5).

Indications for erythropoietin therapy

Recombinant erythropoietin may be given intravenously or, more effectively, subcutaneously. Doses between 50 and 300 units/kg three times weekly are usually needed. The main indication is end-stage renal disease (with or without dialysis). Other uses under trial are pre-autologous blood transfusions; haemopoietic recovery (post-chemotherapy or bone marrow transplantation); anaemia of chronic disorders, e.g. in rheumatoid arthritis or cancer; and anaemia in aplastic anaemia, myelodysplasia and AIDS (see also p. 371).

Other substances needed for erythropoiesis

Because of the very great numbers of new red cells that are produced each day, the marrow requires many precursors to

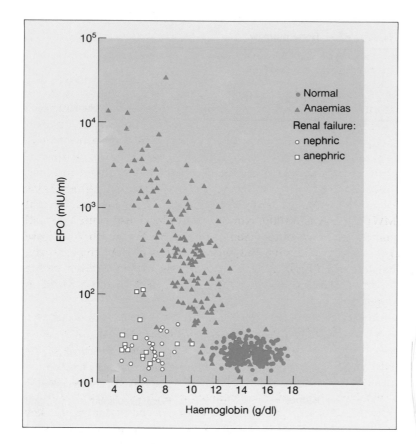

Fig. 2.5 The relation between radioimmunoassay estimates of erythropoietin (EPO) in plasma and haemoglobin concentration. Anaemias exclude conditions shown to be associated with impaired production of EPO. (From Pippard *et al.*, 1992.)

synthesize the new cells and the large amounts of haemoglobin. The following groups of substances are needed:

1 *Metals*: iron, manganese, cobalt.
2 *Vitamins*: vitamin B_{12}, folate, vitamin C, vitamin E, vitamin B_6 (pyridoxine), thiamine, riboflavin and pantothenic acid.
3 *Amino acids.*
4 *Hormones*: stem cell factor (SCF), IL-3, GM-CSF, erythropoietin, androgens and thyroxine.

Well recognized anaemias occur with iron, vitamin B_{12} or folate deficiencies and, in renal disease, with deficiency of erythropoietin. Anaemias also occur with amino acid (protein), thyroxine or androgen deficiency but these may be adaptations to the lower tissue O_2 consumption, rather than a direct effect of the deficiency on erythropoiesis. Anaemia also occurs in the deficiency of vitamin C (scurvy), vitamin E and riboflavin, but it is not clear whether these are purely due to an effect of these deficiencies on erythropoiesis. Vitamin B_6-responsive anaemias also occur but these are not usually due to vitamin B_6 deficiency (see p. 50).

Haemoglobin

Haemoglobin synthesis

The main function of red cells is to carry O_2 to the tissues and to return carbon dioxide (CO_2) from the tissues to the lungs. In order to achieve this gaseous exchange, they contain the specialized protein, haemoglobin. Each red cell contains approximately 640 million haemoglobin molecules. Each molecule of normal adult haemoglobin (Hb) A (the dominant haemoglobin in blood after the age of 3−6 months) consists of four polypeptide chains $\alpha_2\beta_2$, each with its own haem group. The molecular weight (MW) of Hb A is 68 000. Normal adult blood also contains small quantities of two other haemoglobins, Hb F and Hb A_2. These also contain α chains, but with γ and δ chains, respectively, instead of β (Table 2.1). The synthesis of the various globin chains in the foetus and adult is discussed in more detail in Chapter 6.

The major switch from foetal to adult haemoglobin occurs 3−6 months after birth (see Fig. 6.1a). Sixty-five per cent of haemoglobin is synthesized in the erythroblasts and 35% at the reticulocyte stage.

Haem synthesis occurs largely in the mitochondria by a series of biochemical reactions commencing with the condensation of glycine and succinyl coenzyme A under the action of the key rate-limiting enzyme δ-aminolaevulinic acid (ALA) synthetase (Fig. 2.6). Pyridoxal phosphate (vitamin B_6) is a coenzyme for this reaction which is stimulated by erythropoietin and inhibited by haem. Ultimately, protoporphyrin combines with iron in the ferrous (Fe^{2+}) state to form haem (Fig. 2.7), each molecule of which combines with a globin chain made on the polyribosomes (Fig. 2.6). A tetramer of four globin chains each with its own haem group in a 'pocket' is then formed to make up a haemoglobin molecule (Fig. 2.8).

Haemoglobin function

The red cells in systemic arterial blood carry O_2 from the lungs to the tissues and return in venous blood with CO_2 to the lungs. As the haemoglobin molecule loads and unloads O_2, the individual globin chains in the haemoglobin molecule move on

Table 2.1 Normal haemoglobins in adult blood.

	Hb A	Hb F	Hb A_2
Structure	$\alpha_2\beta_2$	$\alpha_2\gamma_2$	$\alpha_2\delta_2$
Normal (%)	96−98	0.5−0.8	1.5−3.2

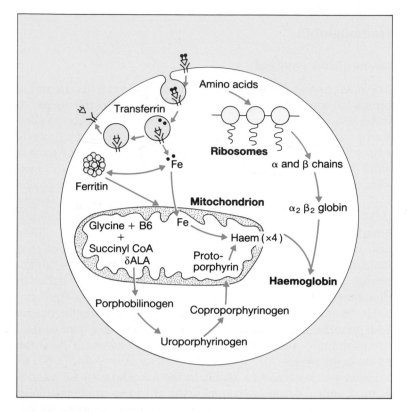

Fig. 2.6 Haemoglobin synthesis in the developing red cell. The mitochondria are the main sites of proto-porphyrin synthesis, iron (Fe) is supplied from circulating transferrin; globin chains are synthesized on ribosomes. δALA, δ-aminolaevulinic acid; CoA, coenzyme A.

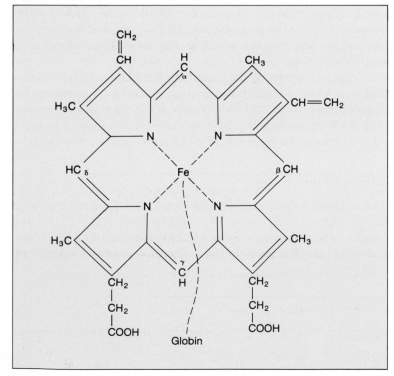

Fig. 2.7 The structure of haem.

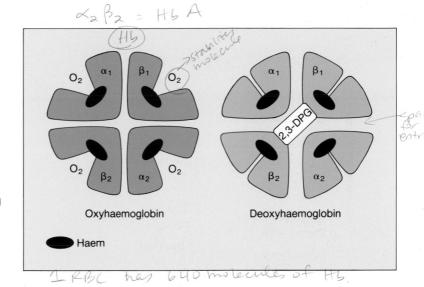

Fig. 2.8 The oxygenated and deoxygenated haemoglobin molecule. α, β, globin chains of normal adult haemoglobin (Hb A); 2,3-DPG, 2,3-diphosphoglycerate.

each other (Fig. 2.8). The $\alpha_1\beta_1$ and $\alpha_2\beta_2$ contacts stabilize the molecule. The β chains slide on the $\alpha_1\beta_2$ and $\alpha_2\beta_1$ contacts during oxygenation and deoxygenation. When O_2 is unloaded, the β chains are pulled apart, permitting entry of the metabolite 2,3-diphosphoglycerate (2,3-DPG) resulting in a lower affinity of the molecule for O_2. This movement is responsible for the sigmoid form of the haemoglobin O_2-dissociation curve (Fig. 2.9). The P_{50} (i.e. the partial pressure of O_2 at which haemoglobin is half saturated with O_2) of normal blood is 26.6 mmHg. With increased affinity for O_2, the curve shifts to the left (i.e. the P_{50} falls) while, with decreased affinity for O_2, the curve shifts to the right (i.e. the P_{50} rises).

Normally *in vivo*, O_2 exchange operates between 95% saturation (arterial blood) with a mean arterial O_2 tension of 95 mmHg and 70% saturation (venous blood) with a mean venous O_2 tension of 40 mmHg.

The normal position of the curve depends on the concentration of 2,3-DPG, H^+ ions and CO_2 in the red cell and on the structure of the haemoglobin molecule. High concentrations of 2,3-DPG, H^+ or CO_2, and the presence of certain haemoglobins, e.g. sickle haemoglobin (Hb S), shift the curve to the right whereas foetal haemoglobin (Hb F)—which is unable to bind 2,3-DPG—and certain rare abnormal haemoglobins associated with polycythaemia shift the curve to the left because they give up O_2 less readily than normal.

Methaemoglobinaemia

This is a clinical state in which circulating haemoglobin is present with iron in the oxidized (Fe^{3+}) state instead of the usual Fe^{2+} state. It may arise because of a hereditary deficiency

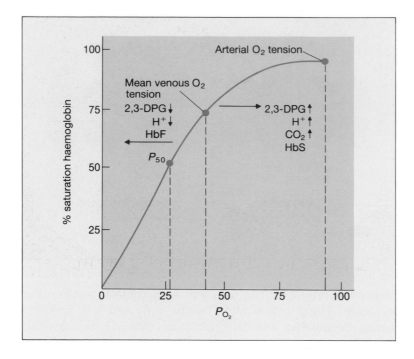

Fig. 2.9 The haemoglobin oxygen (O_2)-dissociation curve.

of NADH (nicotinamide-adenine dinucleotide, reduced), dia-phorase or inheritance of a structurally abnormal haemoglobin (Hb M). These contain an amino acid substitution affecting the haem pocket of the globin chain. Toxic methaemoglobinaemia (and/or sulphaemoglobinaemia) occurs when a drug or other toxic substance oxidizes haemoglobin. In all these states, the patient is likely to show cyanosis.

The red cell

In order to carry haemoglobin into close contact with the tissues and for successful gaseous exchange, the red cell, $8\,\mu m$ in di-ameter, must be able to pass repeatedly through the micro-circulation whose minimum diameter is $3.5\,\mu m$, to maintain haemoglobin in a reduced (ferrous) state and to maintain osmotic equilibrium despite the high concentration of protein (haemo-globin) in the cell. Its total journey throughout its 120-day lifespan has been estimated to be 300 miles. To fulfil these functions, the cell is a flexible, biconcave disc (Fig. 2.10) with an ability to generate energy as ATP by the anaerobic, glycolytic (Embden–Meyerhof) pathway (Fig. 2.11) and to generate reducing power as NADH by this pathway and as NADPH (nicotinamide-adenine-dinucleotide phosphate, reduced) by the hexose monophosphate shunt (Fig. 2.12).

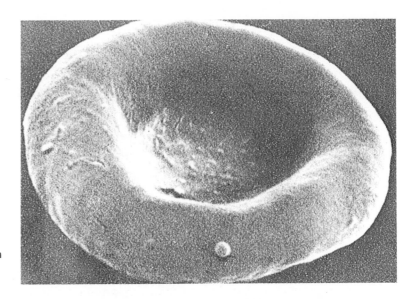

Fig. 2.10 A scanning electron microscopic view of a normal red cell.

Red cell metabolism

Embden–Meyerhof pathway

In this series of biochemical reactions glucose is metabolized to lactate (Fig. 2.11). For each molecule of glucose used, two molecules of ATP (adenosine triphosphate) and thus two high-energy phosphate bonds are generated. This ATP provides energy for maintenance of red cell volume, shape and flexibility. The red cell has an osmotic pressure five times that of plasma and an inherent weakness of the membrane results in continual Na^+ and K^+ movement. A membrane ATPase sodium pump is needed, and this uses one molecule of ATP to move three sodium ions out and two potassium ions into the cell.

The Embden–Meyerhof pathway also generates NADH which is needed by the enzyme methaemoglobin reductase to reduce functionally dead methaemoglobin (oxidized haemoglobin) containing ferric iron (produced by oxidation of about 3% of haemoglobin each day) to functionally active, reduced haemoglobin. 2,3-DPG which is generated in the Luebering–Rapoport shunt, or side-arm, of this pathway (Fig. 2.11b) forms a 1:1 complex with haemoglobin and, as mentioned earlier, is important in the regulation of haemoglobin's oxygen affinity.

Hexose monophosphate (pentose phosphate) pathway

About 5% of glycolysis occurs by this oxidative pathway in which glucose-6-phosphate is converted to 6-phosphogluconate and so to ribulose-5-phosphate (Fig. 2.12). NADPH is generated and is linked with glutathione which maintains sulphydril

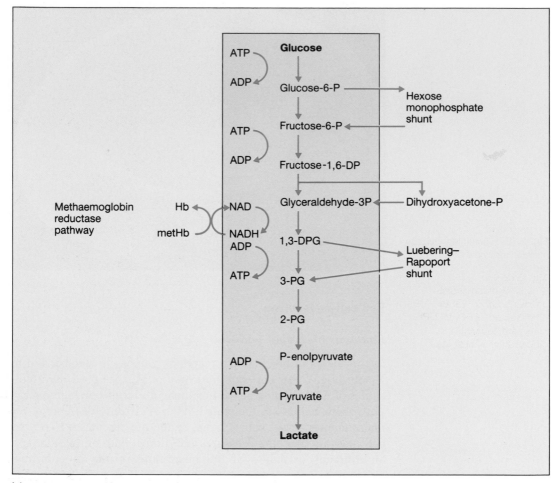

(a)

Fig. 2.11 (a) The Embden–Meyerhof glycolytic pathway. (b) The Luebering–
Rapoport shunt which regulates the concentration of 2,3-DPG (2,3-
diphosphoglycerate) in the red cell. ADP, adenosine diphosphate; ATP,
adenosine triphosphate; NAD, NADH, nicotinamide-adenine dinucleotide; PG,
phosphoglycerate.

(−SH) groups intact in the cell including those in haemoglobin
and the red cell membrane. NADPH is also used by another
methaemoglobin reductase to maintain haemoglobin iron in the
functionally active Fe^{2+} state. In one of the commonest inherited
abnormalities of red cells, glucose-6-phosphate dehydrogenase
(G6PD) deficiency, the red cells are extremely susceptible to
oxidant stress (see p. 83).

Red cell membrane

This is a bipolar lipid layer containing structural and contractile

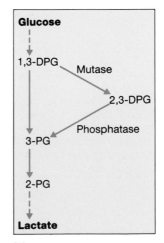

(b)

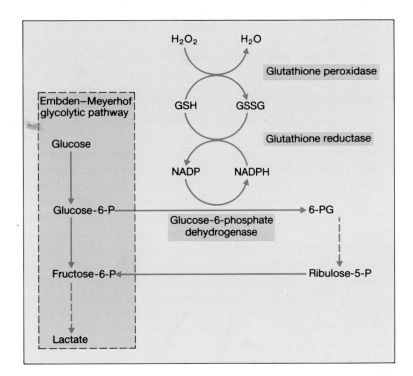

Fig. 2.12 The hexose monophosphate shunt pathway. GSH, GSSG, glutathione; NADP, NADPH, nicotinamide-adenine-dinucleotide phosphate.

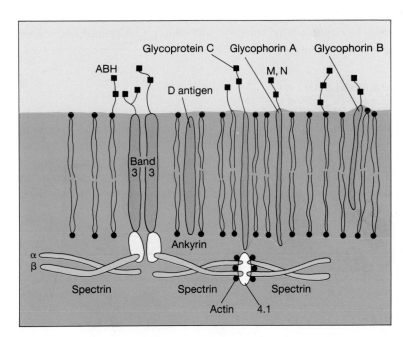

Fig. 2.13 The structure of the red cell membrane. Some of the penetrating and integral proteins carry carbohydrate antigens; other antigens are attached directly to the lipid layer.

proteins and numerous enzymes and surface antigens (Fig. 2.13). About 50% of the membrane is protein, 40% is fat and up to 10% is carbohydrate. The lipids consist of 60% phospholipid,

30% neutral lipids (mainly cholesterol) and 10% glycolipids. The phospho- and glycolipids are structural with polar groups on the external and internal surfaces and non-polar groups at the centre of the membrane. Carbohydrates occur only on the external surface while proteins are either peripheral or integral, penetrating the lipid bilayer. The proteins have been numbered accordingly to their mobility on polyacrylamide gel electrophoresis (PAGE).

Four major proteins (spectrin, actin, protein 4.1 and ankyrin) form a lattice on the internal side of the red cell membrane and are important in maintaining the biconcave shape. Spectrin is the most abundant and consists of two chains, α and β, wound around each other in a heterodimer, connecting at their head ends in a tetramer linked to actin and attached to the integral membrane protein, band 4.1. At the tail end, the β spectrin chains attach to ankyrin which connects to band 3, the transmembrane protein that acts as an anion channel (Fig. 2.13).

Defects of the proteins may explain some of the abnormalities of shape of the red cell membrane, e.g. hereditary spherocytosis and elliptocytosis (see Chapter 5), while alterations in lipid composition due to congenital or acquired abnormalities in plasma cholesterol or phospholipid may be associated with other membrane abnormalities. For instance, an increase in cholesterol and phospholipid has been suggested as one cause of target cells whereas a large selective increase in cholesterol may cause acanthocyte formation (see Fig. 2.16).

Anaemia

This is normally defined as a haemoglobin concentration in the blood of less than 13.5 g/dl in adult males and less than 11.5 g/dl in adult females, although some use 14.0 g/dl and 12.0 g/dl as the adult lower limits of normal. From the age of 3 months to puberty, less than 11.0 g/dl indicates anaemia. As newborn infants have a high haemoglobin level, 15.0 g/dl is

	Male	Female
Haemoglobin (Hb)* (g/dl)	13.5−17.5	11.5−15.5
Haematocrit (PCV) (%)	40−52	36−48
Red cell count (× 10^{12}/l)	4.5−6.5	3.9−5.6
Mean cell haemoglobin (MCH) (pg)	27−34	
Mean cell volume (MCV) (fl)	80−95	
Mean cell haemoglobin concentration (MCHC) (g/dl)	30−35	

Table 2.2 Normal adult red cell values.

* In children normal haemoglobin values are: newborn, 15.0−21.0 g/dl; 3 months, 9.5−12.5 g/dl; 1 year to puberty, 11.0−13.5 g/dl.

taken as the lower limit at birth (Table 2.2). Reduction of haemo-globin is usually accompanied by a fall in red cell count and packed cell volume (PCV) but these may be normal in some patients with subnormal haemoglobin levels (and therefore by definition anaemic). Alterations in total circulating plasma volume as well as of total circulating haemoglobin mass deter-mine the haemoglobin concentration. Reduction in plasma volume (as in dehydration) may mask anaemia or even cause polycythaemia (see p. 292); conversely, an increase in plasma volume (as with splenomegaly or pregnancy) may cause anaemia even with a normal total circulating red cell and haemoglobin mass.

After acute major blood loss, anaemia is not immediately apparent since the total blood volume is reduced. It takes up to a day for the plasma volume to be replaced and so for the degree of anaemia to become apparent (see p. 407). Regeneration of the haemoglobin mass takes substantially longer. The initial clinical features of major blood loss are, therefore, due to reduction in blood volume rather than to anaemia.

Clinical features

The major adaptations to anaemia are in the cardiovascular system (with increased stroke volume and tachycardia) and in the haemoglobin O_2-dissociation curve. In some patients with quite severe anaemia there may be no symptoms or signs, whereas others with mild anaemia may be severely incapacitated. The presence or absence of clinical features can be considered under four major headings:

1 *Speed of onset.* Rapidly progressive anaemia causes more symptoms than anaemia of slow onset because there is less time for adaptation in the cardiovascular system and in the O_2-dissociation curve of haemoglobin.

2 *Severity.* Mild anaemia often produces no symptoms or signs but these are usually present when the haemoglobin is less than $9-10 \, \text{g/dl}$. Even severe anaemia (haemoglobin concentration as low as $6.0 \, \text{g/dl}$) may produce remarkably few symptoms, how-ever, when there is very gradual onset in a young subject who is otherwise healthy.

3 *Age.* The elderly tolerate anaemia less well than the young because of the effect of lack of oxygen on organs when normal cardiovascular compensation (increased cardiac output due to increased stroke volume and tachycardia) is impaired.

4 *Haemoglobin O_2-dissociation curve.* Anaemia, in general, is associated with a rise in 2,3-DPG in the red cells and a shift in the O_2-dissociation curve to the right so that oxygen is given up more readily to tissues. This adaptation is particularly marked in some anaemias which either affect red cell metabolism directly, e.g. in the anaemia of pyruvate kinase deficiency (which causes a rise in 2,3-DPG concentration in the red cells) or which are associated with a low affinity haemoglobin (e.g. Hb S).

Symptoms

If the patient does have symptoms, these are usually shortness of breath (particularly on exercise), weakness, lethargy, palpitation and headaches. In older subjects symptoms of cardiac failure, angina pectoris or intermittent claudication or confusion may be present. Visual disturbances due to retinal haemorrhages may complicate very severe anaemia, particularly of rapid onset.

Signs

These may be divided into general and specific. General signs include pallor of mucous membranes which occurs if the haemoglobin level is less than 9−10 g/dl (Fig. 2.14). Skin colour, on the other hand, is not a reliable sign of anaemia; the state of the skin circulation rather than the haemoglobin content of the blood largely determines skin colour. A hyperdynamic circulation may be present with tachycardia, a bounding pulse, cardiomegaly and a systolic flow murmur especially at the apex. Particularly in the elderly, features of congestive heart failure may be present. Retinal haemorrhages are unusual (Fig. 2.15). Specific signs are associated with particular types of anaemia, e.g. koilonychia (spoon nails) with iron deficiency, jaundice with haemolytic or megaloblastic anaemias, leg ulcers with sickle cell and other haemolytic anaemias, bone deformities with thalassaemia major and other severe congenital haemolytic anaemias.

The association of features of anaemia with excess infections or spontaneous bruising suggest that neutropenia or thrombocytopenia may also be present.

Fig. 2.14 Pallor of the conjunctival mucosa (a) and of the nail bed (b) in two patients with severe anaemia (haemoglobin ≈6.0 g/dl).

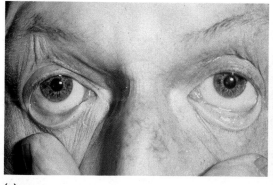

(a)

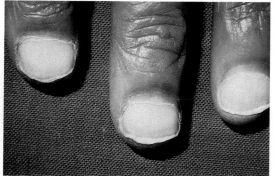

(b)

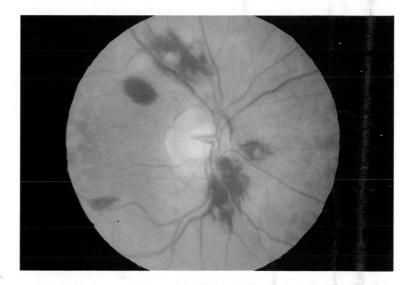

Fig. 2.15 Retinal haemorrhages in a patient with severe anaemia (haemoglobin 2.5 g/dl) due to severe chronic haemorrhage.

Classification and laboratory findings

Red cell indices

Although classification of anaemia based on its cause, e.g. failure of red cell production or excess loss or destruction of red cells, has been used, the most useful classification (now that modern electronic equipment measures accurately a number of parameters of red cell size and haemoglobin content) is that based on red cell indices (Table 2.3). This classification has two major advantages:

1 The type of anaemia (size of the red cells and their haemoglobin content) suggests the nature of the underlying defect and therefore the particular investigations which would be most useful in confirming one or other diagnosis.

2 Abnormal red cell indices may suggest an underlying abnormality before anaemia as defined earlier has developed, e.g. macrocytosis (large red cells) with early vitamin B_{12} or folate deficiency or alcohol excess. Abnormal indices may also point to an important disorder in which anaemia may not occur, e.g. some cases of thalassaemia trait in which the red cells are very small (microcytic) but because of their increased numbers the haemoglobin concentration in blood is normal.

In two common physiological situations, the mean corpuscular volume (MCV) may be outside the normal adult range. In the newborn for a few weeks the MCV is high but, in infancy, it is low (e.g. 70 fl at 1 year of age) and rises slowly throughout childhood to the normal adult range. In normal pregnancy there is a slight rise in MCV, even in the absence of other causes of macrocytosis, e.g. folate deficiency.

Microcytic, hypochromic	Normocytic, normochromic	Macrocytic
MCV < 80 fl	MCV 80–95 fl	MCV > 95 fl
MCH < 27 pg	MCH > 26 pg	
Iron deficiency	Many haemolytic anaemias	Megaloblastic: vitamin B_{12} or folate deficiency
Thalassaemia	Secondary anaemia	
Anaemia of chronic diseases (some cases)	After acute blood loss	Non-megaloblastic: alcohol, liver disease, myelodysplasia, aplastic anaemia, etc.
Lead poisoning	Mixed deficiencies	See p. 72
Sideroblastic anaemia (some cases)	Bone marrow failure, e.g. post-chemotherapy, infiltration by carcinoma, etc. Renal disease	

Table 2.3 Classification of anaemia.

Other laboratory findings

Although the red cell indices will point to the type of anaemia, further useful information can be obtained from the initial blood sample.

Leucocyte and platelet counts

Measurement of these helps to distinguish 'pure' anaemia from 'pancytopenia' (a drop in red cells, granulocytes and platelets) which suggests a more general marrow defect, e.g. due to marrow hypoplasia, infiltration or general destruction of cells (e.g. hypersplenism). In anaemias due to haemolysis or haemorrhage the neutrophil and platelet counts are often raised; in infections and leukaemias the leucocyte count is also often raised and there may be abnormal leucocytes or neutrophil precursors present.

Reticulocyte count

The normal count is 0.5–2.0%, and the absolute count $25-75 \times 10^9/l$. This should rise in anaemia because of erythropoietin increase and be higher the more severe the anaemia. This is particularly so when there has been time for erythroid hyperplasia to develop in the marrow as in chronic haemolysis. After an acute major haemorrhage, there is an erythropoietin response in 6 hours, the reticulocyte count rises within 2–3 days, reaches a maximum in 6–10 days and remains raised until the haemoglobin returns to the normal level—providing iron deficiency or some other additional cause for anaemia is not present. If the reticulocyte count is not raised in an anaemic patient this suggests impaired marrow function or lack of erythropoietin stimulus (Table 2.4).

Blood film
It is essential to examine the blood film in all cases of anaemia. Abnormal red cell morphology (Fig. 2.16) or red cell inclusions (Fig. 2.17) may suggest a particular diagnosis. When causes of both microcytosis and macrocytosis are present, e.g. mixed iron and folate or B_{12} deficiency, the indices may be normal but the blood film reveals a 'dimorphic' appearance (a dual population of large, well haemoglobinized cells and small, hypochromic cells). During the blood film examination the white cell differential count is performed, platelet number and morphology are assessed and the presence or absence of abnormal cells, e.g. normoblasts, granulocyte precursors or blast cells, is noted.

Table 2.4 Factors impairing the normal reticulocyte response to anaemia.

1 Marrow diseases, e.g. hypoplasia, infiltration by carcinoma, lymphoma, myeloma, acute leukaemia, tuberculosis
2 Deficiency of iron, vitamin B_{12} or folate
3 Lack of erythropoietin, e.g. renal disease
4 Reduced tissue O_2 consumption, e.g. myxoedema, protein deficiency
5 Ineffective erythropoiesis, e.g. thalassaemia major, megaloblastic anaemia, myelodysplasia, myelofibrosis, congenital dyserythropoietic anaemia
6 Chronic inflammatory or malignant disease

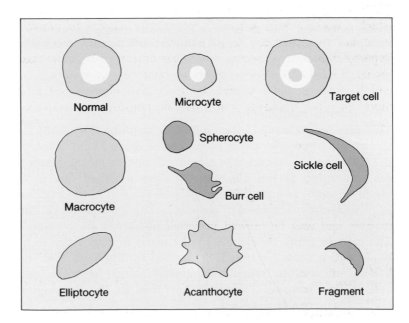

Fig. 2.16 Some of the more frequent variations in size (anisocytosis) and shape (poikilocytosis) that may be found in different anaemias.

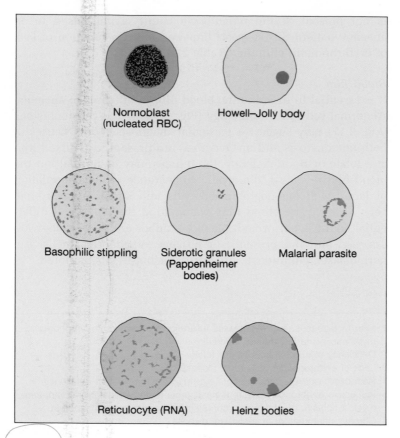

Normoblast (nucleated RBC)

Howell–Jolly body

Basophilic stippling

Siderotic granules (Pappenheimer bodies)

Malarial parasite

Reticulocyte (RNA)

Heinz bodies

Fig. 2.17 Red cell inclusions which may be seen in the peripheral blood film in various conditions. The reticulocyte RNA and Heinz bodies are only demonstrated by supravital staining, e.g. with new methylene blue. Heinz bodies are oxidized denatured haemoglobin. Siderotic granules (Pappenheimer bodies) contain iron. They are purple on conventional staining but blue with Perls' stain. The Howell–Jolly body is a DNA remnant. Basophilic stippling is denatured RNA.

Bone marrow examination

This may be performed by aspiration or trephine (Fig. 2.18).

Aspiration provides a film on which the detail of the developing cells can be examined (e.g. normoblastic or megaloblastic), the proportion of the different cell lines assessed (myeloid : erythroid ratio) and the presence of cells foreign to the marrow (e.g. secondary carcinoma) observed. The cellularity of the marrow can also be viewed provided fragments are obtained. The marrow films are stained by the usual Romanowsky technique and a stain for iron is performed routinely so that the amount of iron in reticulo-endothelial stores (macrophages) and as fine granules ('siderotic' granules) in the developing erythroblasts can be assessed.

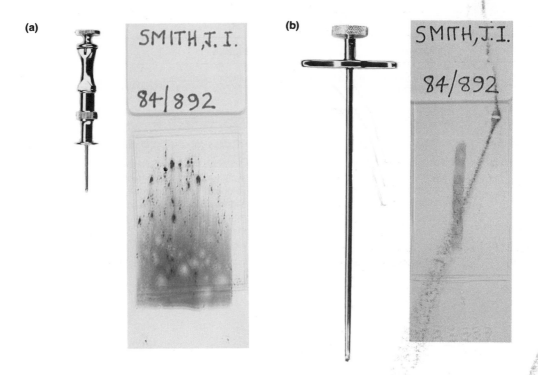

Fig. 2.18 (a) The Salah bone marrow aspiration needle and a smear made from a bone marrow aspirate. (b) The Jamshidi bone marrow trephine needle and normal trephine section.

Bone marrow aspiration is not required in some cases of anaemia, e.g. obvious cases of iron deficiency anaemia where more simple ancillary tests can confirm the diagnosis suspected from the peripheral blood count. But in other cases of anaemia, as well as in many other blood and systemic diseases, bone marrow aspiration provides invaluable diagnostic help. In some conditions, the cells obtained may be used for more detailed special tests (Table 2.5).

Trephine provides a core of bone including marrow and is examined as a histological specimen after fixation in formalin, decalcification and sectioning. With the introduction of simple, reliable needles (e.g. Jamshidi), trephine biopsy is easy to perform. It is less valuable than aspiration when individual cell detail is to be examined (e.g. diagnosis of megaloblastic anaemia or acute leukaemia) but provides a panoramic view of the marrow from which overall marrow architecture, cellularity and presence of abnormal infiltrates can be reliably determined.

Ineffective erythropoiesis

Erythropoiesis is not entirely efficient since about 10−15% of erythropoiesis in a normal bone marrow is ineffective, i.e. the developing erythroblasts die within the marrow without producing mature cells. Together with their haemoglobin, they are ingested by marrow macrophages. This ineffective erythro-

Table 2.5 Comparison of bone marrow aspiration and trephine biopsy.

	Aspiration	Trephine
Site	Sternum or posterior iliac crest (tibia in infants)	Posterior iliac crest
Stains	Romanowsky; Perls' reaction (for iron)	Haematoxylin + eosin; reticulin (silver stain)
Result available	1–2 hours	1–7 days (according to decalcification method)
Main indications	Investigation of anaemia, pancytopenia, suspected leukaemia or myeloma, neutropenia, thrombocytopenia, etc.	Indications for additional trephine: suspicion of polycythaemia vera, myelofibrosis and other myeloproliferative disorders, aplastic anaemia, malignant lymphoma, secondary carcinoma, cases of splenomegaly or pyrexia of undetermined cause. Any case where aspiration gives a 'dry' tap
Special tests	Cytogenetics, microbiological culture, biochemical analysis, immunological and cytochemical markers, immunoglobulin or T cell receptor gene analysis, DNA or RNA analysis for gene abnormalities, progenitor cell culture	

poiesis or 'intramedullary haemolysis' is substantially increased in a number of chronic anaemias (see Table 2.4). The serum unconjugated bilirubin (derived from breaking down haemoglobin) and lactate dehydrogenase (LDH, derived from breaking down cells) are usually raised when ineffective erythropoiesis is marked. Radioactive iron is rapidly cleared from plasma to the marrow but there is poor incorporation into circulating red cells. The reticulocyte count is low in relation to the degree of anaemia and to the proportion of erythroblasts in the marrow.

Quantitative aspects of erythropoiesis

A number of tests can be performed to assess total erythropoiesis, the amount of erythropoiesis that is effective in producing circulating red cells and the lifespan of circulating red cells.

Tests of total erythropoiesis

1 *Marrow cellularity and the myeloid:erythroid ratio* (i.e. the proportion of granulocyte precursors to red cell precursors in the bone marrow, normally 2.5:1 to 12:1). This ratio falls and may be reversed when total erythropoiesis is selectively increased.

2 *Plasma iron turnover.* The extent of erythropoiesis may be

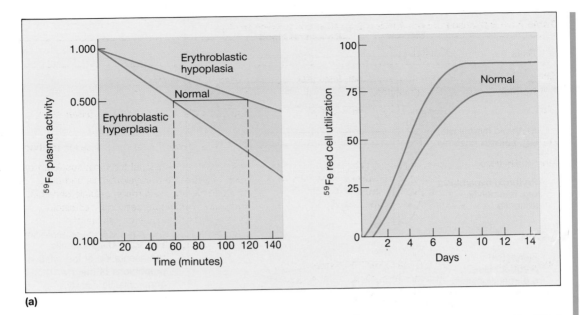

(a)

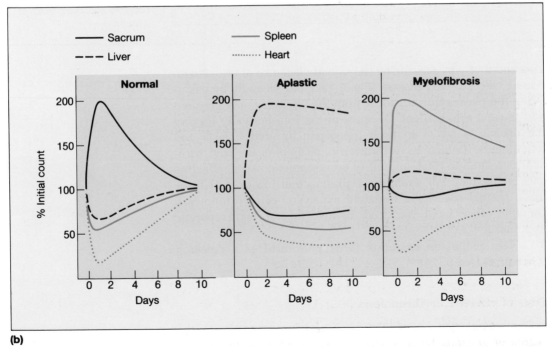

(b)

Fig. 2.19 (a) ^{59}Fe ferrokinetic study. A trace dose of ^{59}Fe is injected intravenously and attaches to transferrin in plasma. The transferrin carries the ^{59}Fe to cells with transferrin receptors, especially marrow erythroblasts. (*Left*) Initial clearance of ^{59}Fe from plasma. This is rapid with a normal half clearance time of 60–120 minutes. Clearance is delayed in erythroblastic hypoplasia and more rapid in erythroblastic hyperplasia. (*Right*) ^{59}Fe red cell utilization or incorporation. In normal subjects this rises steadily from 24 hours to a maximum of 70–80% on the 10–14th day. (b) ^{59}Fe ferrokinetic study; surface counting patterns. (*Left*) Normal; (*centre*) aplastic anaemia (note lack of accumulation in the bone marrow (sacrum)); (*right*) myelofibrosis (pattern of extramedullary erythropoiesis in the liver and spleen).

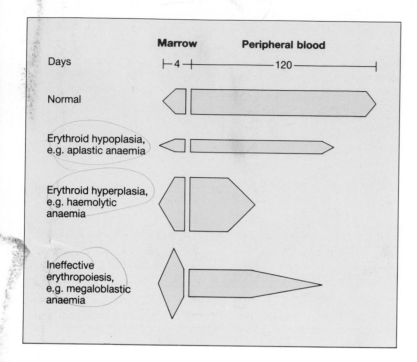

Fig. 2.20 Diagrammatic representation of the relative proportions of marrow erythroblastic activity, circulating red cell mass and red cell lifespan in normal subjects and three types of anaemia.

assessed firstly by measuring the rate of clearance of transferrin-bound ^{59}Fe from the plasma (Fig. 2.19a) and secondly by calculating the plasma iron turnover from the clearance measurement and plasma iron content. As most of the iron normally leaving the plasma is taken up from transferrin by erythroblasts and reticulocytes (which have transferrin receptors), the iron turnover is related to total amount of erythropoietic tissue (effective and ineffective). For example, a plasma iron turnover of three times normal suggests a threefold expansion of erythropoiesis. On the other hand, reduced figures suggest erythropoietic hypoplasia.

3 *Carbon monoxide excretion* (only performed as a research procedure) (see p. 74).

Tests of effective erythropoiesis

1 *The reticulocyte count.* This is raised in proportion to the degree of anaemia when erythropoiesis is effective, but is low when there is ineffective erythropoiesis or an abnormality preventing normal marrow response (see Table 2.4).

2 ^{59}Fe *incorporation into circulating red cells.* The iron incorporated into haemoglobin which reappears in the circulation after the first day of the study is an indication of effective erythropoiesis. This iron has entered erythroblasts from transferrin and has been incorporated into their haemoglobin.

Normally 70–80% of the injected ^{59}Fe is utilized in this manner and reappears in the circulation within 10 days (Fig. 2.19a). Maximum red cell iron incorporation values of less than 70% indicate diminished or ineffective erythropoiesis.

The sites of erythropoiesis (medullary and extramedullary) are demonstrated by counting the radioactivity over the sacrum, liver, spleen and heart (Fig. 2.19b).

Red cell lifespan

This is measured by ^{51}Cr-labelled red cell survival. A sample of the subject's blood is incubated with ^{51}Cr which binds firmly to haemoglobin and the labelled cells are re-injected into the circulation. The disappearance of ^{51}Cr from the blood is measured sequentially over the next 3 weeks. The sites of red cell destruction are determined by surface counting over the spleen, liver and heart (as an index of blood activity). Typical results in a haemolytic anaemia are shown in Fig. 5.2. Figure 2.20 shows typical changes in marrow erythropoiesis and circulating red cell mass in some of the different types of anaemia.

Bibliography

Erslev A.J. & Gabuzda T.G. (1985) *Pathophysiology of Blood*, 3rd Edition. W.B. Saunders, Philadelphia.

Erslev A.J., Schuster S.J. & Caro J. (1989) Erythropoietin and its clinical promise. *European Journal of Haematology*, **43**, 367–373.

Eschbach J.W. (1989) The anemia of chronic renal failure: pathophysiology and the effects of recombinant erythropoietin (Clinical conference). *Kidney International*, **35**, 134–148.

Granick M.B. (ed.) (1990) *Erythropoietin in Clinical Applications*. Marcel Dekker, New York.

Pippard M.J., Hughes R.T. & Cotes P.M. (1992) Erythropoietin. In *Recent Advances in Haematology*, 6 (eds A.V. Hoffbrand & M.K. Brenner). Churchill Livingstone, Edinburgh, pp. 1–18.

Chapter 3
Iron Deficiency and Other Hypochromic Anaemias

Iron deficiency is the commonest cause of anaemia in every country of the world. It is the most important, but not sole, cause of a microcytic, hypochromic anaemia, in which all three red cell indices (the MCV, MCH and MCHC—mean corpuscular volume, haemoglobin and haemoglobin concentration, respectively) are reduced and the blood film shows microcytic, hypochromic red cells. This appearance is due to a defect in haemoglobin synthesis (Fig. 3.1). The thalassaemias, in which globin synthesis is reduced, are considered in Chapter 6. Iron deficiency and the hypochromic anaemias other than thalassaemia, and the approach to the diagnosis of a patient found to have a hypochromic anaemia, are discussed in this chapter.

Iron overload and its treatment are dealt with in Chapter 6.

Nutritional and metabolic aspects of iron

Iron is one of the commonest elements in the earth's crust, yet iron deficiency is the commonest cause of anaemia. This is because the body has a limited ability to absorb iron and excess loss of iron due to haemorrhage is frequent.

Body iron distribution

Haemoglobin contains about two-thirds of body iron (Table 3.1). Iron is incorporated from plasma transferrin into developing erythroblasts in the bone marrow and into reticulocytes (Fig. 3.2). Transferrin obtains iron mainly from reticulo-endothelial (RE) cells (macrophages). Only a small proportion of plasma iron comes from dietary iron absorbed through the duodenum and jejunum. At the end of their life, red cells are broken down in the macrophages of the RE system and their iron is subsequently released into the plasma. Some of the iron is also stored in the RE cells as haemosiderin and ferritin, the amount varying widely according to overall body iron status.

Ferritin is a water-soluble protein—iron complex of molecular weight (MW) 465 000; it is made up of an outer protein shell, apoferritin, consisting of 22 subunits and an iron—phosphate—hydroxide core. It contains up to 20% of its weight as iron and is

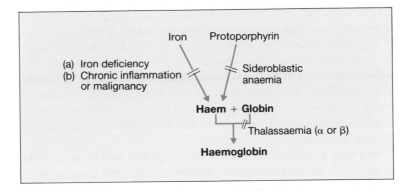

Fig. 3.1 The causes of a hypochromic microcytic anaemia. These include lack of iron (iron deficiency) or of iron release from macrophages to serum (anaemia of chronic inflammation or malignancy), failure of protoporphyrin synthesis (sideroblastic anaemia) or of globin synthesis (α- or β-thalassaemia). Lead also inhibits haem and globin synthesis.

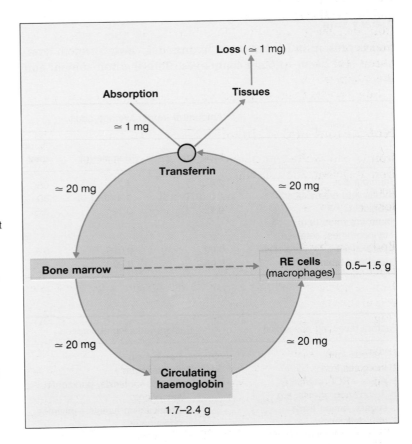

Fig. 3.2 Daily iron cycle. Most of the iron in the body is contained in circulating haemoglobin (Table 3.1) and is re-utilized for haemoglobin synthesis after the red cells die. Iron is transferred from macrophages to plasma transferrin and so to bone marrow erythroblasts. Iron absorption is normally just sufficient to make up for iron loss. The dashed line indicates ineffective erythropoiesis. RE, reticuloendothelial.

not visible by light microscopy. Each molecule of apoferritin may bind up to 4000–5000 atoms of iron and its synthesis is stimulated by iron. *Haemosiderin* is an insoluble protein–iron

complex of varying composition containing about 37% of iron
by weight. It is probably derived from partial lysosomal digestion
of aggregates of ferritin molecules and is visible in macrophages
by light microscopy after staining by Perls' (Prussian blue) reaction. Iron in ferritin and haemosiderin is in the ferric form.
It is mobilized after reduction to the ferrous form, vitamin C
being involved. A copper-containing enzyme, caeruloplasmin,
catalyses oxidation of the iron to the ferric form for binding to
plasma transferrin.

Iron is also present in muscle as myoglobin and in most cells
of the body in iron-containing enzymes, e.g. cytochromes, suc-
cinic dehydrogenase, catalase, etc. (Table 3.1). This tissue iron
is less likely to become depleted than haemosiderin, ferritin and
haemoglobin in states of iron deficiency, but some reduction of
haem-containing enzymes may occur in severe chronic iron
deficiency.

Dietary iron

Iron is present in food as ferric hydroxides, ferric—protein complexes and haem—protein complexes. Both the iron content and

Table 3.1 The distribution of body iron

	Amount of iron in average adult		
	Male (g)	Female (g)	% of total
Haemoglobin	2.4	1.7	65
Ferritin and haemosiderin	1.0 (0.3—1.5)	0.3 (0—1.0)	30
Myoglobin	0.15	0.12	3.5
Haem enzymes (e.g. cytochromes, catalase, peroxidases, flavoproteins)	0.02	0.015	0.5
Transferrin-bound iron	0.004	0.003	0.1

Table 3.2 Iron absorption.

Factors favouring absorption	Factors reducing absorption
1 Ferrous form	1 Ferric form
2 Inorganic iron	2 Organic iron
3 Acids—HCl, vitamin C	3 Alkalis—antacids, pancreatic secretions
4 Solubilizing agents, e.g. sugars, amino acids	4 Precipitating agents—phytates, phosphates
5 Iron deficiency	5 Iron excess
6 Increased erythropoiesis	6 Decreased erythropoiesis
7 Pregnancy	7 Infection
8 Primary haemochromatosis	8 Tea
	9 Desferrioxamine

the proportion of iron absorbed differ from food to food; in general, meat and, in particular, liver is a better source than vegetables, eggs or dairy foods. The average Western diet contains 10−15 mg of iron from which only 5−10% is normally absorbed. The proportion can be increased to 20−30% in iron deficiency or pregnancy (Table 3.2) but, even in these situations, most dietary iron remains unabsorbed.

Iron absorption

This occurs through the duodenum and less through the jejunum; it is favoured by factors such as acid and reducing agents keeping the iron soluble, particularly maintaining it in the Fe^{2+} rather than Fe^{3+} state (Table 3.2). Organic iron is partly broken down to inorganic iron, but some intact haem iron may also enter the mucosal cell to be split within it. The control of the amount of iron entering portal blood lies partly at the brush borders which influence the amount entering the mucosal cell but also within the cell. Excess iron is combined with apoferritin to form ferritin, which is shed into the gut lumen when the mucosal cell reaches the tip of the intestinal villus. In iron deficiency, more iron enters the cell and a greater proportion of this intramucosal iron is transported into portal blood; in iron overload, less iron enters the cell and a greater proportion of this is shed back into the gut lumen. Iron enters plasma in the Fe^{3+} form but, except in rare cases of iron overload, free iron is not present in plasma, since it binds to transferrin in portal blood.

Iron transport

Most internal iron exchange is concerned with providing iron to the marrow for erythropoiesis (Fig. 3.2). Iron is transported in plasma bound to a β-globulin, transferrin (siderophyllin), of MW 80 000. This protein is synthesized in the liver, has a half-life of 8−10 days, and is capable of binding two atoms of iron per molecule. It is re-utilized after it has given up its iron (Fig. 3.2). Normally it is one-third saturated but there is a diurnal variation in serum iron, the highest values occurring in the morning and the lowest in the evening. Transferrin gains iron mainly from the macrophages of the RE system and it is the diurnal variation in their release of iron which explains the diurnal variation in serum iron concentration. The erythroblasts and reticulocytes (and placenta) obtain iron from transferrin because they are particularly rich in specific transferrin receptors (see Fig. 2.6). Each day, 6 g of haemoglobin are synthesized which requires approximately 20 mg of iron (Fig. 3.2). There is also a minor flow of iron from plasma into non-erythroid cells and it has been estimated that the total plasma iron of only 4 mg turns over seven times each day.

When plasma iron is raised and transferrin is saturated, the amount of iron transferred to parenchymal cells, e.g. those of the liver, endocrine organs, pancreas and heart, is increased.

Iron requirements

The amount of iron required each day to compensate for losses from the body and growth varies with age and sex; it is highest in pregnancy and in adolescent and menstruating females (Table 3.3). These groups, therefore, are particularly likely to develop iron deficiency if there is additional iron loss or prolonged reduced intake.

Iron deficiency

Clinical features

When iron deficiency is developing, the RE stores (haemosiderin and ferritin) become completely depleted before anaemia occurs (Fig. 3.3). At an early stage, there are usually no clinical abnormalities. Later, the patient may develop the general symptoms and signs of anaemia and also show a painless glossitis, angular stomatitis, brittle, ridged or spoon nails (koilonychia), dysphagia due to pharyngeal webs (Paterson−Kelly or Plummer−Vinson syndrome (Fig 3.4) and unusual dietary cravings (pica). Atrophic gastritis and reduced gastric secretion, usually reversible with iron therapy, occurs in a proportion of patients. The cause of the epithelial cell changes is not clear but may be related to reduction of iron in iron-containing enzymes.

Table 3.3 Estimated daily iron requirements. Units are mg/day.

	Urine, sweat, faeces	Menses	Pregnancy	Growth	Total
Adult male	0.5−1				0.5−1
Post-menopausal female	0.5−1				0.5−1
Menstruating female*	0.5−1	0.5−1			1−2
Pregnant female*	0.5−1		1−2		1.5−3
Children (average)	0.5			0.6	1.1
Female (age 12−15)*	0.5−1	0.5−1		0.6	1.6−2.6

* These groups more likely to develop iron deficiency.

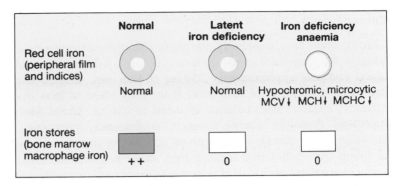

	Normal	Latent iron deficiency	Iron deficiency anaemia
Red cell iron (peripheral film and indices)	Normal	Normal	Hypochromic, microcytic MCV↓ MCH↓ MCHC↓
Iron stores (bone marrow macrophage iron)	++	0	0

Fig. 3.3 The development of iron deficiency anaemia. Reticuloendothelial (macrophage) stores are lost completely before anaemia develops. MCH, mean corpuscular haemoglobin; MCHC, mean corpuscular haemoglobin concentration; MCV, mean corpuscular volume.

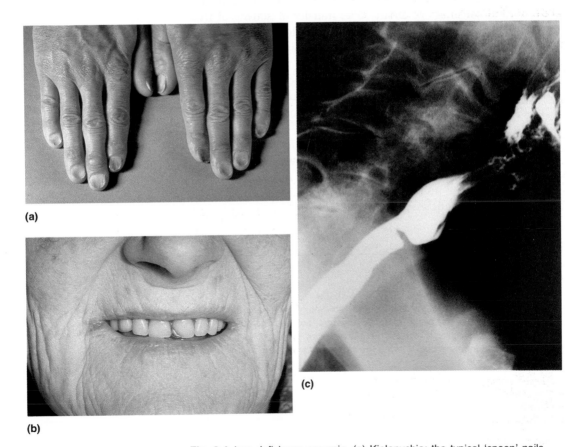

(a)

(b)

(c)

Fig. 3.4 Iron deficiency anaemia. (a) Kiolonychia: the typical 'spoon' nails. (b) Angular cheilosis: fissuring and ulceration of the corner of the mouth. (c) Paterson–Kelly (Plummer–Vinson) syndrome: barium swallow X-ray showing a filling defect due to a post-cricoid web.

Causes

Chronic blood loss, especially uterine or from the gastrointestinal tract is the dominant cause (Table 3.4). Half a litre of whole blood contains approximately 250 mg of iron and, despite the increased absorption of food iron at an early stage of iron deficiency, negative iron balance is usual in chronic blood loss. Increased demands during infancy, adolescence, pregnancy, lactation and in menstruating women account for the prevalence of latent iron deficiency (absent iron stores without anaemia) and a consequent high risk of anaemia in these particular clinical groups. Newborn infants have a store of iron derived from the breakdown of excess red cells. From 3 to 6 months, there is a tendency for negative iron balance to occur due to growth. Mixed feeding, particularly with iron-fortified foods, prevents iron deficiency.

In pregnancy, increased iron is needed for an increased maternal red cell mass of about 35%, transfer of 300 mg of iron to the foetus, and because of blood loss at delivery. Although iron absorption is also increased, prophylactic iron therapy is now given routinely.

Menorrhagia (a loss of 80 ml or more of blood at each cycle) is difficult to assess clinically, although the loss of clots, the use of large numbers of pads or tampons, or prolonged periods all suggest excessive loss.

It has been estimated to take 8 years for a normal adult male to develop iron deficiency anaemia solely due to a poor diet or malabsorption resulting in no iron intake at all. In clinical practice, inadequate intake or malabsorption are only rarely the sole cause of iron deficiency anaemia. Coeliac disease, partial or

---

Table 3.4 Causes of iron deficiency

Chronic blood loss
- Uterine
- Gastrointestinal, e.g. oesophageal varices, hiatus hernia, peptic ulcer, aspirin (or other non-steroidal anti-inflammatory drugs) ingestion, partial gastrectomy, carcinoma of the stomach, caecum, colon or rectum, hookworm, angiodysplasia, colitis, piles, diverticulosis, etc.
- Rarely haematuria, haemoglobinuria, pulmonary haemosiderosis, self-inflicted blood loss

Increased demands (see also Table 3.3)
- Prematurity
- Growth
- Child-bearing

Malabsorption
- For example gastrectomy, coeliac disease

Poor diet
- A contributory factor in many countries but rarely the sole cause

total gastrectomy and atrophic gastritis may, however, predispose to iron deficiency. There is also evidence that iron deficiency may cause or contribute to atrophic gastritis. The poor quality, largely vegetable diet taken in many under-developed countries may also produce a background of latent iron deficiency on which hookworm, repeated pregnancies and prolonged lactation may place additional stress.

Laboratory findings

These are summarized and contrasted with those in other hypochromic anaemias in Table 3.9.

Red cell indices and blood film

Even before anaemia occurs, the red cell indices fall and they fall progressively as the anaemia becomes more severe. The blood film shows hypochromic, microcytic cells with occasional target cells and pencil-shaped poikilocytes (Fig. 3.5). The reticulocyte count is low in relation to the degree of anaemia. When iron deficiency is associated with severe folate or vitamin B_{12} deficiency a 'dimorphic' film occurs with a dual population of red cells of which one is macrocytic and the other microcytic and hypochromic; the indices may be normal. A dimorphic blood film is also seen in patients with iron deficiency anaemia who have received recent iron therapy and produced a population of new well-filled normal-sized red cells (Fig. 3.6) and when the patient has been transfused. The platelet count is often moderately raised in iron deficiency, particularly when haemorrhage is continuing.

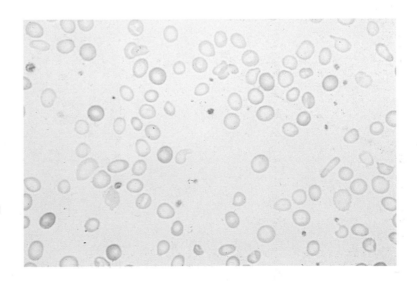

Fig. 3.5 The peripheral blood film in severe iron deficiency anaemia. The cells are microcytic and hypochromic with occasional target cells.

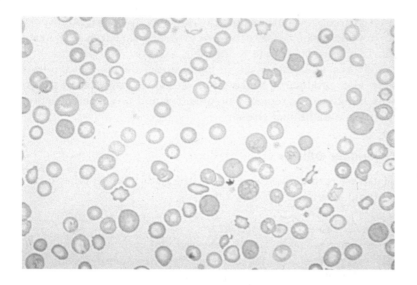

Fig. 3.6 Dimorphic blood film in iron-deficiency anaemia responding to iron therapy. Two populations of red cells are present, one microcytic and hypochromic, the other normocytic and well haemoglobinized.

Bone marrow iron

Bone marrow examination is not essential to assess iron stores except in complicated cases, but iron staining is carried out routinely on all bone marrow aspirations that are performed for any reason. In iron deficiency anaemia there is a complete absence of iron from stores (macrophages) and absence of siderotic iron granules from developing erythroblasts (Fig 3.7). The erythroblasts are small and have a ragged cytoplasm.

Fig. 3.7 Bone marrow iron assessed by Perls' stain. (a) Normal iron stores indicated by blue staining in the macrophages. Inset: normal siderotic granule in erythroblast. (b) Absence of blue staining (absence of haemosiderin) in iron deficiency. Inset: absence of siderotic granules in erythroblasts.

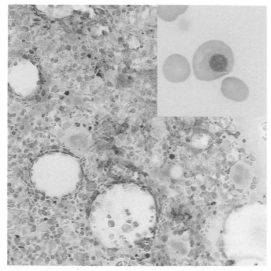

(a)

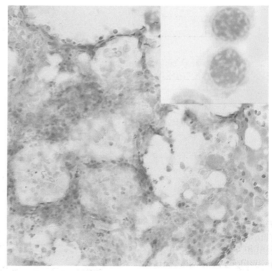

(b)

Serum iron and total iron-binding capacity (TIBC)

The serum iron falls and TIBC rises so that the IBC is less than 10% saturated (Fig. 3.8). This contrasts both with the anaemia of chronic disorders (see below) when the serum iron and the TIBC are both reduced and with other hypochromic anaemias where the serum iron is normal or even raised.

Serum ferritin

A small fraction of body ferritin circulates in the serum, the concentration being related to tissue, particularly RE, iron stores. The normal range in men is higher than in women (Fig. 3.8). In iron deficiency anaemia, the serum ferritin is very low while a raised serum ferritin indicates iron overload or excess release of ferritin from damaged tissues, e.g. acute hepatitis. The serum ferritin is normal or raised in the anaemia of chronic disorders.

Free erythrocyte protoporphyrin (FEP)

This increases early in iron deficiency before anaemia develops. Raised FEP levels are, however, also found in lead poisoning, some cases of sideroblastic anaemia and in erythropoietic porphyria. The test is not carried out routinely.

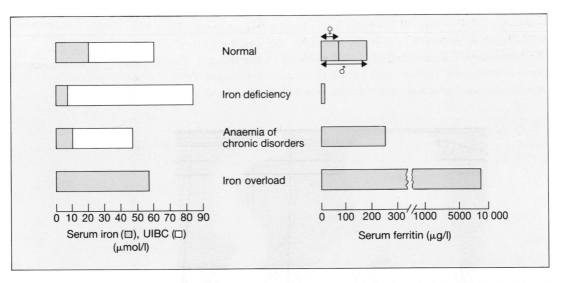

Fig. 3.8 The serum iron, unsaturated serum iron-binding capacity (UIBC) and serum ferritin in normal subjects and in those with iron deficiency, anaemia of chronic disorders and iron overload. The total iron-binding capacity (TIBC) is made up of the serum iron and the UIBC. In some laboratories, the transferrin content of serum is measured directly by immunodiffusion, rather than by its ability to bind iron, and is expressed as g/l. Normal serum contains 2–4 g/l of transferrin (1 g/l transferrin≃20 μmol/l binding capacity). Normal ranges for serum iron are 10–30 μmol/l; for TIBC, 40–75 μmol/l; for serum ferritin, male, 40–340 μg/l; and for serum ferritin, female, 14–150 μg/l.

Investigation of the cause of iron deficiency (see Table 3.4)

In premenopausal women, menorrhagia and/or repeated pregnancies are the usual causes of the deficiency although other causes must be sought if these are not present. In men and postmenopausal women, gastrointestinal blood loss is the main cause and the exact site is sought from the clinical history, physical and rectal examination, by occult blood tests, and by appropriate use of upper gastrointestinal endoscopy, sigmoidoscopy or colonoscopy and X-rays of the oesophagus, stomach, small and large intestine (Fig. 3.9). Hookworm ova are looked for in stools of subjects from areas where this infestation occurs. Rarely, a coeliac axis angiogram is needed to demonstrate angiodysplasia.

Occult blood tests depend on chemical detection of the intact haem ring with guaiac reagents or by the pseudoperoxidase test. Kits are of varying sensitivity, the more sensitive (e.g. to 2–3 ml daily blood loss) require dietary control of animal haemoproteins to avoid false-positive results while the less sensitive (e.g. to 10–12 ml daily blood loss) may give false-negative results. Oral iron therapy should not affect the result. Cr-labelling of red cells with a 5-day collection of stools is a more accurate method of assessing faecal blood loss.

If these tests are negative and intermittent gastrointestinal blood loss is excluded, loss of iron in the urine as haematuria or haemosiderinuria (due to chronic intravascular haemolysis) is considered. A normal chest X-ray excludes the rare condition of pulmonary haemosiderosis. Self-induced haemorrhage is more common in nurses and other medically associated but psychiatrically disturbed individuals. A whole-body counter is

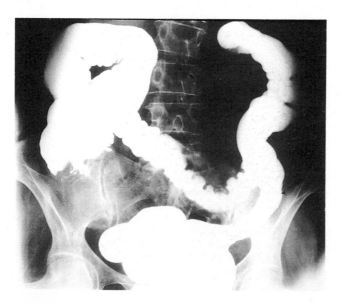

Fig. 3.9 Barium enema of a male patient aged 63 years who presented with iron-deficiency anaemia. There is a filling defect of the caecum and barium does not enter the terminal ileum. Carcinoma of the caecum was found at laparotomy.

useful for demonstrating loss of ^{51}Cr-labelled red cells from the body, without loss in urine or stools. A long-continued poor diet or malabsorption are considered, but are rarely the sole cause of deficiency in the UK.

Treatment

The underlying cause is treated as far as possible. In addition, iron is given to correct the anaemia and replenish iron stores (Table 3.5).

Oral iron
The best preparation is ferrous sulphate which is cheap, contains 67 mg in each 200 mg (anhydrous) tablet and is preferably given in doses spaced by at least 6 hours since the duodenum is refractory to iron absorption for a few hours after a single dose. Optimal absorption is obtained by giving iron to patients who are fasting. If side effects occur (e.g. nausea, abdominal pain, constipation or diarrhoea), these can be reduced by giving iron with food or by using a preparation of lower iron content, e.g. ferrous gluconate, which is also cheap but contains less iron (37 mg) per 300 mg tablet. Ferrous succinate, lactate and fumarate are equally good preparations but more expensive. An elixir is available for children. Combinations of iron with vitamins should not be used (except iron−folic acid combinations in pregnancy) as these are more expensive. Slow-release preparations release most of their iron in the lower small intestine where it cannot be absorbed.

Oral iron therapy should be given for long enough both to correct the anaemia and to replenish body iron stores, which usually means for 4−6 months. The haemoglobin should rise at the rate of about 2 g/dl every 3 weeks. There is a reticulocyte response related to the degree of anaemia. Failure of response to oral iron has several possible causes (Table 3.6) which should all be considered before parenteral iron is used.

Prophylactic iron therapy
This is given throughout pregnancy, often as a single daily tablet of ferrous sulphate combined with folic acid. Patients undergoing regular haemodialysis and premature babies also receive iron prophylactically.

Table 3.5 Treatment of iron deficiency

1 Determine underlying cause and treat this
2 Correct anaemia and replenish stores by oral iron, e.g. daily ferrous sulphate or ferrous gluconate (4−6 months). Rarely parenteral iron (intravenous or intramuscular) is needed, e.g. iron-dextran or iron-sorbitol-citrate

- Continuing haemorrhage
- Failure to take tablets
- Wrong diagnosis — especially thalassaemia trait, sideroblastic anaemia
- Mixed deficiency — associated folate or vitamin B_{12} deficiency
- Another cause for anaemia — e.g. malignancy, inflammation
- Malabsorption — this is a rare cause
- Use of slow-release preparation

Table 3.6 Failure of response to oral iron.

Parenteral iron

This may be given as a total dose infusion of iron-dextran, or by repeated injections of iron-dextran (Imferon) or iron-sorbitol-citrate (Jectofer). There may be hypersensitivity or anaphylactoid reactions and parenteral iron is therefore only given when it is considered necessary to replenish body iron rapidly, in, for example, late pregnancy or when oral iron is ineffective (e.g. severe malabsorption) or impractical (e.g. severe gastric or intestinal inflammatory disease). The haematological response to parenteral iron is no faster than to adequate doses of oral iron but the stores are replenished much faster.

Anaemia of chronic disorders

One of the most common anaemias occurs in patients with a variety of chronic inflammatory and malignant diseases (Table 3.7). The characteristic features are:
1 normochromic, normocytic or mildly hypochromic indices and red cell morphology;
2 mild and non-progressive anaemia (haemoglobin rarely less than 9.0 g/dl) — the severity being related to the severity of the disease;
3 both the serum iron and TIBC are reduced;
4 the serum ferritin is normal or raised; and
5 bone marrow storage (RE) iron is normal but erythroblast iron is reduced (see Table 3.9).

The pathogenesis of this anaemia appears to be related to decreased release of iron from macrophages to plasma, reduced

Chronic inflammatory diseases
- Infections, e.g. pulmonary abscess, tuberculosis, osteomyelitis, pneumonia, bacterial endocarditis
- Non-infectious, e.g. rheumatoid arthritis, SLE (systemic lupus erythematosus) and other connective tissue diseases, sarcoidosis, Crohn's disease

Malignant diseases
- For example carcinoma, lymphoma, sarcoma

Table 3.7 Causes of the anaemia of chronic disorders.

red cell lifespan and an inadequate erythropoietin response to anaemia. The anaemia is only corrected by successful treatment of the underlying disease and does not respond to iron therapy despite the low serum iron. Recombinant erythropoietin has been found to improve the anaemia in some cases. In many conditions this anaemia is complicated by anaemia due to other causes, e.g. iron, vitamin B_{12} or folate deficiency, renal failure, bone marrow failure, hypersplenism, endocrine abnormality, leucoerythroblastic anaemia, etc. and these are discussed in Chapter 20.

Sideroblastic anaemia

This is a refractory anaemia with hypochromic cells in the peripheral blood and increased marrow iron; it is defined by the presence of many pathological ring sideroblasts in the bone marrow (Fig. 3.10). These are abnormal erythroblasts containing numerous iron granules arranged in a ring or collar around the nucleus instead of the few randomly distributed iron granules seen when normal erythroblasts are stained for iron. The anaemia is classified into different types (Table 3.8). There is probably always a defect in haem synthesis. In the hereditary forms, the anaemia is characterized by a markedly hypochromic and microcytic blood picture. This is due to a congenital enzyme defect, e.g. of δ-aminolaevulinic acid synthetase or haem synthetase. The much more common primary acquired form, is one subtype of myelodysplasia. It is also termed 'refractory anaemia with ring sideroblasts'. This condition is discussed together with the other types of myelodysplasia in Chapter 12.

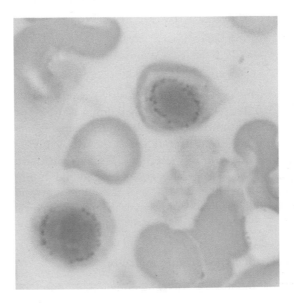

Fig. 3.10 Ring sideroblasts with a perinuclear ring of iron granules in sideroblastic anaemia.

Table 3.8 Classification of sideroblastic anaemia

Hereditary
- Usually occurs in males, transmitted by females; also occurs rarely in females

Acquired
- Primary
  Myelodysplasia FAB Type 2
- Secondary
  Other malignant diseases of the marrow, e.g. other types of myelodysplasia, myelosclerosis, myeloid leukaemia, myeloma
  Drugs, e.g. antituberculous (isoniazid, cycloserine), alcohol, lead
  Other benign conditions, e.g. haemolytic anaemia, megaloblastic anaemia, malabsorption

In the hereditary and primary acquired diseases, 15% or more of marrow erythroblasts are ring sideroblasts. Ring sideroblasts also occur with lesser frequency in other marrow disorders, especially the other types of myelodysplasia, the myelo-proliferative diseases, acute myeloid leukaemia (see p. 214) and myeloma. They may also occur in the bone marrow of patients taking certain drugs, excess alcohol or with lead poisoning. Vitamin B_6 (pyridoxine) deficiency or vitamin B_6 antagonists (e.g. isoniazid) are rare causes.

In some patients, particularly with the hereditary type, there is a response to pyridoxine therapy. Folate deficiency may occur and folic acid therapy should also be tried. In many severe cases, however, repeated blood transfusions are the only method of maintaining a satisfactory haemoglobin concentration and transfusional iron overload becomes a major problem. Other treatments which have been tried in myelodysplasia may be tried in the primary acquired (refractory anaemia with ring sideroblasts) form (Chapter 12).

Lead poisoning

Lead inhibits both haem and globin synthesis at a number of points. In addition it interferes with the breakdown of RNA by inhibiting the enzyme pyrimidine 5′ nucleotidase, causing ac-cumulation of denatured RNA in red cells, the RNA giving an appearance called basophilic stippling on the ordinary (Romanowsky) stain (Fig. 2.17). The anaemia may be hypo-chromic or predominantly haemolytic, and the bone marrow may show ring sideroblasts. Free erythrocyte protoporphyrin is raised.

Differential diagnosis of hypochromic anaemia

Table 3.9 lists the laboratory investigations that may be

necessary. The clinical history is particularly important as the source of the haemorrhage leading to iron deficiency or the presence of a chronic disease may be revealed. The country of origin and the family history may suggest a possible diagnosis of thalassaemia or other haemoglobinopathy. Physical examination may also be helpful in determining a site of haemorrhage, features of a chronic inflammatory or malignant disease, koilonychia, or, in some haemoglobinopathies, an enlarged spleen or bony deformities.

In the thalassaemia trait, the red cells tend to be small, often with an MCV of 60 fl or less, even when anaemia is mild or absent, the red cell count being over $5.0 \times 10^{12}/l$. On the other hand, in iron deficiency anaemia the indices fall progressively with the degree of anaemia, and when anaemia is mild the indices are often only just reduced below normal (e.g. MCV 75−80 fl). In the anaemia of chronic disorders, the indices are also not markedly low, an MCV in the range 75−82 fl being usual.

It is usual to perform a serum iron and TIBC measurement or, alternatively, serum ferritin estimation to confirm a diagnosis of iron deficiency. Haemoglobin electrophoresis with an estimation of Hb A_2 and Hb F is carried out in all patients suspected of thalassaemia or a haemoglobinopathy because of the family history, country of origin, red cell indices and blood film. Clearly iron deficiency or the anaemia of chronic disorders may

Table 3.9 Laboratory diagnosis of a hypochromic anaemia

	Iron deficiency	Chronic inflammation or malignancy	Thalassaemia trait (α or β)	Sideroblastic anaemia
MCV MCH MCHC*	All reduced in relation to severity of anaemia	Low normal or mild reduction	All reduced; very low for degree of anaemia	Very low in congenital type but MCV often raised in acquired type
Serum iron	Reduced	Reduced	Normal	Raised
TIBC	Raised	Reduced	Normal	Normal
Serum ferritin	Reduced	Normal or raised	Normal	Raised
Bone marrow iron stores	Absent	Present	Present	Present
Erythroblast iron	Absent	Absent	Present	Ring forms
Haemoglobin electrophoresis	Normal	Normal	Hb A_2 raised in β form[†]	Normal

* With modern electronic counters, the MCHC is not a reliable index of a hypochromic anaemia.
[†] Other types including major forms (see Chapter 6).
MCH, mean corpuscular haemoglobin; MCHC, mean corpuscular haemoglobin concentration; MCV, mean corpuscular volume; TIBC, total iron-binding capacity.

also occur in these subjects. Beta-thalassaemia trait is characterized by a raised Hb A_2 percentage above 3.5, but in α-
thalassaemia trait there is no abnormality on simple haemoglobin
studies. The diagnosis of α-thalassaemia trait is usually made by
exclusion of all other causes of hypochromic red cells and by
the presence of a red cell count $>5.0 \times 10^{12}/l$. Globin chain
synthesis or DNA studies can be used to confirm the diagnosis.
In some patients, however, occasional red cells show deposits of
Hb H (β^4) in reticulocyte preparations (Chapter 6).

Bone marrow examination is essential if a diagnosis of sideroblastic anaemia is suspected, but is not usually needed in diagnosis of the other hypochromic anaemias.

The investigation of a hypochromic anaemia is not complete
if a diagnosis of iron deficiency is confirmed. As discussed
on p. 46, it is then mandatory to determine the cause of the
deficiency—in nearly every case chronic haemorrhage. In
females of childbearing age, uterine haemorrhage is the most
frequent cause, but in males and post-menopausal females the
gastrointestinal tract is the usual source of bleeding; faecal occult
blood tests, endoscopy, barium meal, follow-through and enema
X-rays and tests for hookworm ova usually reveal the diagnosis
(Table 3.4).

Bibliography

Brittenham G.M. (1991) Disorders of iron metabolism: iron deficiency and overload. In *Hematology: Basic Principles and Practice* (eds R. Hoffman, E.J. Benz, S.J. Shattil, B. Furie & H.J. Cohen). Churchill Livingstone, New York, pp. 329–349.

Cox T.M. & Lord D.K. (1989) Hereditary haemochromatosis. *European Journal of Haematology*, **42**, 113–125.

Fairbanks V.F. & Beutler E. (1990a) Iron metabolism. In *Hematology*, 4th Edition (eds W.J. Williams, E. Beutler, A.J. Erslev & M.A. Lichtman). McGraw Hill, New York, pp. 329–339.

Fairbanks V.F. & Beutler E. (1990b) Iron deficiency. In *Hematology*, 4th Edition (eds W.J. Williams, E. Beutler, A.J. Erslev & M.A. Lichtman). McGraw Hill, New York, pp. 482–505.

Huebers H.A. & Finch C.A. (1987) The physiology of transferrin and transferrin receptors. *Physiology Reviews*, **67**, 520–582.

Jacobs A. (1985) Iron deficiency and iron overload. *CRC Critical Reviews in Oncology/Hematology*, **3**, 143–186.

Kuhn L.C. (1991) mRNA–protein interactions regulate critical pathways in cellular iron metabolism. *British Journal of Haematology*, **79**, 1–6.

Worwood M. (1990) Ferritin. *Blood Reviews*, **4**, 259–269.

Chapter 4
Megaloblastic Anaemias and Other Macrocytic Anaemias

Megaloblastic anaemias

This is a group of anaemias in which the erythroblasts in the bone marrow show a characteristic abnormality, maturation of the nucleus being delayed relative to that of the cytoplasm. The nuclear chromatin maintains an open, stippled, lacy appearance despite normal haemoglobin formation in the cytoplasm of the erythroblasts as they mature. The underlying defect accounting for the asynchronous maturation of the nucleus is defective DNA synthesis and, in clinical practice, this is usually due to deficiency of vitamin B_{12} (B_{12}) or folate. Less commonly, abnormalities of metabolism of these vitamins or other lesions in DNA synthesis may cause an identical haematological appearance (Table 4.1). Dietary and metabolic aspects of the two vitamins are reviewed before considering the anaemia.

Vitamin B_{12}

This vitamin is synthesized in nature by microorganisms; animals acquire it by eating other animal foods, by internal production due to intestinal bacteria (not in humans) or by eating bacterially contaminated foods. The vitamin consists of a small group of compounds, the cobalamins, which have the same basic structure, with a cobalt atom at the centre of a corrin ring which is attached to a nucleotide portion (Fig. 4.1). Methyl (CH_3-) and ado (deoxadenosyl) groups are attached to the cobalt in the two main natural forms, while cyano (CN) and hydroxoyl ($-OH$) groups are present in the two more stable pharmacological forms (Fig. 4.1). The vitamin is found in foods of animal

Table 4.1 Causes of megaloblastic anaemias.

1 Vitamin B_{12} deficiency

2 Folate deficiency

3 Abnormalities of vitamin B_{12} or folate metabolism, transcobalamin deficiency, nitrous oxide, anti-folate drugs

4 Other defects of DNA synthesis:
congenital enzyme deficiencies, e.g. orotic aciduria
acquired, e.g. alcohol, therapy with hydroxyurea, cytosine arabinoside

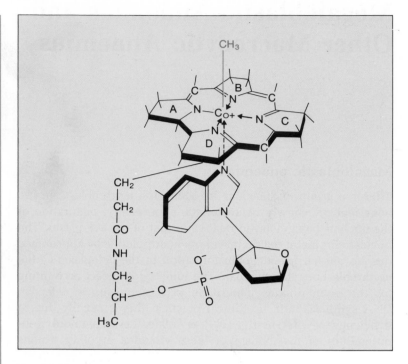

Fig. 4.1 The structure of methylcobalamin (methyl B_{12}), the main form of vitamin B_{12} in human plasma. Other forms include deoxyadenosylcobalamin (ado B_{12}), the main form in human tissues; hydroxocobalamin (hydroxo B_{12}), the main form in treatment; and cyanocobalamin (cyano B_{12}), the radioactively labelled (^{57}Co or ^{58}Co) form used to study vitamin B_{12} absorption or metabolism.

origin such as liver, fish and dairy produce but does not occur in fruit, cereals or vegetables unless these have been contaminated by bacteria. Table 4.2 considers nutritional aspects of B_{12} and folate.

Absorption

A normal diet contains a large excess of B_{12} compared with daily needs (Table 4.2). B_{12} is released from protein complexes in food, and ultimately combined, molecule to molecule, with the glycoprotein intrinsic factor (IF). Peptic digestion at low pH assists in the release of B_{12} from food. IF (MW 45 000) binds cobalamin but not non-physiological analogues of B_{12}. A second B_{12}-binding protein ('R') initially attaches to B_{12} in gastric juice but this B_{12} is released from the R protein by pancreatic digestion, and then is able to attach to IF.

IF is synthesized by the gastric parietal cells and the IF$-B_{12}$ complex is attached to specific surface receptors for IF in the distal ileum (Fig. 4.2). IF also binds B_{12} in bile, forming an enterohepatic circulation.

Table 4.2 Vitamin B_{12} and folate: nutritional aspects.

	Vitamin B_{12}	Folate
Normal daily dietary intake	7–30 μg	200–250 μg
Main foods	Animal produce only	Most, especially liver, greens and yeast
Cooking	Little effect	Easily destroyed
Minimal adult daily requirement	1–2 μg	150 μg
Body stores	2–3 mg (sufficient for 2–4 years)	10–12 mg (sufficient for 4 months)
Absorption		
Site	Ileum	Duodenum and jejunum
Mechanism	Intrinsic factor	Conversion to methyltetrahydrofolate
Limit	2–3 μg daily	50–80% of dietary content
Enterohepatic circulation	5–10 μg/day	90 μg/day
Transport in plasma	Most bound to TC I; TC II essential for cell uptake	Weakly bound to albumin
Major intracellular physiological forms	Methyl- and deoxyadenosyl-cobalamin	Reduced polyglutamate derivatives
Usual therapeutic form	Hydroxocobalamin	Folic (pteroylglutamic) acid

Transport: the transcobalamins

Vitamin B_{12} is absorbed into portal blood where it appears attached to a plasma-binding protein, transcobalamin II (TC II) which is a polypeptide (MW 38 000) synthesized in the liver, macrophages and the ileum. IF itself is not absorbed. TC II delivers B_{12} to bone marrow and other tissues by a process of receptor-mediated endocytosis; TC II being broken down.

Although TC II is the essential plasma protein for transferring B_{12} into the cells of the body, the amount of B_{12} on TC II is normally very low (<50 ng/l). TC II deficiency causes megaloblastic anaemia because of failure of B_{12} to enter marrow (and other cells) from plasma but the serum B_{12} level in TC II deficiency is normal. This is because most B_{12} in plasma is bound to another transport protein, TC I. This is a glycoprotein thought to be largely synthesized by granulocytes. In myeloproliferative diseases where granulocyte production is greatly increased, the TC I and B_{12} levels in serum both rise considerably.

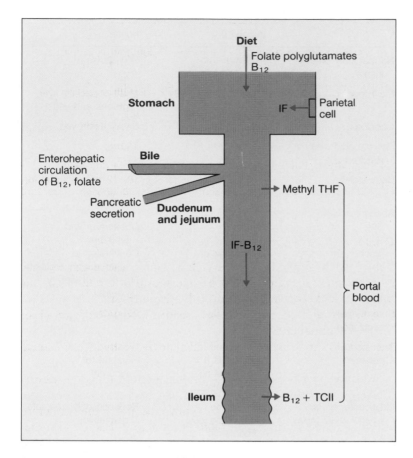

Fig. 4.2 The absorption of dietary vitamin B_{12} after combination with intrinsic factor (IF), through the ileum. Folate absorption occurs through the duodenum and jejunum after conversion of all dietary forms to methyltetra-hydrofolate (methyl THF). TC II, transcobalamin II.

B_{12} bound to TC I does not transfer readily to marrow; it appears to be functionally 'dead'. An identical plasma protein to TC I with a slightly different structure in the sugar moiety has been termed TC III. TC I and III can bind analogues of B_{12} and transport them to the liver for excretion in bile.

Biochemical function

Vitamin B_{12} is a coenzyme for two biochemical reactions in the body: firstly as methyl B_{12} as a co-factor in the methylation of homocysteine to methionine by methyl THF (tetrahydrofolate) (Fig. 4.3a) and secondly as deoxyadenosyl B_{12} (ado B_{12}) in conversion of methylmalonyl CoA (coenzyme A) to succinyl CoA (Fig. 4.3b). Assay of homocysteine in plasma and of methylmalonic acid in urine or plasma have been used as tests for B_{12} deficiency but have not entered regular clinical use.

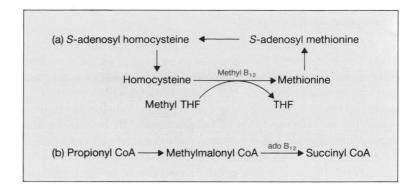

Fig. 4.3 The biochemical reactions of vitamin B_{12} in humans. ado B_{12}, deoxyadenosylcobalamin; CoA, coenzyme A; THF, tetrahydrofolate.

Folate

Folic (pteroylglutamic) acid is yellow, stable and water soluble. It is the parent compound of a large group of compounds, the folates, which are derived from it by three means.

1 Addition of extra glutamic acid residues, so-called pteroyl- or folate-polyglutamates.

2 Reduction to dihydrofolates (DHFs) or the metabolically active THFs.

3 Addition of single carbon units, e.g. methyl (CH_3-), formyl ($CHO-$) or methylene ($CH_2 =$) (Fig. 4.4).

Human beings are unable to synthesize the folate structure and thus require preformed folate as a vitamin. Bacteria synthesize folate *de novo* from pteridine, *p*-amino benzoic acid and glutamic acid. Sulphonamides block the incorporation of *p*-amino benzoic acid and thus inhibit bacterial folate synthesis.

Fig. 4.4 The structure of folic (pteroylglutamic) acid. Dietary folates may contain: (a) additional hydrogen atoms at positions 7 and 8 (dihydrofolate) or 5, 6, 7 and 8 (tetrahydrofolate); (b) a formyl group at N_5 or N_{10}, a methyl group at N_5 or other 1-carbon groups; and (c) additional glutamate moiety attached to the γ-carboxyl group of the glutamate moiety.

Absorption and transport

Folate polyglutamates are the main intracellular forms but, in body fluids, folate is transported as the monoglutamate methyl THF and is loosely bound to proteins. During absorption through the upper small intestine, all dietary folates are converted to methyl THF (Fig. 4.5). Dietary folate polyglutamates are hydrolysed by an enzyme 'pteroyl polyglutamate hydrolase' to the monoglutamate form which is then fully reduced and methylated in the intestinal cell. Bilary folate is reabsorbed by the same mechanism. Folate-binding proteins are present on the intestinal cell (as well as in milk, placenta, liver and other tissues) but their physiologic significance is not well understood.

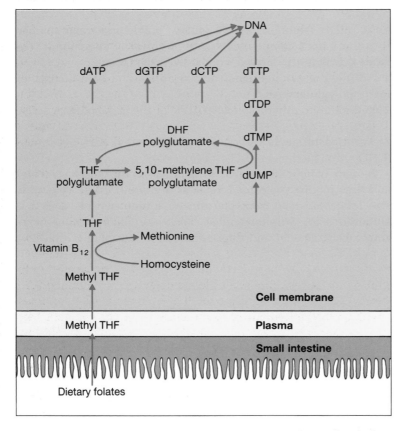

Fig. 4.5 The biochemical basis of megaloblastic anaemia due to vitamin B_{12} or folate deficiency. Folate is required in one of its coenzyme forms, 5,10-methylene tetrahydrofolate (THF) polyglutamate, in the synthesis of thymidine monophosphate from its precursor deoxyuridine monophosphate. Vitamin B_{12} is needed to convert methyl THF, which enters the cells from plasma, to THF, from which polyglutamate forms of folate are synthesized. Dietary folates are all converted to methyl THF (a monoglutamate) by the small intestine. A, adenine; C, cytosine; d, deoxyribose; DHF, dihydrofolate; DP, diphosphate; G, guanine; MP, monophosphate; T, thymine; TP, triphosphate; U, uracil.

Biochemical reactions

Folates are needed in a variety of biochemical reactions in the body involving single carbon unit transfer. Three of these are in DNA synthesis, two in the synthesis of purines and the third, thymidylate synthesis, is a key reaction in pyrimidine synthesis (Fig. 4.5). The other folate-dependent reactions are largely concerned in amino acid interconversions, e.g. homocysteine conversion to methionine and serine to glycine.

Biochemical basis for megaloblastic anaemia

DNA is formed by polymerization of four precursors, the deoxyribonucleoside triphosphates (Fig. 4.5). Each provides a base: thymine or cytidine (pyrimidine) or adenine or guanine (purine), a sugar (deoxyribose) and a phosphate group. The sugar and phosphate moieties form the backbones of the double helix. Folate deficiency is thought to cause megaloblastic anaemia by inhibiting thymidylate synthesis, a rate-limiting step in DNA synthesis in which thymine, one of the two pyrimidine bases of DNA, is synthesized as its nucleotide-derivative thymidine monophosphate from deoxyuridine monophosphate (Fig. 4.5). This reaction needs 5,10-methylene THF polyglutamate as coenzyme.

All body cells including those of the bone marrow, receive folate from plasma as methyl THF. B_{12}, by its involvement in the methylation of homocysteine to methionine, is needed in the conversion of this methyl THF to THF. This is a substrate for folate polyglutamate synthesis inside cells. Formyl THF, derived from THF may also act as substrate for folate polyglutamate synthesis but methyl THF itself cannot. The folate polyglutamates act as intracellular folate coenzymes, including 5,10-methylene THF polyglutamate, the coenzyme form of folate involved in the thymidylate synthetase reaction (Fig. 4.5). Lack of B_{12}, therefore, slows the demethylation of methyl THF thus depriving cells of THF needed for folate polyglutamate synthesis and so of the 5,10-methylene THF polyglutamate coenzyme form needed for DNA synthesis. Other folate biochemical reactions (e.g. in purine synthesis) are also impaired in B_{12} (or folate) deficiency due to lack of the appropriate folate polyglutamate coenzyme.

Other congenital or acquired causes of megaloblastic anaemia (e.g. anti-metabolite drug therapy) inhibit purine or pyrimidine synthesis at one or other step. The result is a reduced supply of one or other of the four precursors needed for DNA synthesis.

Replication of chromosomal DNA in the presence of reduced concentration of one or other of the four deoxyribonucleotide precursors is incomplete, and in many cells chromosomal breaks are formed with death of cells in the 'S' phase of the cell cycle resulting in ineffective haemopoiesis.

Folate reduction

During thymidylate synthesis, the folate polyglutamate coenzyme becomes oxidized from the THF state to the functionally dead DHF (Fig. 4.5). Regeneration of active THF requires the enzyme DHF reductase. Inhibitors of this enzyme (e.g. methotrexate) therefore inhibit all folate coenzyme reactions, and so DNA synthesis, and are useful drugs mainly in the treatment of malignant disease or other diseases, e.g. of the skin, with excessive cell turnover. The weaker antagonist, pyrimethamine, is used primarily against malaria. Trimethoprim, active against bacterial DHF reductase but only very weakly against the human enzyme, is used in antibacterial combination with a sulphonamide, as co-trimoxazole. Toxicity due to methotrexate or pyrimethamine is reversed by giving the patient the stable fully reduced folate, folinic acid (5-formyl THF).

Vitamin B$_{12}$ deficiency

In Western countries, the deficiency is usually due to (Addisonian) pernicious anaemia (Table 4.3). Much less commonly the deficiency may be caused by veganism in which the diet lacks B$_{12}$ (usually in Hindu Indians), gastrectomy or small intestinal lesions. There is no syndrome of B$_{12}$ deficiency due to increased utilization or loss of the vitamin, so the deficiency

---

Table 4.3 Causes of vitamin B$_{12}$ deficiency.

NUTRITIONAL, especially vegans

MALABSORPTION

Gastric causes
- Adult (Addisonian) pernicious anaemia
- Congenital lack or abnormality of intrinsic factor
- Total or partial gastrectomy

Intestinal causes
- Intestinal stagnant loop syndrome — jejunal diverticulosis, blind-loop, stricture, etc.
- Chronic tropical sprue
- Ileal resection and Crohn's disease
- Congenital selective malabsorption with proteinuria
- Fish tapeworm

Other causes of malabsorption of B$_{12}$ (e.g. severe pancreatitis, gluten-induced enteropathy, therapy with metformin or phenformin, HIV infection, irradiation and chronic graft-vs-host disease) do not usually lead to clinically important B$_{12}$ deficiency.

inevitably takes at least 2 years to develop, i.e. the time needed for body stores to deplete at the rate of $1-2\,\mu g$ each day when there is no new B_{12} entering the body from the diet. Nitrous oxide, however, may rapidly inactivate body B_{12} (p. 71).

Pernicious anaemia

The common adult form consists of atrophy of the stomach, probably autoimmune in origin. The wall of the stomach is thin, with a plasma cell and lymphoid infiltrate of the lamina propria. There is achlorhydria and secretion of IF is absent or almost absent. Corticosteroid therapy can improve the gastric lesion with a return of acid secretion but, because of the side effects, pernicious anaemia (PA) is not treated in this way.

More females than males are affected (1.6 : 1) with a peak occurrence at 60 years, and there may be associated autoimmune disease, e.g. myxoedema, Hashimoto's disease, Addison's disease, vitiligo, hypoparathyroidism and hypogammaglobulinaemia (Table 4.4). The disease (most common in northern Europeans but found in all races) tends to occur in families and there is an association with blood group A, blue eyes and early greying, and there is an increased incidence of carcinoma of the stomach (about $2-3\%$ of all cases of PA). There is no overall association with any HLA (human leucocyte antigen).

Antibodies

Ninety per cent of patients show parietal cell antibody in the serum, and 50% type I or blocking antibody to IF which inhibits IF binding to B_{12}. Thirty-five per cent show a second (type II or precipitating) antibody to IF which inhibits its ileal binding site. IF antibodies are virtually specific for PA but occur in the serum of only half the patients, whereas the more common parietal cell antibody is less specific and occurs quite commonly in older subjects (e.g. 16% of normal women over 60 years). Both types of antibody may also occur in gastric juice. If present, IF antibody inhibits the function of small amounts of remaining IF in gastric juice and this may contribute to the malabsorption of B_{12}.

Table 4.4 Pernicious anaemia: associations.

Female	Vitiligo
Blue eyes	Myxoedema
Early greying	Hashimoto's disease
Northern European	Thyrotoxicosis
Familial	Addison's disease
Blood group A	Hypoparathyroidism
	Hypogammoglobulinaemia
	Carcinoma of the stomach

Childhood PA consists either of congenital lack or abnormality of IF (with an otherwise normal stomach and normal acid secretion) or an early onset of the adult, autoimmune form. Congenital lack of IF usually presents at about 2 years of age when stores of B_{12} which were derived from the mother *in utero* have been used up.

Folate deficiency

This is most often due to a poor dietary intake of folate alone or in combination with a condition of increased folate utilization or malabsorption (Table 4.5). Excess cell turnover of any sort, including pregnancy, is the main cause of an increased need for folate. The mechanism by which anticonvulsants and barbiturates cause the deficiency is still controversial. Alcohol, sulphasalazine and other drugs may have multiple effects on folate metabolism.

Clinical features

The onset is usually insidious with gradually progressive symptoms and signs of anaemia (Chapter 2). Sometimes an intermittent infection causes the patient to seek medical help. The

Table 4.5 Causes of folate deficiency.

NUTRITIONAL
Especially old age, institutions, poverty, famine, special diets, goat's milk anaemia, etc.

MALABSORPTION
Tropical sprue, coeliac disease (adult or child). Possible contributory factor to folate deficiency in some patients with partial gastrectomy, extensive jejunal resection or Crohn's disease

EXCESS UTILIZATION

Physiological
• Pregnancy and lactation, prematurity

Pathological
• Haematological diseases: haemolytic anaemias, myelosclerosis
• Malignant disease: carcinoma, lymphoma, myeloma
• Inflammatory diseases: Crohn's disease, tuberculosis, rheumatoid arthritis, psoriasis, exfoliative dermatitis, malaria

EXCESS URINARY FOLATE LOSS
Active liver disease, congestive heart failure

DRUGS
Anticonvulsants, sulphasalazine

MIXED
Liver disease, alcoholism, intensive care

Table 4.6 Definite effects of vitamin B$_{12}$ or folate deficiency.

Megaloblastic anaemia
Macrocytosis of epithelial cell surfaces
Neuropathy (for vitamin B$_{12}$ only)*
Sterility
Rarely, reversible melanin skin pigmentation
Decreased osteoblast activity

* Neural tube defects in the foetus may be related to folate deficiency.

patient may be mildly jaundiced (lemon yellow tint) (Fig. 4.6) from the excess breakdown of haemoglobin mainly due to increased ineffective erythropoiesis in the bone marrow. Glossitis (a beefy-red, sore tongue) (Fig. 4.7), angular stomatitis (Fig. 4.8) and mild symptoms of malabsorption with loss of weight may be present due to the epithelial abnormality. Purpura due to thrombocytopenia and widespread melanin pigmentation (the cause for which is unclear) are less frequent presenting features (Table 4.6). Many symptomless patients are diagnosed when a blood count that has been performed for another reason reveals macrocytosis.

Vitamin B$_{12}$ neuropathy (subacute combined degeneration of the cord)

Severe B$_{12}$ deficiency may cause a progressive neuropathy affecting the peripheral sensory nerves, and posterior and lateral columns (Fig. 4.9). The neuropathy is symmetrical and affects the lower limbs more than the upper limbs. The patient, more often male, notices tingling in the feet, difficulty in walking and may fall over in the dark. Rarely, optic atrophy or severe

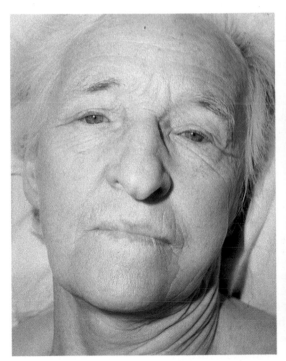

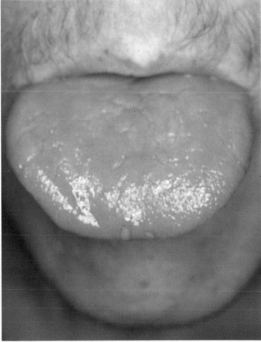

Fig. 4.6 Megaloblastic anaemia: pallor and mild icterus in a patient with a haemoglobin count of 7.0 g/dl and a MCV of 132 fl.

Fig. 4.7 Megaloblastic anaemia: glossitis—the tongue is beefy-red and painful.

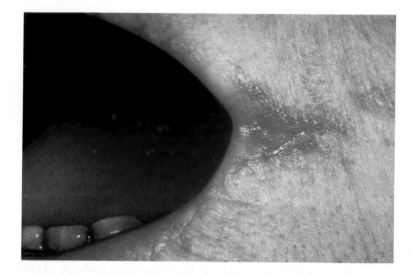

Fig. 4.8 Megaloblastic anaemia: angular cheilosis (stomatitis).

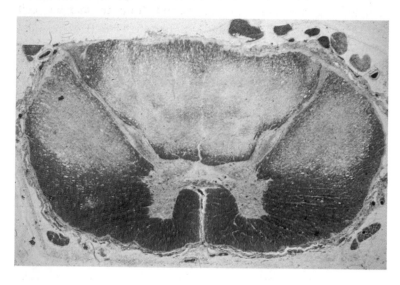

Fig. 4.9 A cross-section of the spinal cord in a patient who died with subacute combined degeneration of the cord (Weigert–Pal stain). There is demyelination of dorsal and dorsolateral columns.

psychiatric symptoms are present. Anaemia may be severe, mild or even absent, but the blood film and bone marrow appearances are always abnormal. The cause of the neuropathy is uncertain, but accumulation of S-adenosyl homocysteine due to excessive entry of homocysteine without an adequate mechanism for disposal of its end products of metabolism, has been postulated.

The evidence that folate deficiency in the adult can cause a neuropathy is conflicting. Methotrexate (an antifolate drug) can damage the brain. Folic acid therapy has been shown to reduce the incidence of neural tube defects (anencephaly, encephalocoele and spina bifida) in the foetus.

Laboratory findings

The anaemia is macrocytic (MCV > 95 fl and often as high as 120–140 fl in severe cases) and the macrocytes are typically oval in shape (Fig. 4.10). The reticulocyte count is low in relation to the degree of anaemia and the total white cell and platelet counts may be moderately reduced, especially in severely anaemic patients. A proportion of the neutrophils show hypersegmented nuclei (with six or more lobes). The bone marrow is usually hypercellular and the erythroblasts are large and show failure of nuclear maturation maintaining an open, fine, primitive chromatin pattern but normal haemoglobinization (Fig. 4.11). Many dying erythroblasts may be seen. Giant and abnormally shaped metamyelocytes are present. The changes correlate with the severity of anaemia so that, in mildly anaemic patients, the abnormalities may be quite difficult to recognize.

The serum unconjugated bilirubin, hydroxybutyrate and LDH (lactate dehydrogenase) are all raised (due to marrow cell breakdown—ineffective erythropoesis and leucopoiesis). The serum iron and ferritin are normal or raised.

Diagnosis of vitamin B_{12} or folate deficiency

It is usual to assay serum B_{12}, serum and red cell folate (Table 4.7). Either microbiological or radioisotope dilution assays are used. The serum B_{12} is usually very low in megaloblastic anaemia or neuropathy due to B_{12} deficiency. The serum and red cell folate are both low in megaloblastic anaemia due to folate deficiency. In B_{12} deficiency the serum folate tends to rise but the red cell folate (largely folate polyglutamates) falls due to failure of folate polyglutamate synthesis. In the absence

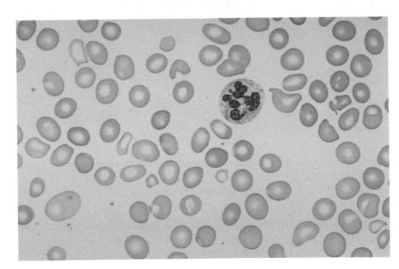

Fig. 4.10 Megaloblastic anaemia: peripheral blood film showing oval macrocytes.

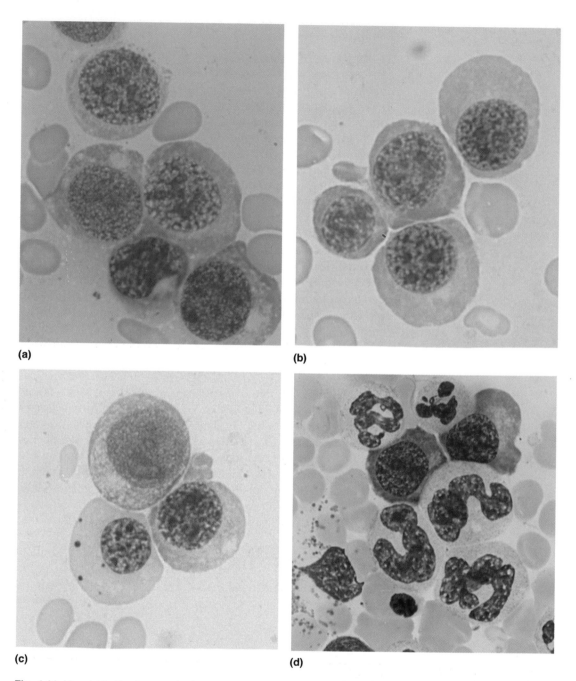

(a)

(b)

(c)

(d)

Fig. 4.11 Megaloblastic changes in the bone marrow in a patient with severe megaloblastic anaemia. (a–c) Erythroblasts showing fine, open stippled (primitive) appearance of the nuclear chromatin even in late cells (pale cytoplasm with some haemoglobin formation). (d) Abnormal giant metamyelocytes and band forms.

of B_{12} deficiency, however, the red cell folate is a more accurate guide than the serum folate of tissue folate status. Combined deficiencies may be difficult to sort out. The haematological

Table 4.7 Laboratory tests for vitamin B_{12} and folate deficiency.

Test	Normal value*	Result in Vitamin B_{12} deficiency	Result in Folate deficiency
Serum B_{12}	160–925 ng/l	Low	Normal or borderline
Serum folate	3.0–15.0 µg/l	Normal or raised	Low
Red cell folate	160–640 µg/l	Normal or low	Low

* Normal values differ slightly with different commercial kits.

response of the patient to specific therapy is particularly helpful in those cases with low serum levels of both vitamins providing that daily physiological doses (1 µg B_{12} or 100 µg folic acid) are used, since a response will only occur if there is deficiency of the appropriate vitamin. Large doses of folic acid (e.g. 5 mg daily) cause a haematological response (but may aggravate the neuropathy) in B_{12} deficiency and thus should not be given alone unless B_{12} deficiency has been excluded, e.g. by showing a normal serum B_{12} level.

The deoxyuridine (dU) suppression test may be used to diagnose megaloblastic anaemia (Fig. 4.12). It measures the degree to which unlabelled dU suppresses uptake of radioactive thymidine into the DNA of bone marrow cells *in vitro*. The test is abnormal (less suppression of thymidine uptake by dU) in megaloblastic anaemia due to B_{12} or folate deficiency.

Tests for cause of vitamin B_{12} or folate deficiency

For B_{12} deficiency, absorption tests (Table 4.8) using an oral dose of radioactive cobalt (^{57}Co)-labelled cyanocobalamin are valuable in distinguishing malabsorption from an inadequate diet. When the test is repeated with an active IF preparation gastric lesions such as PA can be distinguished from intestinal lesions; IF correcting absorption in PA and other gastric lesions

Table 4.8 Tests for cause of vitamin B_{12} or folate deficiency.

Vitamin B_{12}	Folate
1 Diet history	1 Diet history
2 B_{12} absorption — IF	2 Tests for intestinal malabsorption
3 IF, parietal cell antibodies	3 Jejunal biopsy
4 Endoscopy or barium meal and follow through	4 Underlying disease
5 Gastric function — acid, IF	

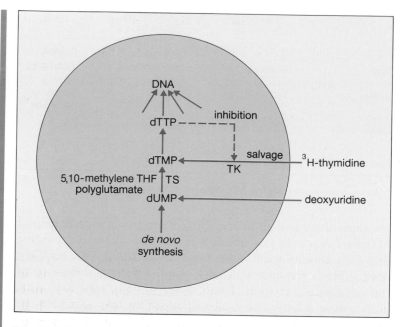

Fig. 4.12 The deoxyuridine (dU) suppression test. Excess unlabelled dU suppresses the incorporation of ³H-thymidine into DNA. Incorporation of ³H-thymidine alone with no dU equals 100%. The results show the following dU suppressed values: normal <10%; B_{12} deficiency >10%, corrected by B_{12} *not* by methyl-THF; folate deficiency >10%, corrected by methyl THF *not* by B_{12}; megaloblastic anaemia not due to B_{12} or folate deficiency or to another fault of the thymidylate synthetase <10%. d, deoxyribose; MP, monophosphate; T, thymine; THF, tetrahydrofolate; TK, thymidine kinase; TP, triphosphate; TS, thymidylate synthetase; U, uridine.

	Dose of labelled B_{12} given alone	Dose of labelled B_{12} given with IF
Vegan	Normal	Normal
Pernicious anaemia or gastrectomy	Low	Normal
Ileal lesion	Low	Low
Intestinal blind-loop syndrome	Low*	Low*

Table 4.9 Results of absorption tests of radioactive vitamin B_{12}.

* Corrected by antibiotic therapy.

but not in intestinal diseases (Table 4.9). Absorption is most frequently measured indirectly by the urinary excretion (Schilling) technique in which absorbed labelled B_{12} is 'flushed' into a 24-hour urine sample by a large (1000 µg) dose of non-radioactive B_{12} given simultaneously with the labelled oral dose. Whole body counting is also used to measure radioactive B absorption in some centres. Tests using labelled B_{12} given with food are also used.

Other useful tests are listed in Table 4.8. These are mainly concerned with assessing gastric function and testing for antibodies to gastric antigens. In all cases of pernicious anaemia, X-ray or endoscopy studies should be performed to confirm the presence of gastric atrophy and exclude carcinoma of the stomach.

For folate deficiency, the diet history is most important, although it is difficult to estimate folate intake accurately. Unsuspected coeliac disease or other underlying conditions (see Table 4.5) should also be considered.

Treatment

Most cases only need therapy with the appropriate vitamin (Table 4.10). In severely anaemic patients in whom there is no clear indication which deficiency is present, but who need treatment urgently, it may be safer to initiate treatment with both vitamins after blood has been taken for B_{12} and folate examinations and a bone marrow test has been performed. In the elderly, the presence of heart failure should be corrected with diuretics and oral potassium supplements given for 10 days (since hypokalaemia has been found to occur during the response in some cases). Infection should be sought and treated. Blood transfusion should be avoided since it may cause circulatory overload. If it is essential (because of anoxia) $1-2$ units of packed cells should be given slowly, possibly with removal of blood from the other arm.

Table 4.10 Treatment of megaloblastic anaemia.

	Vitamin B_{12} deficiency	Folate deficiency
Compound	Hydroxocobalamin	Folic acid
Route	Intramuscular	Oral
Dose	1000 µg	5 mg
Initial	6 × 1000 µg over 2–3 weeks	Daily for 4 months
Maintenance	1000 µg every 3 months	Depends on underlying disease; life-long therapy may be needed in chronic inherited haemolytic anaemias, myelosclerosis, renal dialysis
Prophylactic	Total gastrectomy Ileal resection	Pregnancy, severe haemolytic anaemias, dialysis, prematurity

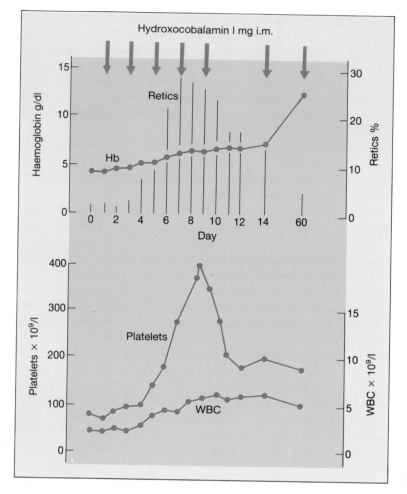

Fig. 4.13 A typical haematological response to vitamin B_{12} (hydroxo-cobalamin) therapy in pernicious anaemia. Retics, reticulocytes; WBC, white blood cells.

Response to therapy

The patient feels better after 24–48 hours of correct vitamin therapy with increased appetite and well being. A reticulocyte response begins on the second or third day with a peak at 6–7 days—its height is inversely proportional to the initial red cell count (Fig. 4.13). The haemoglobin should rise by 2–3 g/dl each fortnight. The white cell and platelet counts become normal in 7–10 days and the marrow is normoblastic in about 48 hours, although giant metamyelocytes persist for up to 12 days. The serum iron falls over the first day and the LDH and ferritin more slowly.

The peripheral neuropathy may partly improve but spinal cord damage is irreversible.

Inadequate response

This may be because the wrong vitamin has been given, because the patient has an associated cause for anaemia (e.g. iron deficiency, infection or malignancy), or because the diagnosis is incorrect.

Prophylactic therapy

Vitamin B_{12} is given to patients who have total gastrectomy or ileal resection. Folic acid is given in pregnancy at a recommended dose of 400 µg daily. For women who have had a previous pregnancy with a foetus with a neural tube defect, folic acid 4 mg daily is advised preconception and continued for the first 12 weeks of the pregnancy. All women of child-bearing age are recommended to have an intake of at least 400 µg daily (by increased intake of folate-rich or folate-supplemented foods or as folic acid) to prevent a first occurrence of a neural tube defect in the foetus.

Folic acid is also given to patients undergoing chronic dialysis and with severe haemolytic anaemias and chronic myelosclerosis, and to premature babies.

Other megaloblastic anaemias

See Table 4.1.

Abnormalities of vitamin B_{12} or folate metabolism

These are unusual and include congenital deficiencies of enzymes concerned in B_{12} or folate metabolism or of the serum transport protein for B_{12}, TC II, which is needed for serum B_{12} to enter bone marrow cells. Nitrous oxide (N_2O) anaesthesia causes rapid inactivation of body B_{12} by oxidizing the reduced cobalt atom of methyl B_{12}. Megaloblastic marrow changes occur with several days of N_2O administration and can cause pancytopenia. Chronic exposure (as in dentists and anaesthetists) has been associated with neurological damage resembling B_{12}-deficiency neuropathy. Anti-folate drugs, particularly those which inhibit DHF reductase (e.g. methotrexate and pyrimethamine) may also cause megaloblastic change. Trimethoprim, which inhibits bacterial DHF reductase, has only a slight action against the human enzyme and causes megaloblastic change only in patients already B_{12}- or folate-deficient.

Defects of DNA synthesis not related to vitamin B_{12} or folate

Congenital deficiency of one or other enzyme concerned in purine or pyrimidine synthesis may cause megaloblastic anaemia identical in appearance to that due to a deficiency of B_{12} or folate. The best known is orotic aciduria. Therapy with drugs which inhibit purine or pyrimidine synthesis (such as hydroxyurea, cytosine arabinoside, 6-mercaptopurine and zidovudine (AZT)) also causes megaloblastic anaemia. Megaloblastic changes may also occur in association with erythroleukaemia and acquired sideroblastic anaemia, but the site of the defect in DNA synthesis in these conditions is unknown and the anaemia does not respond to B_{12} or folate therapy. The dU suppression test gives a normal result.

Other macrocytic anaemias

Big circulating red cells can be caused by a variety of conditions other than B_{12} or folate deficiency. In some of these situations the bone marrow shows normoblastic rather than megaloblastic erythropoiesis (Table 4.11). The exact mechanisms creating the large red cells in each of these conditions is not clear although, in some, increased lipid deposition on the red cell membrane and, in others, alterations in blast maturation time in the marrow, have been suggested. Reticulocytes are bigger than mature red cells. The red cells in the macrocytic but normoblastic anaemias are usually round rather than oval and the neutrophils are not hypersegmented. Alcohol is the most frequent cause of a raised MCV (mean corpuscular volume) in the absence of anaemia. In some severe alcoholics, however, megaloblastic anaemia is due to a direct toxic action of alcohol on the marrow or to an associated dietary deficiency of folate. The other underlying conditions listed in Table 4.11 are usually easily diagnosed provided that they are considered and the appropriate investigations to exclude B_{12} or folate deficiency (e.g. serum B_{12} and folate assay and bone marrow examination) are carried out.

Differential diagnosis of macrocytic anaemias

The clinical history and physical examination may suggest B_{12} or folate deficiency as the cause. Diet and drugs, alcohol intake, family history, history suggestive of malabsorption, presence of autoimmune diseases or other associations with PA (Table 4.4), previous gastrointestinal disease or operations, are all important. The presence of jaundice, glossitis or a neuropathy are also valuable pointers to megaloblastic anaemia.

   The laboratory features of particular importance are the shape of macrocytes (oval in megaloblastic anaemia), the presence of hypersegmented neutrophils and of leucopenia and thrombocytopenia and the bone marrow appearance, whether megaloblastic or not. Serum B_{12}, serum and red cell folate (and in some the dU suppression test), and special tests for causes of these

Table 4.11 Causes of macrocytosis other than megaloblastic anaemia.

1 Alcohol
2 Liver disease
3 Myxoedema
4 Reticulocytosis
5 Cytotoxic drugs
6 Aplastic anaemia
7 Pregnancy
8 Myelodysplastic syndromes
9 Myeloma
10 Neonatal

deficiencies are used to complete the diagnosis of megaloblastic anaemia. Exclusion of alcoholism (particularly if the patient is not anaemic), liver and thyroid function tests and bone marrow examination for myelodysplasia, aplasia or myeloma are important in the investigation of macrocytosis not due to B_{12} or folate deficiency.

Bibliography

Antony A.C. (1991) Megaloblastic anemias. In *Hematology: Basic Principles and Practice* (eds R. Hoffman, E.J. Benz, S.J. Shattil, B. Furie & H.J. Cohen). Churchill Livingstone, New York, pp. 392–422.

Babior B. (1990a) Metabolic aspects of folic acid and vitamin B_{12}. In *Hematology*, 4th Edition (eds W.J. Williams, E. Beutler, A.J. Erslev & M.A. Lichtman). McGraw Hill, New York, pp. 339–354.

Babior B. (1990b) The megaloblastic anaemias. In *Hematology*, 4th Edition (eds W.J. Williams, E. Beutler, A.J. Erslev & M.A. Lichtman). McGraw Hill, New York, pp. 453–481.

Blakley R.L. & Whitehead V.M. (1986) *Folates and Pteridines, Vol. 3. Nutritional, Pharmacological and Physiological Aspects*. John Wiley, New York.

Chanarin I. (1969, 1979, 1990) *The Megaloblastic Anaemias*, 1st, 2nd, 3rd Editions. Blackwell Scientific Publications, Oxford.

Cooper B.A. & Zittoun J. (eds) (1987) *Cobalamin and Folate*. Progress en Hematologie, Doin, Paris.

Crellin R., Bottiglieri T. & Reynolds E.H. (1993) Folates and psychiatric disorders: clinical potential. *Drugs*, **45**, 623–636.

Fenton W.A. & Rosenberg L.E. (1989) Inherited disorders of cobalamin transport and metabolism. In *Metabolic Basis of Inherited Disease*, 6th Edition (eds C.R. Scriver, A.L. Beaudet, W.S. Sly & D. Valle). McGraw Hill, New York, pp. 2065–2082.

Hoffbrand A.V. (1983) Pernicious anaemia. *Scottish Medical Journal*, **28**, 218–227.

Kapadia C.R. & Donaldson R.M. (1985) Disorders of cobalamin (vitamin B_{12}) absorption and transport. *Annual Review of Medicine*, **36**, 93–110.

Rosenblatt D.S. (1989) Inherited disorders of folate metabolism. In *Metabolic Basis of Inherited Disease*, 6th Edition (eds C.R. Scriver, A.L. Beaudet, W.S. Sly & D. Valle). McGraw Hill, New York, pp. 2049–2064.

Shane B. & Stokstad E.L.R. (1985) Vitamin B_{12}–folate inter-relationships. *Annual Review of Nutrition*, **5**, 115–141.

Weir D.G., Keating S., Molloy A. *et al.* (1988) Methylation deficiency causes vitamin B_{12}-associated neuropathy in the pig. *Journal of Neurochemistry*, **51**, 1949–1952.

Wickramasinghe S.N. & Matthews J.H. (1988) Deoxyuridine suppression: biochemical basis and diagnostic applications. *Blood Reviews*, **2**, 168–177.

Chapter 5
Haemolytic Anaemias

Normal red cell destruction

Red cell destruction usually occurs after a mean lifespan of 120 days when the cells are removed extravascularly by the macrophages of the reticuloendothelial (RE) system, especially in the marrow but also in the liver and spleen. Red cell metabolism gradually deteriorates as enzymes are degraded and not replaced, until the cells become non-viable, but the exact reason why the red cells die is obscure. The breakdown of red cells liberates iron for recirculation via plasma transferrin to marrow erythroblasts, and protoporphyrin which is broken down to bilirubin. This circulates to the liver where it is conjugated to glucuronides which are excreted into the gut via bile and converted to stercobilinogen and stercobilin (excreted in faeces) (Fig. 5.1). Stercobilinogen and stercobilin are partly reabsorbed and excreted in urine as urobilinogen and urobilin. A small fraction of protoporphyrin is converted to carbon monoxide (CO) and excreted via the lungs. Globin chains are broken down to amino acids which are reutilized for general protein synthesis in the body. Haptoglobins are proteins present in normal plasma capable of binding haemoglobin. The haemoglobin–haptoglobin complex is removed from plasma by the RE system. Intravascular haemolysis (breakdown of red cells within blood vessels) plays little or no part in normal red cell destruction.

Haemolytic anaemias

Haemolytic anaemias are defined as those anaemias which result from an increase in the rate of red cell destruction. Because of erythropoietic hyperplasia and anatomical extension of bone marrow, red cell destruction may be increased several-fold before the patient becomes anaemic (compensated haemolytic disease). The normal adult marrow, after full expansion, is able to produce red cells at six to eight times the normal rate. Reticulocytes are raised, particularly in the more anaemic cases and those in which erythropoiesis is effective (as in hereditary spherocytosis) compared to those haemolytic anaemias in which red cell production is largely ineffective (as in β-thalassaemia major). The reticulocytes appear as larger, slightly blue-staining (poly-

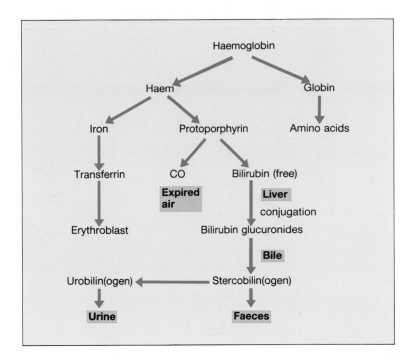

Fig. 5.1 Normal red cell breakdown. This takes place extravascularly in the macrophages of the reticuloendothelial system.

chromatic) cells in the ordinary peripheral blood film but can be counted accurately after supravital staining.

The lifespan of the normal red cell is 120 days; in severe haemolysis the cells survive only a few days. ^{51}Chromium (^{51}Cr)-labelled red cell survival studies may be needed to confirm haemolysis and to determine sites of destruction by surface counting over the different organs (Fig. 5.2). Diagnosis of the type of anaemia in any particular case requires a full clinical history, including family history and drug history, as well as clinical examination and appropriate laboratory tests.

Table 5.1 is a simplified classification of the haemolytic anaemias. Hereditary haemolytic anaemias are usually the result of 'intrinsic' red cell defects; normal transfused blood survives as long in these patients as in healthy recipients. Acquired haemolytic anaemias are usually the result of an 'extracorpuscular' or 'environmental' change. Normal transfused blood in these patients will have the same short survival as the patient's own red cells. Paroxysmal nocturnal haemoglobinuria (PNH), an acquired disorder, is an exception. PNH reds cells have an intrinsic defect.

Clinical features

The patient may show pallor of the mucous membranes, mild fluctuating jaundice and splenomegaly. There is no bile in the urine but this may turn dark on standing because of excess

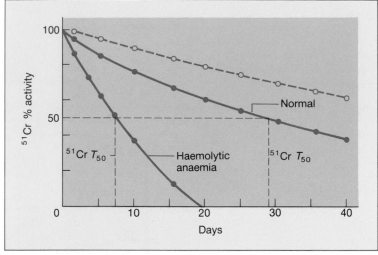

(a)

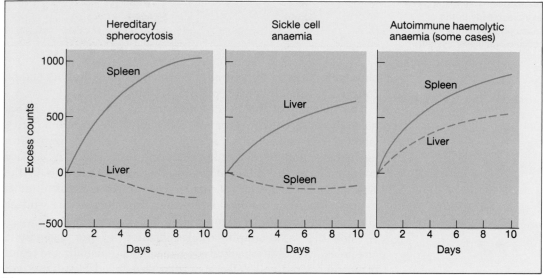

(b)

Fig. 5.2 (a) ^{51}Cr red cell survival studies. The ^{51}Cr T_{50} (half-life) in normal subjects is 30 ± 2 days. When data are corrected for elution of ^{51}Cr from red cells (dashed line), the mean cell life is 50 ± 5 days. In haemolytic anaemia, the ^{51}Cr T_{50} is usually less than 15 days. (b) Surface counting patterns in haemolytic anaemia during ^{51}Cr red cell survival studies: (*left*) dominant splenic destruction, e.g. hereditary spherocytosis; (*centre*) dominant liver destruction, e.g. sickle cell disease; (*right*) combined pattern of destruction, e.g. some cases of autoimmune haemolytic anaemia.

urobilinogen. Pigment gallstones may complicate the condition (Fig. 5.3) and some patients (particularly with sickle cell disease) develop ulcers around the ankle. Aplastic crises may occur, usually precipitated by infection with parvovirus which

Table 5.1 Classification of haemolytic anaemia.

Hereditary	Acquired
MEMBRANE For example hereditary spherocytosis, hereditary elliptocytosis	IMMUNE *Autoimmune* • Warm antibody type • Cold antibody type }see Table 5.5
METABOLISM For example G6PD deficiency, pyruvate kinase deficiency	*Alloimmune* • Haemolytic transfusion reactions • Haemolytic disease of the newborn • Allografts, especially marrow transplantation
HAEMOGLOBIN Abnormal (HbS, HbC, unstable); see Chapter 6	*Drug associated*
	RED CELL FRAGMENTATION SYNDROMES *Arterial grafts, cardiac valves* *Microangiopathic* • Thrombotic thrombocytopenic purpura • Haemolytic uraemic syndrome • Meningococcal sepsis • Pre-eclampsia • Disseminated intravascular coagulation
	MARCH HAEMOGLOBINURIA
	INFECTIONS For example malaria, clostridia
	CHEMICAL AND PHYSICAL AGENTS Especially drugs, industrial/domestic substances, burns
	SECONDARY For example liver and renal disease
	PAROXYSMAL NOCTURNAL HAEMO-GLOBINURIA (PNH)

'switches off' erythropoiesis, and are characterized by a sudden increase in anaemia and drop in reticulocyte count.

Folate deficiency is also likely to occur in chronic haemolytic anaemias because of increased utilization of the vitamin by the rapidly proliferating (DNA-synthesizing) bone marrow. If severe, this may cause an aplastic crisis in which the bone marrow is megaloblastic.

Laboratory findings

The laboratory findings are conveniently divided into three groups.

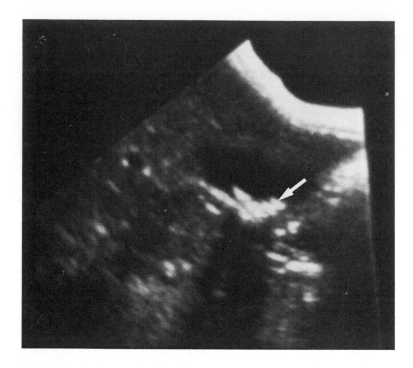

Fig. 5.3 Ultrasound of pigment gallstones (arrowed) in a 16-year-old male patient with hereditary spherocytosis (courtesy of L. Berger).

1 *Features of increased red cell breakdown*:
   (a) serum bilirubin raised, unconjugated and bound to albumin;
   (b) urine urinobilinogen increased;
   (c) faecal stercobilinogen increased;
   (d) serum haptoglobins absent because the haptoglobins become saturated with haemoglobin and the complex is removed by RE cells.
2 *Features of increased red cell production*:
   (a) reticulocytosis;
   (b) bone marrow erythroid hyperplasia; the normal marrow myeloid:erythoid ratio of 2:1 to 12:1 is reduced to 1:1 or reversed.
3 *Damaged red cells*:
   (a) morphology—microspherocytes, elliptocytes, fragments, etc.;
   (b) osmotic fragility, autohaemolysis, etc.;
   (c) red cell survival shortened. Best shown by ^{51}Cr labelling with study of sites of destruction (see Fig. 5.2).

Particular features of intravascular haemolysis

In some situations the red cells may be destroyed directly in the circulation (Table 5.2). The free haemoglobin released rapidly saturates plasma haptoglobins, the haemoglobin—haptoglobin

Table 5.2 Causes of intravascular haemolysis.

1 Mismatched blood transfusion (usually ABO)
2 G6PD deficiency with oxidant stress
3 Red cell fragmentation syndromes
4 Some autoimmune haemolytic anaemias
5 Some drug- and infection-induced haemolytic anaemias
6 Paroxysmal nocturnal haemoglobinuria
7 March haemoglobinuria
8 Unstable haemoglobin

complex being removed by the RE cells. The excess free haemoglobin is filtered by the glomerulus, rapidly saturates the renal tubular reabsorptive capacity and enters urine (Fig. 5.4). The renal tubules become loaded with haemosiderin, the iron derived from breaking down haemoglobin. Some of the free plasma haemoglobin is removed by hepatic macrophages and the iron in the haem released from this haemoglobulin is oxidized to the trivalent form. When released from the cell it binds to plasma albumin, forming methaemalbumin. Haem is also bound in plasma to another protein, haemopexin, which is then mainly removed by the liver.

The main laboratory features of intravascular haemolysis are as follow.
1 Haemoglobinaemia and haemoglobinuria.
2 Haemosiderinuria (iron storage protein in the spun deposit of urine; it is derived from the break down of haemoglobin in the renal tubular cells).
3 Methaemalbuminaemia (detected spectrophotometrically by Schumm's test).

Hereditary haemolytic anaemias

Membrane defects

Hereditary spherocytosis

Hereditary spherocytosis (HS) is the commonest hereditary haemolytic anaemia in North Europeans.

Pathogenesis
HS is usually due to a defect in the main structural protein (spectrin) of the red cell membrane. The most consistent membrane abnormality is a reduction in spectrin content, the degree correlating with the severity of the haemolytic anaemia (Table 5.3). A variety of genetic lesions in the spectrin genes is likely to

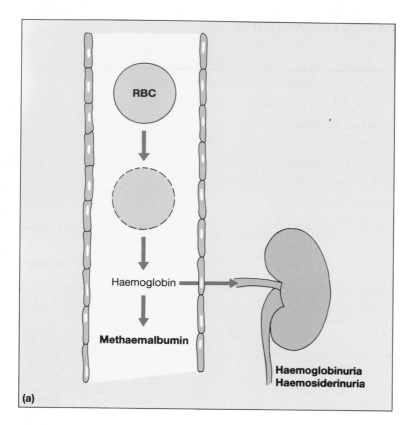

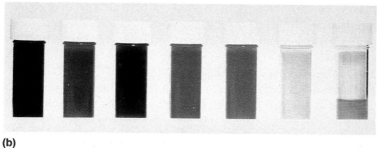

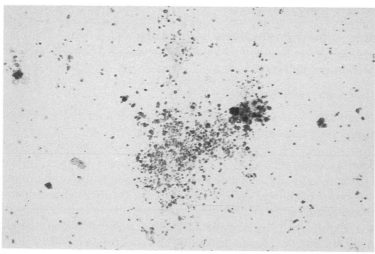

Fig. 5.4 (a) Intravascular haemolysis: the red blood cells (RBC) burst within the circulation and free haemoglobin is liberated into plasma. Some is oxidized and the methaem liberated binds to albumin. The pigments may cause plasma to appear dark brown or black. Some haemoglobin enters the urine and is reabsorbed, degrading in the renal tubules to form haemosiderin. (b) Progressive urine samples in an acute episode of intravascular haemolysis showing haemoglobinuria of decreasing severity. (c) Prussian blue positive deposits of haemosiderin in a urine spun deposit (Perls' stain).

Table 5.3 Molecular basis of hereditary spherocytosis and elliptocytosis.

Hereditary spherocytosis
Mild spectrin deficiency
   Reduced synthesis
   Unstable spectrin
Rarely defective spectrin binding to ankyrin

Hereditary elliptocytosis
α- or β-spectrin mutants leading to defective spectrin dimer formation
α- or β-spectrin mutants leading to defective spectrin ankyrin associations
Abnormal band 4.1
Glycophorin C deficiency

underlie the disease. The loss of membrane may be due to the release of parts of the lipid bilayer that are not supported by the skeleton. The marrow produces red cells of normal biconcave shape but these lose membrane as they circulate through the spleen and the rest of the RE system. The ratio of surface area to volume decreases and the cells become more spherical. Ultimately the spherocytes are unable to pass through the splenic microcirculation where they die prematurely. *In vitro*, glucose helps to reduce haemolysis by preventing undue loss of sodium from the cells through the leaky membrane; and glucose deprivation has been postulated to occur particularly when the cells circulate to the spleen, perhaps because of stasis and plasma skimming.

Inheritance
Dominant, variable expression; rarely autosomal recessive.

Clinical features
The anaemia may present at any age from infancy to old age. Jaundice is typically fluctuating and is particularly marked if the haemolytic anaemia is associated with Gilbert's disease (a defect of hepatic conjugation of bilirubin); splenomegaly occurs in most patients. Pigment gallstones are frequent (see Fig. 5.3); aplastic crises (usually precipitated by infection, nearly always parvovirus) may cause a sudden increase in severity of anaemia.

Haematological findings
Anaemia is usual but not invariable; its severity tends to be similar in members of the same family. Reticulocytes are usually 5–20%. The blood film shows microspherocytes (Fig. 5.5a) which are densely staining with smaller diameters than normal red cells, particularly reticulocytes.

Special tests
1 *Osmotic fragility is increased* (Fig. 5.6). The abnormality may require 24 hours' incubation at 37°C to become obvious.

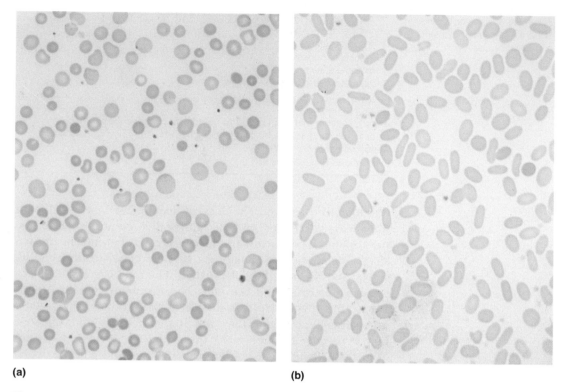

(a)   **(b)**

Fig. 5.5 (a) Blood film in hereditary spherocytosis. The spherocytes are deeply staining and of small diameter. Larger polychromatic cells are reticulocytes (confirmed by supravital staining). (b) Blood film in hereditary elliptocytosis.

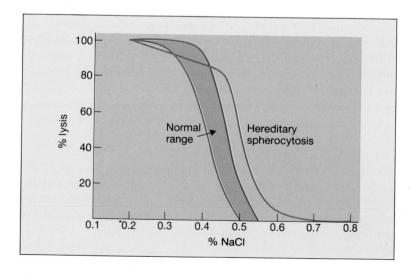

Fig. 5.6 The osmotic fragility in hereditary spherocytosis. The curve is shifted to the right of the normal range (in blue), but a tail of more resistant cells (reticulocytes) is also present.

2 *Autohaemolysis is increased* and corrected by glucose. In this test, the cells are incubated in their own plasma with or without added glucose for 48 hours and the degree of haemolysis is measured.

3 *Direct antiglobulin (Coombs) test is negative.* This excludes autoimmune haemolysis in which spherocytes are also common in the peripheral blood.

4 *^{51}Cr studies* may be used to assess the severity and document dominant splenic destruction (see Fig. 5.2).

Treatment

The principal form of treatment is splenectomy. This is avoided in early childhood, if possible, because of the increased risk of infection (particularly pneumococcal) post-splenectomy at this age. Splenectomy should always produce a rise in the haemoglobin level to normal, even though microspherocytes (formed in the rest of the RE system) remain. In mild cases splenectomy may be avoided unless gallstones develop. Folic acid is given in severe cases. Pneumococcal and haemophilus vaccination is also given before splenectomy is undertaken and oral penicillin prophylaxis is given post-splenectomy (see p. 388).

Hereditary elliptocytosis

This has similar clinical and laboratory features to hereditary spherocytosis except for the appearance of the blood film (Fig. 5.5b), but it is usually a clinically milder disorder. Occasional patients require splenectomy. Defective spectrin dimer—dimer association in the red cell membrane, a deficit in the interaction of spectrin with other membrane proteins or defects in protein 4.1 or glycophorin C have been detected in different cases (Table 5.3). Homozygous or doubly heterozygous elliptocytosis presents with a severe haemolytic anaemia with microspherocytes, poikilocytes and splenomegaly (hereditary pyropoikilocytosis).

Defective red cell metabolism

G6PD deficiency

G6PD (glucose-6-phosphate dehydrogenase) functions to reduce NADP (nicotinamide-adenine-dinucleotide phosphate) while oxidizing glucose-6-phosphate. It is the only source of NADPH in red cells. There are a wide variety of normal genetic variants of the enzyme G6PD, the commonest being type B (Western) and type A in Africans. More than 400 variants of the enzyme G6PD have been characterized which show less activity than normal. It has been estimated that over 200 million people are deficient

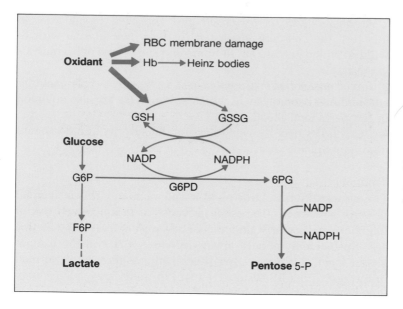

Fig. 5.7 Haemoglobin and red blood cell (RBC) membranes are usually protected from oxidant stress by reduced glutathione (GSH). In G6PD deficiency, NADPH and GSH synthesis is impaired. FP, fructose phosphate; GP, glucose phosphate; G6PD, glucose-6-phosphate dehydrogenase; GSSG, glutathione (oxidized form); NADP, NADPH, nicotinamide-adenine-dinucleotide phosphate.

of the enzyme. These abnormalities are due to a deficiency of the enzyme protein or to a functional inadequacy of the enzyme. There is impaired reduction of glutathione (Fig. 5.7). G6PD deficiency is usually asymptomatic. Although G6PD is present in all cells the main syndromes which occur are acute haemolytic anaemia in response to oxidant stress (drugs, fava beans) or haemolysis due to infections, but neonatal jaundice and, rarely, a congenital non-spherocytic haemolytic anaemia result from different types of enzyme deficiency.

The inheritance is sex-linked, affecting males, and carried by females who show approximately half normal red cell G6PD values. The female heterozygotes have an advantage of resistance to *Falciparum* malaria. The main races affected are in West Africa, the Mediterranean, the Middle East and South-East Asia. The degree of deficiency varies, often being mild (10–15% of normal activity) in black Africans, more severe in Orientals and most severe in Mediterraneans. Severe deficiency occurs occasionally in Caucasians. Most of the mutations causing mild disease are located at the amino end of the gene whereas those associated with non-spherocytic haemolytic anaemia are at the carboxy end.

Clinical features

These are of rapidly developing intravascular haemolysis with haemoglobinuria, precipitated by infection and other acute illness, drugs or the ingestion of the fava bean (Table 5.4). In Blacks, the anaemia is self-limiting because the new young red cells have near normal G6PD activity, the enzyme level

Table 5.4 Agents which may cause haemolytic anaemia in G6PD deficiency.

1 *Infections and other acute illnesses*, e.g. diabetic ketoacidosis

2 *Drugs*
   • anti-malarials, e.g. primaquine, pamaquine, chloroquine, fansidar, maloprim
   • sulphonamides and sulphones, e.g. co-trimoxazole, sulphanilamide, dapsone, salazopyrine
   • other antibacterial agents, e.g. nitrofurans, chloramphenicol
   • analgesics, e.g. aspirin (moderate doses are safe), phenacetin
   • anti-helminths, e.g. β-naphthol, stibophen, nitrodazole
   • miscellaneous, e.g. vitamin K analogues, naphthalene (moth balls), probenecid

3 *Fava beans* (possibly other vegetables)

NB Many common drugs have been reported to precipitate haemolysis in G6PD deficiency, e.g. aspirin, quinine, penicillin, but not at conventional doses.

falling as the cells age in the circulation. In contrast, in the Mediterranean type of deficiency, haemolysis is not necessarily self-limiting.

Diagnosis

Between crises the blood count is normal. The enzyme deficiency is detected by one of a number of screening tests or by direct enzyme assay on red cells. During a crisis, the blood film may show contracted and fragmented cells, 'bite' cells and 'blister' cells (Fig. 5.8) which have had Heinz bodies removed by the

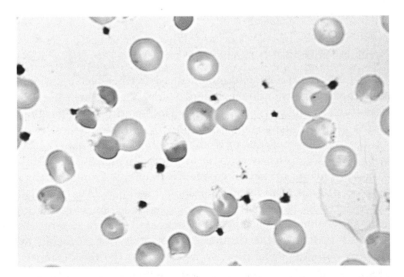

Fig. 5.8 Blood film in G6PD deficiency with acute haemolysis after an oxidant stress. Some of the cells show loss of cytoplasm with separation of remaining haemoglobin from the cell membrane ('blister' cells). There are also numerous contracted and deeply staining cells. Supravital staining (as for reticulocytes) showed the presence of Heinz bodies (see Fig. 2.17).

spleen. Heinz bodies (oxidized, denatured haemoglobin) may be seen in the reticulocyte preparation, particularly if the spleen is absent. There are also features of intravascular haemolysis. Because of the higher enzyme level in young red cells, red cell enzyme assay may give a 'false' normal level in the phase of acute haemolysis with a reticulocyte response. Subsequent assay after the acute phase reveals the low G6PD level when the red cell population is of normal age distribution.

Treatment

The offending drug is stopped, a high urine output is maintained, and blood transfusion undertaken where necessary for severe anaemia. G6PD-deficient babies are prone to neonatal jaundice and in severe cases phototherapy and exchange transfusion may be needed. The jaundice is usually not due to excess haemolysis but to deficiency of G6PD affecting neonatal liver function.

Glutathione deficiency and other syndromes

Other defects in the pentose phosphate pathway leading to similar syndromes to G6PD deficiency have been described — particularly glutathione deficiency.

Glycolytic (Embden–Meyerhof) pathway defects

These are all uncommon and lead to a congenital non-spherocytic haemolytic anaemia. The most frequently encountered is pyruvate kinase deficiency.

Pyruvate kinase (PK) deficiency

This is inherited as an autosomal recessive, the affected patients being homozygous or doubly heterozygous. The red cells become rigid due to reduced ATP formation. The severity of the anaemia varies widely (haemoglobin 4–10 g/dl) and causes relatively mild symptoms because of a shift to the right in the O_2-dissociation curve caused by a rise in intracellular 2,3-DPG. Clinically jaundice is usual and gallstones frequent. Frontal bossing may be present. The blood film shows poikilocytosis and distorted 'prickle' cells, particularly post-splenectomy. Laboratory tests show that autohaemolysis is increased but, in contrast to the finding in hereditary spherocytosis, it is not corrected by glucose; direct enzyme assay is needed to make the diagnosis. The enzyme often shows abnormal characteristics as well as reduced activity. Splenectomy may alleviate the anaemia but does not cure it. It is indicated in those patients who need frequent transfusions.

Acquired haemolytic anaemias

Immune haemolytic anaemias

Autoimmune haemolytic anaemias (AIHA)

These anaemias are due to antibody production by the body against its own red cells. They are characterized by a positive direct antiglobulin test (DAT) (see Fig. 21.3) and divided into 'warm' and 'cold' types (Table 5.5) according to whether the antibody reacts better with red cells at 37°C or 4°C.

Warm AIHA

The red cells are usually coated with IgG alone, IgG and complement or complement alone, but a minority of cases show IgA or IgM coating alone or combined with IgG antibody. The complement component detectable is C3d, the degraded fragment of C3. The AIHA in SLE is typically of the IgG + complement type. Red cells coated with IgG are taken up by RE macrophages, especially in the spleen, which have receptors for the Fc fragment. Part of the coated membrane is lost so the cell becomes progressively more spherical to maintain the same volume and is ultimately prematurely destroyed, usually predominantly in the spleen. Red cells with complement coating alone or in addition to IgG are destroyed more generally in the RE system, and not particularly in the spleen.

Clinical features

The disease may occur at any age in either sex and presents as a haemolytic anaemia of varying severity. The spleen is often enlarged. The disease tends to remit and relapse. It may occur alone or in association with other diseases or arise in some patients as a result of methyl dopa therapy (Table 5.5). When associated with ITP (idiopathic thrombocytopenic purpura),

Table 5.5 Autoimmune haemolytic anaemias: classification.

Warm type	Cold type
• Idiopathic	• Idiopathic

• Secondary
SLE, other 'autoimmune'
  diseases
CLL, lymphomas
Drugs, e.g. methyl dopa
	• Secondary
	Infections—*Mycoplasma*
	  pneumonia, infectious
	  mononucleosis
	Lymphoma

	• Paroxysmal cold haemoglobinuria Rare, sometimes associated with infections, e.g. syphilis

which is a similar condition affecting platelets (see p. 320), it is known as Evans' syndrome.

Laboratory findings

The haematological and biochemical findings are typical of a haemolytic anaemia with spherocytosis prominent in the peripheral blood (Fig. 5.9a). The DAT is positive due to IgG, IgG and complement, IgA or, rarely, IgM on the cells. In some cases, the autoantibody shows specificity within the rhesus system, e.g. anti-c or anti-e (see Chapter 21). The antibodies both on the cell surface and free in serum are best detected at 37°C.

Treatment

1 Remove the underlying cause (e.g. methyl dopa).
2 Corticosteroids. Prednisolone in high, subsequently reducing, doses may be tried (60 mg daily is a usual starting dose in adults).
3 Splenectomy may be of value in those who fail to respond

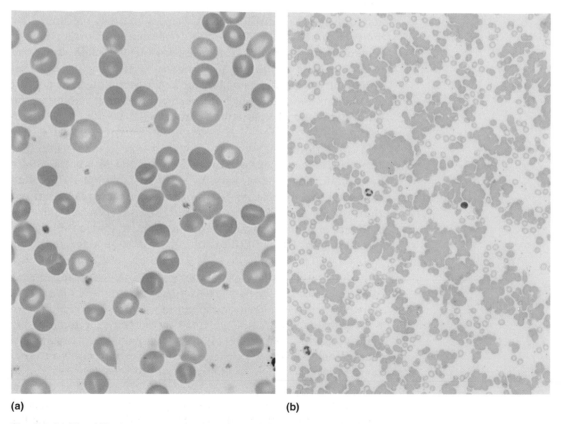

(a)   (b)

Fig. 5.9 (a) Blood film in warm autoimmune haemolytic anaemia. Numerous microspherocytes are present and larger polychromatic cells (reticulocytes). (b) Blood film in cold autoimmune haemolytic anaemia. Marked red cell agglutination is present in films made at room temperature. The blue background is due to the raised plasma protein concentration.

well or fail to maintain a satisfactory haemoglobin level on an acceptably small steroid dosage. ^{51}Cr organ uptake studies pre-operatively confirm whether or not the spleen is the dominant site of destruction (see Fig. 5.2b) and thus may be used to predict the value of splenectomy. Patients with IgG only on the red cells usually respond better to steroid therapy and to splenectomy than those with IgG and complement or with IgA.

4 Immunosuppression may be tried after other measures have failed but is not always of great value. Azathioprine, cyclo-phosphamide, chlorambucil and cyclosporin have been tried.

5 Folic acid is given to severe cases.

6 Blood transfusion may be needed if anaemia is severe and causing symptoms. The blood should be the least incompatible and if the specificity of the autoantibody is known, donor blood is chosen which lacks the relevant antigen(s). The presence of alloantibodies due to previous transfusion or pregnancy should be excluded.

7 High-dose immunoglobulin has been used but with less success than in ITP (see p. 323).

Cold AIHA

In these syndromes the autoantibody, whether monoclonal (as in the idiopathic cold haemagglutinin syndrome or associated with lymphoproliferative disorders) or polyclonal (as following infection, e.g. infectious mononucleosis or *Mycoplasma* pneumonia) attaches to red cells mainly in the peripheral circulation where the blood temperature is cooled. The antibody is usually IgM and binds to red cells best at 4°C. Haemolytic syndromes of varying severity may occur depending on the titre of the antibody in the serum, its affinity for red cells, its ability to bind complement, and its thermal amplitude (whether or not it binds to red cells at 37°C). Agglutination of red cells by the antibody often causes peripheral circulation abnormalities. The antibody may then detach from red cells when they pass to the warmer central circulation but, if complement has been bound, the direct antiglobulin test remains positive—of complement-only type—and the cells are liable to be destroyed in the whole RE system, especially the liver, giving rise to a chronic haemolytic anaemia. Intravascular haemolysis occurs in some of the syndromes, in which the complement sequence is completed on the red cell surface. Low serum levels of complement in other cases may help to protect the patient from a more severe clinical disease.

In nearly all these cold AIHA syndromes, the antibody is directed against the 'I' antigen on the red cell surface or the foetal equivalent of this, the 'i' antigen.

Paroxysmal cold haemoglobinuria is a rare syndrome of acute intravascular haemolysis after exposure to the cold in those with the Donath–Landsteiner antibody, which binds to red

cells in the cold but causes lysis with complement in warm
conditions. Viral infections and syphilis are predisposing causes.

Clinical features
The patient may have a chronic haemolytic anaemia aggravated
by the cold and often associated with intravascular haemolysis.
Mild jaundice and splenomegaly may be present. The patient
may develop acrocyanosis (purplish skin discolouration), e.g. at
the tip of the nose, ears, fingers and toes, due to the agglutination
of red cells in small vessels. Some secondary cases are transient
after an infection, particularly *Mycoplasma* pneumonia or infectious mononucleosis (see Table 5.5).

Laboratory findings
These are similar to those of warm AIHA, except that spherocytosis is less marked, red cells agglutinate in the cold, e.g. on
the blood film made at room temperature (Fig. 5.9b), and the
DAT reveals complement (C_3) only on the red cell surface. Serum
antibodies often present in high titre are IgM, react best at 4°C,
and usually show specificity to antigen 'I' or 'i'. In the rare cold
AIHA, paroxysmal cold haemoglobinuria, the antibodies are IgG
and have specificity for the P blood group antigens.

Treatment
This consists of keeping the patient warm and treating the underlying cause, if present. Alkylating agents (e.g. chlorambucil)
may be helpful in the chronic varieties. Splenectomy does not
usually help unless massive splenomegaly is present, and
steroids are not helpful.

Alloimmune haemolytic anaemias

In these anaemias, antibody produced by one individual reacts
with red cells of another. Two important situations are transfusion of ABO incompatible blood and rhesus disease of the
newborn which are considered in Chapter 21. The increased use
of allogeneic transplantation for renal, hepatic, cardiac and bone
marrow diseases has led to the recognition of alloimmune
haemolytic anaemia due to the production of donor-derived red
cell antibodies in the recipient caused by donor lymphocytes
transferred in the allograft.

Drug-induced immune haemolytic anaemias

Drugs may cause immune haemolytic anaemias by three different
mechanisms (Fig. 5.10): antibody directed against a drug–red
cell membrane complex (e.g. penicillin or cephalothin), deposition of complement via drug–protein (antigen)–antibody

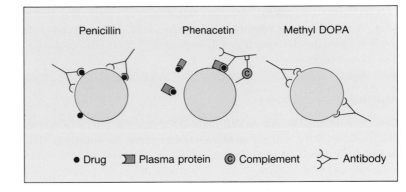

Penicillin Phenacetin Methyl DOPA

● Drug ▱ Plasma protein ⓒ Complement ⋋> Antibody

Fig. 5.10 Three different mechanisms of drug-induced immune haemolytic anaemia. In each case the coated (opsonized) cells are destroyed in the reticulo-endothelial system. DOPA, dihydroxyphenylalanine.

complex onto the red cell surface (e.g. quinidine or chlorpropamide), or an autoimmune haemolytic anaemia in which the role of the drug is mysterious (e.g. methyl dopa). In each case, the haemolytic anaemia gradually disappears when the drug is discontinued but with methyl dopa the autoantibody may persist for several months. The penicillin-induced immune haemolytic anaemias only occur with massive doses of the antibiotic.

Red cell fragmentation syndromes

These arise through physical damage to red cells either on abnormal surfaces (e.g. artificial heart valves or arterial grafts) or as a microangiopathic haemolytic anaemia caused by red cells passing through fibrin strands deposited in small vessels due to disseminated intravascular coagulation (DIC; see p. 344) or through damaged small vessels in malignant hypertension, the haemolytic uraemic syndrome, thrombotic thrombocytopenic purpura, pre-eclampsia or meningococcal sepsis. The peripheral

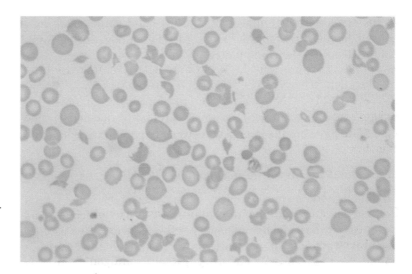

Fig. 5.11 Blood film in microangiopathic haemolytic anaemia (in this patient Gram-negative septicaemia). Numerous contracted and deeply staining cells and cell fragments are present.

blood contains many deeply staining red cell fragments (Fig. 5.11). Clotting abnormalities typical of DIC (see p. 345) with a low platelet count are also present when DIC underlies the haemolysis.

March haemoglobinuria

This is due to damage to red cells between the small bones of the feet, usually during prolonged marching or running. The blood film does not show fragments.

Infections

Infections may cause haemolysis in a variety of ways. They may precipitate an acute haemolytic crisis in G6PD deficiency or cause microangiopathic haemolytic anaemia, e.g. with meningo-coccal or pneumococcal septicaemia. Malaria causes haemolysis due to extravascular destruction of parasitized red cells as well as direct intravascular lysis. Blackwater fever is an acute intra-vascular haemolysis accompanied by acute renal failure due to falciparum malaria. *Clostridium perfringens* septicaemia may cause intravascular haemolysis with marked microspherocytosis.

Chemical and physical agents

Certain drugs, e.g. dapsone and salazopyrine, in high doses cause oxidative intravascular haemolysis with Heinz body for-mation in normal subjects. In Wilson's disease an acute haemo-lytic anaemia may occur due to high levels of copper in the blood. Chemical poisoning, e.g. with lead, chlorate or arsine, may cause severe haemolysis. Severe burns damage red cells causing acanthocytosis or bizarre forms with spherocytes, frag-ments and dumb-bell appearances. Snake and spider bites may cause haemolysis, as may hypophosphataemia (e.g. during intra-venous feeding) due to impaired glycolysis.

Secondary haemolytic anaemias

In many systemic disorders red cell survival is shortened. This may contribute to anaemia (see Chapter 20).

Paroxysmal nocturnal haemoglobinuria (PNH)

This is a rare acquired defect of marrow stem cells which produce an abnormality of the red cell membrane which renders it sensitive to lysis by complement causing chronic intravascular haemolysis. A defect in synthesis of a phosphatidyl inositol which anchors several surface proteins to the membrane is present. The cells lack the enzyme α-1,6-N-acetylglucosaminyl-transferase involved in synthesis of the anchor. The proteins consequently deficient include decay accelerating factor (DAF), membrane inhibitor of reactive lysis (MIRL) and other proteins involved in complement degradation. The lack of MIRL explains the sensitivity of the cells to complement lysis. A number of enzymes including acetylcholinesterase, alkaline phosphatase, ecto-nucleotidase and other proteins (e.g. Fc receptor III) are absent from blood cells. PNH sometimes occurs in association with aplastic anaemia, especially in the recovery phase. The white cell and platelet counts are also often low in PNH because these cells share the red cells' undue sensitivity to complement.

As well as the problem of anaemia, the patient may develop recurrent thromboses of large veins including portal and hepatic veins. PNH is diagnosed by demonstration of red cell lysis in serum at low pH (acid lysis or Ham's test). Low pH activates complement by the alternative pathway. Haemosiderinuria is a feature and can give rise to iron deficiency which may exacerbate the anaemia. The reticulocyte count is lower in relation to the degree of anaemia than in other chronic haemolytic anaemias.

Treatment is unsatisfactory. Iron therapy is used for iron deficiency. In time, the disease occasionally remits but it may transform into aplastic anaemia or acute leukaemia.

Bibliography

Beutler E. (1984) *Red Cell Metabolism*, 3rd Edition. Grune & Stratton, New York.

Beutler E. (1991) Glucose-6-phosphate-dehydrogenase deficiency. *New England Journal of Medicine*, **324**, 169–174.

Dacie J.V. (1988) *The Haemolytic Anaemias. Vol. 2, The Hereditary Haemolytic Anaemias; Vol. 3, The Haemolytic Anaemias of Immune Origin*, 3rd Edition. Churchill Livingstone, Edinburgh.

Lestas A.M. & Bellingham A.J. (1990) A logical approach to the investigation of red cell enzymopathies. *Blood Reviews*, **4**, 148–157.

Mentzer W.C. & Wagner G.M. (eds) (1989) *The Hereditary Haemolytic Anaemias*. Churchill Livingstone, Edinburgh.

Palek J. (1991) Red cell membrane disorders. In *Haematology: Basic Principles and Practice* (eds R. Hoffman, E.J. Benz, S.J. Shahil, B. Furie & H.J. Cohen). Churchill Livingstone, New York, pp. 472–503.

Palek J. & Lambert J. (1990) Genetics of the red cell membrane skeleton. *Seminars in Hematology*, **27**, 290–332.

Rosse W.F. (1989) Paroxysmal nocturnal haemoglobinuria: the biochemical defect and the clinical syndrome. *Blood Reviews*, **3**, 192–200.

Rosse W.F. (1990) *Clinical Immunohaematology: Basic Concepts and Clinical Applications*. Blackwell Scientific Publications, Oxford.

Von dem Borne A.E.G.Kr. (ed.) (1991) Molecular immunohaematology. *Clinical Haematology*, **4**, 793–1014.

Vulliamy T., Mason P. & Luzzatto L. (1992) The molecular basis of glucose-6-phosphate dehydrogenase deficiency. *Trends in Genetics*, **8**, 138–143.

WHO Working Group (1989) Glucose-6-phosphate dehydrogenase deficiency. *Bulletin of the World Health Organisation*, **67**, 601–611.

Chapter 6
Genetic Defects of Haemoglobin

This chapter deals with diseases caused by reduced or abnormal synthesis of normal globin (the haemoglobinopathies). The synthesis of normal haemoglobin both in the foetus and adult is described first.

Haemoglobin synthesis

Normal adult blood contains three types of haemoglobin (Table 2.1, p. 17). The major component is haemoglobin A with the molecular structure $\alpha_2\beta_2$. The minor haemoglobins contain γ (foetal Hb or Hb F) or δ (Hb A_2) chains instead of β chains. In the embryo and foetus, Gower 1, Portland, Gower 2 and foetal Hb dominate at different stages (Fig. 6.1). The genes for the globin chains occur in two clusters, ε, δ and β on chromosome 11 and ζ and α on chromosome 16. Two types of γ chain, G_γ and A_γ, occur depending on whether there is a glycine or alanine amino acid at position 136 in the polypeptide chain. The α chain gene is duplicated and both α genes (α_1 and α_2) on each chromosome are active. In both gene clusters, the genes are arranged in the order in which they are expressed during foetal development (Fig. 6.1).

Molecular aspects

All the globin genes have three exons (coding regions) and two introns (non-coding regions whose DNA is not represented in the finished protein). The initial RNA is transcribed from both introns and exons, and from this transcript the RNA derived from introns is removed by a process known as splicing (Fig. 6.2) The introns always begin with a G-T dinucleotide and end with an A-G dinucleotide. The splicing machinery recognizes these sequences as well as neighbouring conserved sequences. The RNA in the nucleus is also 'capped' (by addition of structure at the 5′ end which contains a 7-methyl guanosine group). The cap structure may be important for attachment of the mRNA to ribosomes. The newly formed mRNA is also polyadenylated at the 3′ end (Fig. 6.2). This stabilizes it. Thalassaemia may arise from mutations or deletions of any of these sequences.

A number of other conserved sequences are important in

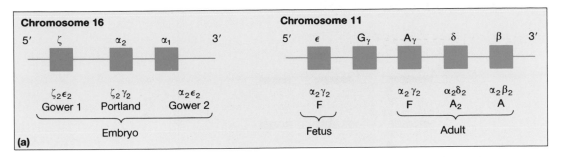

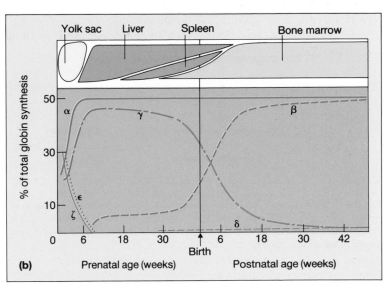

Fig. 6.1 (a) The globin gene clusters on chromosomes 16 and 11. In embryonic, foetal and adult life different genes are activated or suppressed. The different globin chains are synthesized independently and then combine with each other to produce the different haemoglobins. The γ gene may have two sequences, differing by whether there is a glutamic acid or alanine residue at position 136 (G$_\gamma$ or A$_\gamma$, respectively).
(b) Synthesis of individual globin chains in prenatal and postnatal life.

globin synthesis and mutations at these sites may also give rise to thalassaemia. These sequences influence gene transcription, ensure its fidelity and specify sites for the initiation and termination of translation, and ensure the stability of newly synthesized mRNA. Promoters are found 5′ of the gene, either close to the initiation site or more distally. They are the sites where RNA polymerases bind to catalyse gene transcription. Enhancers occur either 5′ or 3′ to the gene (Fig. 6.2). Enhancers are important in the tissue-specific regulation of globin gene expression, and in regulation of the synthesis of the various globin chains during foetal and postnatal life. GATA-1 (GF-1) and NF-E2 transcription factors expressed mainly in erythroid precursors, are important in determining the expression of globin genes in erythroid cells. A locus control region (LCR) is a genetic regulatory element situated 5′ of the β-globin cluster, controlling the genetic activity of the β-globin domain. The LCR determines the very high level of β-globin expression in erythroid progenitors.

Messenger RNA enters the cytoplasm and attaches to ribo-

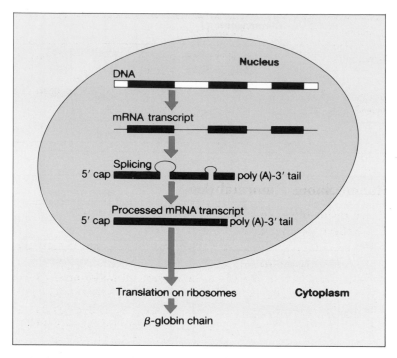

Fig. 6.2 The expression of a human globin gene from transcription, excision of introns, splicing of exons and translation to ribosomes. The primary transcript is cut 20 nucleotides downstream from this sequence 'capped' at the 5′ end, and a poly A tail is then added.

somes (translation) where the synthesis of globin chains takes place. This occurs by attachment of transfer RNAs, each with its individual amino acid by codon/anticodon base pairing to an appropriate position on the mRNA template.

Switch from foetal to adult haemoglobin

The globin genes are arranged on chromosomes 11 and 16 in the order in which they are expressed (see Fig. 6.1). Certain embryonic haemoglobins are usually only expressed in yolk sac erythroblasts. The β-globin gene is expressed at a low level in early foetal life, but the main switch to adult haemoglobin occurs 3–6 months after birth when synthesis of the γ chain is largely replaced by the β chain. How this switch comes about is largely unknown. It is clear, however, that the methylation state of the gene (expressed genes tend to be hypomethylated, non-expressed hypermethylated), the state of the chromosome packaging and various enhancer sequences all play a role in determining whether a particular gene will be transcribed.

Table 6.1 The clinical syndromes produced by haemoglobin abnormalities.

Syndrome	Abnormality
Haemolysis	Crystalline haemoglobins (Hb S, C, D, E, etc.) Rarely unstable haemoglobin
Thalassaemia	α or β due to reduced globin chain synthesis
Familial polycythaemia	Altered oxygen affinity
Methaemoglobinaemia	Failure of reduction (Hb M's)

Haemoglobin abnormalities

These result from the following.

1 Synthesis of an abnormal haemoglobin.

2 Reduced rate of synthesis of normal α- or β-globin chains (the α- and β-thalassaemias).

Table 6.1 shows some of the first group of syndromes which arise from synthesis of an α or β chain with an amino acid substitution. In many cases, however, the abnormality is completely silent. The clinically most important abnormality is sickle cell anaemia. Haemoglobin (Hb) C, D and E like Hb S are substitutions in the β chain and are also common. Unstable haemoglobins are rare and cause a chronic haemolytic anaemia of varying severity with intravascular haemolysis (p. 79). Abnormal haemoglobins may also cause (familial) polycythaemia (p. 293) or one type of congenital methaemoglobinaemia (p. 19).

The genetic defects of haemoglobin are the most common genetic disorders worldwide. They occur in tropical and sub-tropical areas (Fig. 6.3). Sickle cell trait affords protection against *Falciparum* malaria which explains the selection of carriers for survival in areas where malaria is endemic. It is likely that the thalassaemia traits also afford protection against malaria, perhaps by allowing an enhanced immune response.

Thalassaemias

These are a heterogeneous group of genetic disorders which result from a reduced rate of synthesis of α or β chains. Clinically they are divided into hydrops foetalis, β-thalassaemia major, which is transfusion dependent, thalassaemia intermedia characterized by moderate anaemia usually with splenomegaly and iron overload, and thalassaemia minor, the usually symptomless carrier.

Alpha-thalassaemia syndromes

These are usually due to gene deletions and are listed in Table 6.2. As there is duplication of the α-globin gene, deletion

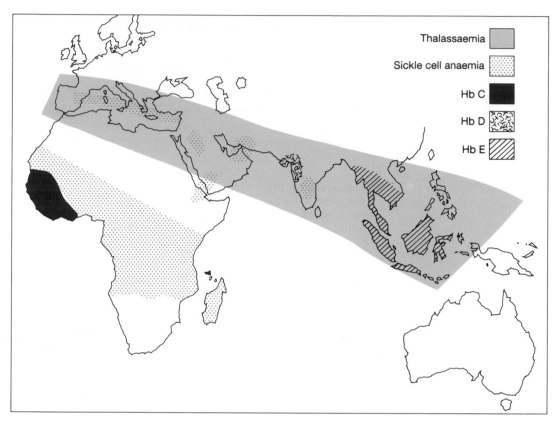

| Thalassaemia |
| Sickle cell anaemia |
| Hb C |
| Hb D |
| Hb E |

Fig. 6.3 The geographical distribution of the thalassaemias and the more common, inherited structural haemoglobin abnormalities.

of four genes is needed to completely suppress α chain synthesis (Fig. 6.4). Since the α chain is essential in foetal as well as in adult haemoglobin, deletion of both α genes on both chromosomes leads to failure of foetal haemoglobin synthesis with death *in utero* (hydrops foetalis, Fig. 6.5). Three α gene deletions leads to a moderately severe (haemoglobin 7−11 g/dl) microcytic, hypochromic anaemia (Fig. 6.6) with splenomegaly (Hb H disease). Haemoglobin H (β_4) can be detected in red cells of these patients by electrophoresis or in reticulocyte preparations (Fig. 6.6). In foetal life, Hb Bart's (γ_4) occurs.

The α-thalassaemia traits are usually not associated with anaemia, but the MCV and MCH are low and the red cell count is over 5.5×10^{12}/l. Haemoglobin electrophoresis is normal but occasionally Hb H bodies may be observed in reticulocyte preparations. α/β chain synthesis studies or DNA analysis are needed to be certain of the diagnosis. The normal α/β synthesis ratio is 1 : 1 and this is reduced in the α-thalassaemias and raised in β-thalassaemias. Uncommon non-deletion forms of α-thalassaemia are due to point mutations producing dysfunction of the genes or rarely to mutations affecting termination of translation which give rise to an elongated chain, e.g. Hb Constant Spring.

Table 6.2 Classification of thalassaemia.

(a) Clinical.

Hydrops foetalis
Four gene deletion α-thalassaemia

Thalassaemia major
Transfusion dependent, homozygous
β^0-thalassaemia or other combinations of β-thalassaemia trait

Thalassaemia intermedia
See Table 6.6

Thalassaemia minor
β^0-thalassaemia trait
β^+-thalassaemia trait
Hereditary persistence of foetal haemoglobin
$\delta\beta$-thalassaemia trait
α^0-thalassaemia trait
α^+-thalassaemia trait

(b) Genetic.

Type	Haplotype	Heterozygous thalassaemia trait (minor)*	Homozygous
α-*thalassaemias*[†]			
α^0	$--/$	MCV, MCH low	Hydrops foetalis
α^+	$-\alpha/$	MCV, MCH minimally reduced	As heterozygous α^0-thalassaemia
β-*thalassaemias*			
β^0		MCV, MCH low (Hb A$_2$ >3.5%)	Thalassaemia major (Hb F 98%, Hb A$_2$ 2%)
β^+		MCV, MCH low (Hb A$_2$ >3.5%)	Thalassaemia major or intermedia (Hb F 70–80%, Hb A 10–20%, Hb A$_2$ variable)
$\delta\beta$ and hereditary persistence of foetal haemoglobin		MCV, MCH low (Hb F 5–20%, Hb A$_2$ normal)	Thalassaemia intermedia (Hb F 100%)
Hb Lepore		MCV, MCH low (Hb A 80–90%, Hb Lepore 10%, Hb A$_2$ reduced)	Thalassaemia major or intermedia (Hb F 80%, Hb Lepore 10–20%, Hb A, Hb A$_2$ absent)

* Occasionally, heterozygous β-thalassaemia is dominant (associated with the clinical picture of thalassaemia intermedia). There are several explanations.
[†] Compound heterozygote $\alpha^0\ \alpha^+$ $(--/-\alpha)$ is haemoglobin H disease.
MCH, mean corpuscular haemoglobin; MCV, mean corpuscular volume.

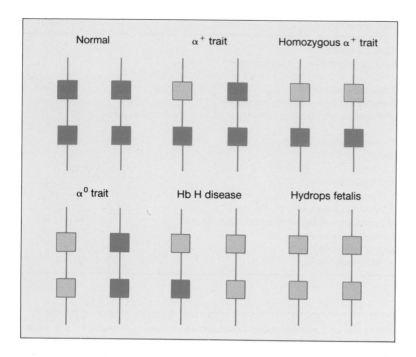

Fig. 6.4 The genetics of α-thalassaemia. Each α gene may be deleted or (less frequently) dysfunctional. The pink boxes represent normal genes, and the blue boxes represent gene deletions or dysfunctional genes.

Beta-thalassaemia syndromes

Beta-thalassaemia major

This condition is also known as Mediterranean or Cooley's anaemia and occurs on average in one in four offspring if both parents are carriers of β-thalassaemia trait. Either no β chain (β^0) or small amounts (β^+) are synthesized. Excess α chains precipitate in erythroblasts and in mature red cells causing severe

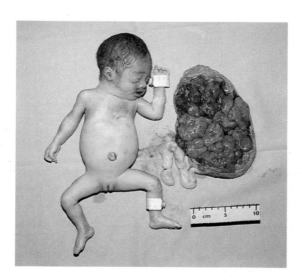

Fig. 6.5 Alpha-thalassaemia: hydrops foetalis, the result of deletion of all four α-globin genes (homozygous α^0-thalassaemia). The main haemoglobin present is Hb Bart's (γ_4). The condition is incompatible with life beyond the foetal stage. (Courtesy of Professor D. Todd.)

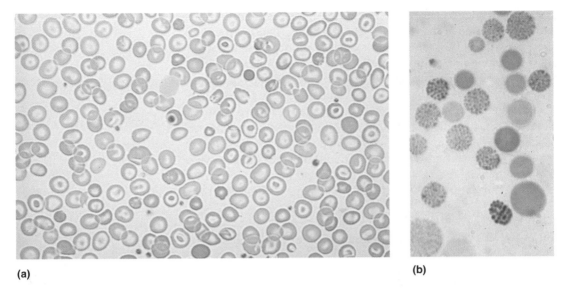

(a)   (b)

Fig. 6.6 (a) Alpha-thalassaemia: haemoglobin H disease (3 α-globin gene deletion). The blood film shows marked hypochromic, microcytic cells with target cells and poikilocytosis. (b) Alpha-thalassaemia: haemoglobin H disease. Supravital staining with brilliant cresyl blue reveals multiple fine, deeply stained deposits ('golf ball' cells) due to precipitation of aggregates of β-globin chains. Hb H can also be detected as a fast-moving band on haemoglobin electrophoresis (see Fig. 6.13).

ineffective erythropoiesis and haemolysis. The greater the α chain excess, the more severe the anaemia. Production of γ chains helps to 'mop up' excess α chains and to ameliorate the condition. Over 100 different genetic defects have now been detected (Figs 6.7 & 6.8).

Fig. 6.7 Distribution of different mutations of β-thalassaemia major round the Mediterranean area (courtesy of Professor A. Cao). IVS, intervening sequences; 1, 6, 110, 745 are mutations of corresponding codons.

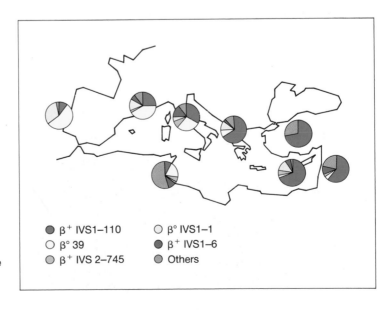

● β⁺ IVS1–110   ○ β° IVS1–1
○ β° 39   ● β⁺ IVS1–6
○ β⁺ IVS 2–745   ● Others

Unlike α-thalassaemia, the majority of genetic lesions are
point mutations rather than gene deletions. These mutations
may be within the gene complex itself or in promoter or enhancer regions. Certain mutations are particularly frequent
in some communities (Fig. 6.7). This may simplify antenatal
diagnosis aimed at detecting the mutations in foetal DNA.
Thalassaemia major is often due to inheritance of two different
mutations, each affecting β-globin synthesis (compound heterozygotes). In some cases deletion of the β gene, δ and β genes or
even δ, β and γ genes occurs. In others, unequal crossing-over
has produced δβ fusion genes (so called Lepore syndrome named
after the first family in which this was diagnosed) (see p. 110).

Clinical features
1 Severe anaemia becomes apparent at 3−6 months after birth
when the switch from α- to β-chain production should take
place.
2 Enlargement of the liver and spleen occurs due to excessive
red cell destruction, extramedullary haemopoiesis and later to
iron overload. The large spleen increases blood requirements by
increasing red cell destruction and pooling, and by causing
expansion of the plasma volume.
3 Expansion of bones due to intense marrow hyperplasia leads
to a thalassaemic facies (Fig. 6.9), and to thinning of the cortex

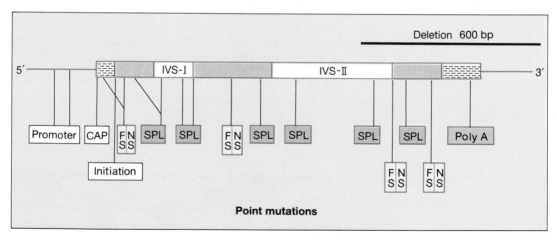

Fig. 6.8 Examples of mutations which produce β-thalassaemia. These include
single base changes, small deletions and insertions of one or two bases
affecting introns, exons or the flanking regions of the β globin gene. FS,
'frameshifts': deletion of nucleotide(s) which places the reading frame out of
phase downstream of the lesion; NS, 'nonsense': premature chain termination
due to a new translational stop codon (e.g. UAA); SPL, 'splicing': inactivation of
splicing or new splice sites generated (aberrant splicing) in exons or introns;
promoter, CAP, initiation: reduction of transcription or translation due to lesion
in promoter, CAP or initiation regions; Poly A: mutations on the Poly-A addition
signal resulting in failure of Poly-A addition and an unstable mRNA.

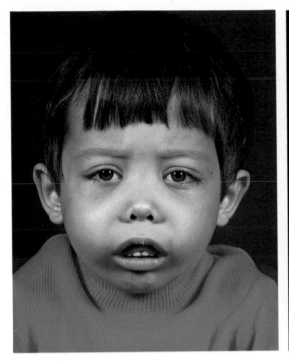

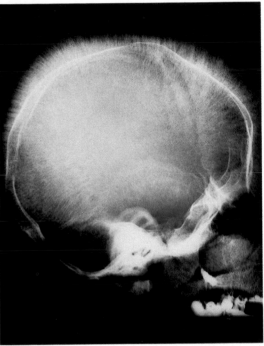

Fig. 6.9 The facial appearance of a child with β-thalassaemia major. The skull is bossed with prominent frontal and parietal bones; the maxilla is enlarged.

Fig. 6.10 The skull X-ray in β-thalassaemia major. There is a 'hair-on-end' appearance due to expansion of the bone marrow into cortical bone.

of many bones with a tendency to fractures and bossing of the skull with a 'hair-on-end' appearance on X-ray (Fig. 6.10).

4 Iron overload due to repeated transfusions (Table 6.3); each 500 ml of transfused blood contains about 250 mg iron. Iron damages the liver (Fig. 6.11), the endocrine organs (with failure of growth, delayed or absent puberty, diabetes mellitus, hypothyroidism, hypoparathyroidism), and the myocardium. Death occurs in the absence of intensive iron chelation in the second or third decade, usually from congestive heart failure or cardiac arrhythmias. Clinical abnormalities usually appear after 50 units (12 g) of iron have been transfused, but organ damage will have occurred earlier than this. Skin pigmentation due to excess

Table 6.3 Causes of refractory anaemia which may lead to transfusional iron overload.

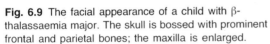

Congenital	*Acquired*
β-thalassaemia major	Myelodysplasia
β-thalassaemia/Hb E disease	Red cell aplasia
Sickle cell anaemia (some cases)	Aplastic anaemia
Red cell aplasia (Diamond–Blackfan)	Myelosclerosis
Sideroblastic anaemia	
Dyserythropoietic anaemia	

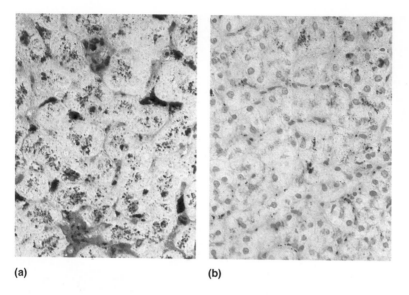

(a)   (b)

Fig. 6.11 Beta-thalassaemia major: needle biopsy of liver. (a) Grade IV siderosis with iron deposition in the hepatic parenchymal cells, bile duct epithelium, macrophages and fibroblasts (Perls' stain). (b) Reduction of iron excess in liver after intensive chelation therapy.

melanin and haemosiderin gives a slatey grey appearance at an early stage of iron overload.

5 Infections may occur for a variety of reasons. In infancy, without adequate transfusion, the anaemic child is prone to bacterial infections. Pneumococcal and meningococcal infections are likely if splenectomy has been carried out and prophylactic penicillin is not taken. *Yersinia enterocolitica* occurs particularly in iron-loaded patients being treated with desferrioxamine; it may cause severe gastroenteritis. Transmission of viruses or other infections by blood transfusion or during subcutaneous infusions of desferrioxamine may occur. Liver disease in thalassaemia major may be due to viral hepatitis transmitted by blood transfusion. Hepatitis C is the most common but hepatitis B is also frequent where this infection is endemic. HIV has been transmitted to some patients by blood transfusion.

Laboratory diagnosis

1 There is a severe hypochromic microcytic anaemia with raised reticulocyte percentage with normoblasts, target cells and basophilic stippling in the blood film (Fig. 6.12).

2 Haemoglobin electrophoresis reveals absence or almost complete absence of Hb A with almost all the circulating haemoglobin being Hb F. The Hb A_2 per cent is normal, low or slightly raised (Fig. 6.13). α/β-chain synthesis studies on circulating reticulocytes show marked increase in the α/β ratio with reduced or absent β-chain synthesis. DNA analysis using restriction enzymes and Southern blotting or the PCR (polymerase chain reaction) reaction with restriction enzyme analysis (see p. 118) can be used to identify the defect on each allele.

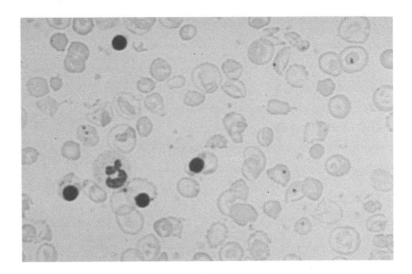

Fig. 6.12 Blood film in thalassaemia major.

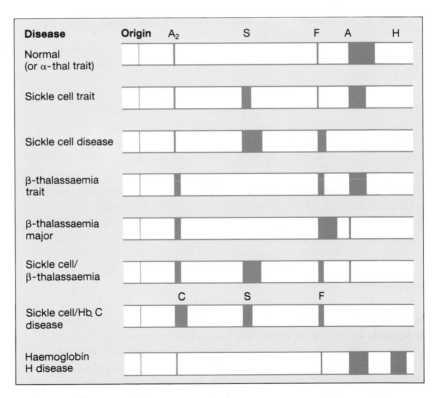

Fig. 6.13 Haemoglobin electrophoretic patterns in normal adult human blood and in subjects with sickle cell (Hb S) trait or disease, β-thalassaemia trait, β-thalassaemia major, Hb S/β-thalassaemia or Hb S/Hb C disease and Hb H disease.

Table 6.4 Assessment of iron overload.

Assessment of iron stores

Serum ferritin

Serum iron and percentage saturation of transferrin (iron-binding capacity)

Bone marrow biopsy (Perls' stain) for reticuloendothelial stores

Liver biopsy (parenchymal and reticuloendothelial stores)

Liver CT scan or NMR

Desferrioxamine iron excretion test (chelatable iron)

Repeated phlebotomy until iron deficiency occurs

Assessment of tissue damage due to iron overload

Cardiac	Clinical; chest X-ray; ECG; 24-hour monitor; echocardiography; radionuclide (MUGA) scan to check left ventricular ejection fraction at rest and with stress
Liver	Liver function tests; liver biopsy; CT scan
Endocrine	Clinical examination (growth and sexual development); glucose tolerance test; pituitary gonadotrophin release tests; thyroid, parathyroid, gonadal, adrenal function, growth hormone assays; X-rays for bone age

CT, computerized tomography; ECG, electrocardiography; NMR, nuclear magnetic resonance.

Assessment of iron status. The tests that may be performed to assess iron overload are listed in Table 6.4. Tests may also be carried out to determine the degree of organ damage caused by iron. The serum ferritin is most widely used to measure iron stores, and it is usual in thalassaemia major to attempt to keep the level between 1000 µg/l and 1500 µg/l, when the body iron stores are about 5−10 times normal. However, the serum ferritin is raised in relation to iron status in viral hepatitis and other inflammatory disorders and should therefore be interpreted in conjunction with other tests (e.g. liver biopsy (Fig. 6.11), urine iron excretion in response to desferrioxamine) and the clinical picture.

Treatment
1 Regular blood transfusions are needed to maintain the haemoglobin over 10g/dl at all times. This usually requires 2−3 units every 4−6 weeks. Fresh blood, filtered to remove white cells, gives the best red cell survival with the fewest reactions. The patients should be genotyped at the start of the transfusion programme in case red cell antibodies against transfused red cells develop.
2 Regular folic acid (e.g. 5mg daily) is given if the diet is poor.
3 Iron chelation therapy is used to prevent iron overload. Des-

ferrioxamine is inactive by mouth and may be given by a separate infusion bag 1−2 g with each unit of blood transfused. It is mainly given by subcutaneous infusion 20−40 mg/kg over 8−12 hours, 5−7 days weekly (Fig. 6.14). It is commenced in infants after 10−15 units of blood have been transfused. Chelated iron is largely excreted in urine as ferrioxamine but up to a third of chelated iron is lost in the stools. In heavily iron-loaded cases, excretion rates of up to 200 mg or more of iron daily can be achieved. Iron intake from blood transfusions with severe refractory anaemias usually averages 0.5 mg/kg/day. If patients comply with this intensive iron chelation regime, life expectancy for patients with thalassaemia major and other chronic refractory anaemias receiving regular blood transfusion (see Table 6.3) improves considerably. In some cases, intensive chelation therapy can reverse heart damage caused by iron overload. Lack of compliance, however, is frequent, especially in teenagers. Moreover, the cost of the drug precludes its use in many countries where thalassaemia is common.

With good compliance with subcutaneous desferrioxamine normal growth and sexual development also occurs but excess desferrioxamine in high doses especially in children has led to high tone deafness, retinal damage with night blindness and loss of visual acuity, and to growth retardation.

Clinical trials with oral iron chelation agents are now in progress. The α-ketohydroxypyridines are the most promising group of compounds and 1,2-dimethyl-3-hydroxypyrid-4-one (L_1) has been found in short-term trials as effective as desferrioxamine in increasing urinary iron excretion. Long-term trials with this drug are in progress.

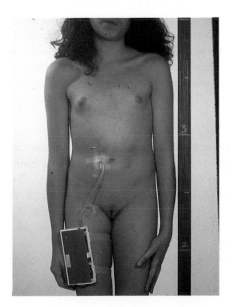

Fig. 6.14 Beta-thalassaemia major: subcutaneous infusion of desferrioxamine infusion in progress using a portable, battery-driven pump.

4 Vitamin C, 200 mg daily, increases excretion of iron produced by desferrioxamine.

5 Splenectomy may be needed to reduce blood requirements. This is delayed until the patient is over 6 years old because of the high risk of dangerous infections post-splenectomy earlier in life. Pneumococcal vaccine is given pre-operatively and prophylactic penicillin therapy (e.g. 250 mg b.d. orally) for life after splenectomy.

6 Endocrine therapy is given either as replacement because of end organ failure or to stimulate the pituitary if puberty is delayed. Diabetes mellitus if present will require insulin therapy. It does not reverse even with intensive iron chelation. Calcium and vitamin D may be needed for hypoparathyroidism.

7 Immunization against hepatitis B should be carried out in all non-immune patients.

8 Bone marrow transplantation has been carried out successfully in patients, usually less than 16 years old, from an HLA-matching sibling or, rarely, HLA-matching parent. The success rate (long-term thalassaemia major-free survival) is about 80%. Failures are due to reconstitution of thalassaemic marrow, acute or chronic graft-vs-host disease (GVHD) or to other transplant-related complications. There is a 5−10% mortality during the procedure. Patients without liver fibrosis or hepatomegaly (good compliers with desferrioxamine) have been found to do best.

Thalassaemia intermedia

Cases of thalassaemia of moderate severity (haemoglobin 7.0−10.0 g/dl) who do not need regular transfusions are called thalassaemia intermedia (Table 6.5). This is a clinical syndrome, therefore, which may be due to a variety of genetic defects. It may be due to homozygous β-thalassaemia with production of more Hb F than usual or with mild defects in β-chain synthesis, or to β-thalassaemia trait alone but of unusual severity, or β-thalassaemia trait in association with other mild globin abnormalities, e.g. Hb Lepore. The coexistence of α-thalassaemia trait improves the haemoglobin level in homozygous β-thalassaemia by reducing the degree of chain imbalance and thus of α-chain precipitation and ineffective erythropoiesis. On the other hand, patients with β-thalassaemia trait who also have excess (5 or 6) α genes tend to be more anaemic than usual. The patient with thalassaemia intermedia may show bone deformity, enlarged liver and spleen, extramedullary erythropoiesis (Fig. 6.15) and features of iron overload due to increased iron absorption. Hb H disease, three-gene deletion α-thalassaemia, is a type of thalassaemia intermedia without iron overload or extramedullary haemopoiesis.

Table 6.5 Thalassaemia intermedia.

Homozygous β-thalassaemia
Homozygous mild β⁺-thalassaemia
Coinheritance of α-thalassaemia
Enhanced ability to make foetal haemoglobin (γ-chain production)

Heterozygous β-thalassaemia
Coinheritance of additional α-globin genes (ααα/αα or ααα/ααα)

δβ-thalassaemia and hereditary persistence of foetal haemoglobin
Homozygous δβ-thalassaemia
Heterozygous δβ-thalassaemia/β-thalassaemia
Homozygous Hb Lepore (some cases)

Haemoglobin H disease

Beta-thalassaemia trait (minor)

This is a common, usually symptomless abnormality character-ized like α-thalassaemia trait by a hypochromic, microcytic blood picture (MCV and MCH very low but red cell count high) and mild or no anaemia (haemoglobin 10−15 g/dl). It is usually more severe than α trait and a raised Hb A_2 (>3.5%) confirms the diagnosis. The body iron content is normal unless iron therapy has mistakenly been given. There is a 25% chance of a child being born with thalassaemia major if both parents have β-thalassaemia trait. Antenatal diagnosis and abortion can prevent this (p. 116). On average 50% of their offspring will be carriers and 25% normal.

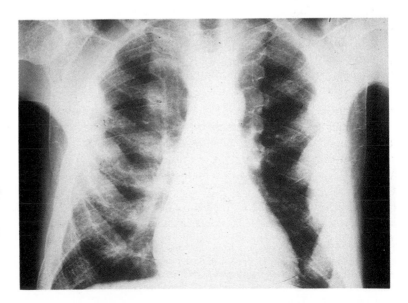

Fig. 6.15 Chest radiograph of a patient with β-thalassaemia intermedia showing hilar shadows due to paravertebral extramedullary haemopoietic deposits. There is also marked medullary expansion within the ribs.

Hereditary persistence of foetal haemoglobin

These are a heterogenous group of conditions due to deletions or cross-overs affecting the production of β and γ chains or in non-deletion forms to point mutations upstream from the γ-globin genes.

Delta, beta-thalassaemia

This involves failure of production of both β and δ chains. Foetal haemoglobin production is increased to 5–20% in the heterozygous state which resembles thalassaemia minor haematologically. In the homozygous state, only Hb F is present, and haematologically the picture is of thalassaemia intermedia.

Haemoglobin Lepore

This is an abnormal haemoglobin due to unequal crossing-over of the β and δ genes to produce a polypeptide chain consisting of the δ chain at its amino end and β chain at its carboxyl end. The δβ-fusion chain is synthesized inefficiently and normal δ- and β-chain production is abolished. The homozygotes show thalassaemia intermedia and the heterozygotes thalassaemia trait.

Association of β-thalassaemia trait with other haemoglobinopathies

The combination of β-thalassaemia trait with Hb E trait usually causes a transfusion-dependent thalassaemia major syndrome, but some cases are intermediate. β-thalassaemia trait with Hb S trait produces the clinical picture of sickle cell anaemia rather than of thalassaemia (p. 111). β-thalassaemia trait with Hb D trait causes a mild hypochromic microcytic anaemia.

Normal β-chain	Amino acid	pro	glu	glu
	Base composition	CCT	G(A)G	GAG
Sickle β-chain	Base composition	CCT	G(T)G	GAG
	Amino acid	pro	val	glu

Fig. 6.16 Molecular pathology of sickle cell anaemia. There is a single base change in the DNA coding for the amino acid in the sixth position in the β-globin chain (adenine is replaced by thymine). This leads to an amino acid change from glutamic acid to valine. A, adenine; C, cytosine; G, guanine; glu, glutamic acid; pro, proline; T, thymine; val, valine.

Sickle cell anaemia

Hb S (Hb $\alpha_2\beta_2^s$) is insoluble and forms crystals when exposed to low oxygen tension. Deoxygenated sickle haemoglobin polymerizes into long fibres, each consisting of seven intertwined double strands with cross-linking. The red cells sickle and may block different areas of the microcirculation causing infarcts of various organs. The abnormality is due to substitution of valine for glutamic acid in position 6 in the β chain (Fig. 6.16).

Homozygous disease

Clinical features

These are of a severe haemolytic anaemia punctuated by crises. The symptoms of anaemia are often mild in relation to the severity of the anaemia since Hb S gives up oxygen (O_2) to tissues relatively easily compared with Hb A, its O_2-dissociation curve being shifted to the right (p. 20). The clinical expression of Hb SS is very variable, some patients having an almost normal life, free of crises but others develop severe crises even as infants and may die in early childhood or as young adults. Crises may be painful, visceral, aplastic or haemolytic.

Painful vascular–occlusive crises. Painful crises are the most frequent and are precipitated by such factors as infection, acidosis, dehydration or deoxygenation (e.g. altitude, operations, obstetric delivery, stasis of the circulation, exposure to cold, violent exercise, etc). Infarcts may occur in a variety of organs including bones (hips, shoulders and vertebrae are commonly affected) (Fig. 6.17), the lungs and the spleen. The most serious

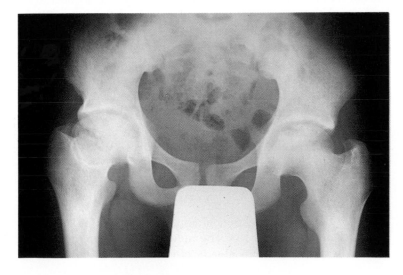

Fig. 6.17 Sickle cell anaemia: radiograph of the pelvis of a young man of West Indian origin which shows avascular necrosis with flattening of the femoral heads, more marked on the right, coarsening of the bone architecture and cystic areas in the right femoral neck due to previous infarcts.

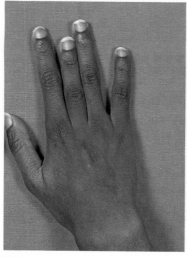
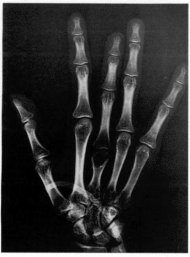

(a)   (b)

Fig. 6.18 (a) Sickle cell anaemia: the hand of an 18-year-old Nigerian boy with the 'hand–foot' syndrome. There is marked shortening of the right middle finger because of dactylitis in childhood affecting the growth of the epiphysis. (b) X-ray of hand shown in (a). There is shortening of the right middle metacarpal bone due to infarction of the growing epiphysis in childhood.

vascular–occlusive crisis is of the brain (a stroke occurs in 7% of all patients) or spinal cord. In children the 'hand–foot' syndrome (painful dactylitis due to infarcts of the small bones) is frequent and may lead to digits of varying lengths (Fig. 6.18).

Visceral sequestration crises. These are due to sickling within organs and pooling of blood, often with a severe exacerbation of anaemia. A severe chest syndrome with infiltrates on X-ray is the commonest cause of death. Hepatic and girdle sequestration crises and splenic sequestration all may lead to severe illness requiring exchange transfusions.

Aplastic crises. These may occur due to infection with parvovirus and/or folate deficiency and are characterized by a sudden fall in haemoglobin usually requiring transfusion. They are characterized by a fall in reticulocytes as well as haemoglobin.

Haemolytic crises. These are characterized by an increased rate of haemolysis with a fall in haemoglobin but rise in reticulocytosis and usually accompany a painful crisis.

Other clinical features
Ulcers of the lower legs are common, due to vascular stasis and local ischaemia (Fig. 6.19). The spleen is enlarged in infancy and early childhood but later is often reduced in size due to

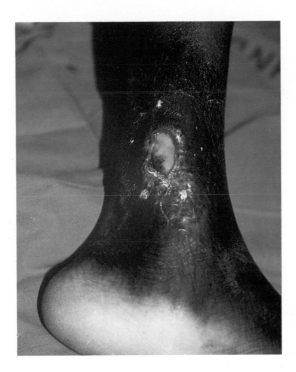

Fig. 6.19 Sickle cell anaemia: medial aspect of the ankle of a 15-year-old Nigerian boy showing necrosis and ulceration.

infarcts (autosplenectomy). A proliferative retinopathy and priapism are other clinical complications. Chronic damage to the liver may occur through micro-infarcts. Pigment (bilirubin) gall stones are frequent. The kidneys are vulnerable to infarctions of the medulla with papillary necrosis. Failure to concentrate urine aggravates the tendency to dehydration and crisis and nocturnal enuresis is common. Glomerulosclerosis is an uncommon severe complication.

Laboratory findings
1 The haemoglobin is usually 6−9 g/dl − low in comparison to symptoms of anaemia.
2 Sickle cells and target cells occur in the blood (Fig. 6.20a). Features of splenic atrophy (e.g. Howell−Jolly bodies) may also be present.
3 Screening tests for sickling are positive when the blood is deoxygenated (e.g. with dithionate and Na_2HPO_4).
4 *Haemoglobin electrophoresis* (see Fig. 6.13). In Hb SS, no normal Hb A is detected. The amount of Hb F is variable and is usually 5−15%, larger amounts are normally associated with a milder disorder, e.g. so-called benign sickle cell anaemia in Saudi Arabia.

Treatment
1 Prophylactic − avoid those factors known to precipitate crises,

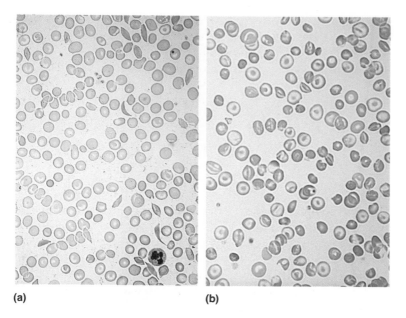

(a)   (b)

Fig. 6.20 (a) Sickle cell anaemia: peripheral blood film showing deeply staining sickle cells, target cells and polychromasia (a Howell—Jolly body is seen in a red cell in the top right portion of the field). (b) Homozygous Hb C disease: peripheral blood film showing many target cells, deeply staining rhomboidal and spherocytic cells.

especially dehydration, anoxia, infections, stasis of the circulation, and cooling of the skin surface.

2 Folic acid, e.g. 5 mg daily.

3 Good general nutrition and hygiene.

4 Pneumococcal vaccination and regular oral penicillin to reduce the frequency of crises precipitated by infections.

5 Crises — rest, rehydrate by oral fluids and/or intravenous normal saline, give antibiotics if infection is present and bicarbonate only if the patient is acidotic. Strong analgesics are usually needed including opiates. Blood transfusion is given only if there is very severe anaemia with symptoms. Exchange transfusion may be needed particularly if there is neurological damage or a visceral sequestration crisis or repeated painful crises. This is repeated to achieve a Hb S percentage of less than 30 in severe cases.

6 Particular care is needed in pregnancy and anaesthesia. Before delivery or operations, patients may be transfused repeatedly with normal blood to reduce the proportion of circulating Hb S to less than 30%. Careful anaesthetic and recovery techniques must be used to avoid hypoxaemia or acidosis. Routine transfusions throughout pregnancy are given to those with a bad obstetric history or a history of frequent crises.

7 Transfusions — these are also sometimes given repeatedly prophylactically to patients having frequent crises or who have had major organ damage, e.g. of the brain, to suppress Hb S production completely over a period of several months or even years. Iron overload may become a problem and iron chelation therapy may then be needed.

8 Bone marrow transplantation—the risks of this procedure generally outweigh the possible benefits, but for carefully selected patients it does offer a potential cure.

9 Research into a drug to enhance Hb F synthesis or to stabilize the red cell membrane or to increase the solubility of Hb S is taking place. No drug has yet emerged that is sufficiently effective and safe for general use although trials of hydroxyurea therapy to enhance Hb F production are in progress. 'Gene therapy' is a distant prospect not yet available (see p. 120).

Sickle cell trait

This is a benign condition with no anaemia and normal appearance of red cells on a blood film but crises can be caused by extreme stress, e.g. anoxia and severe infections. Haematuria is the most common symptom and is thought to be due to minor infarcts of the renal papillae. Hb S varies from 25% to 45% of the total haemoglobin (see Fig. 6.13). Care must be taken with anaesthesia and in pregnancy.

Combination of Hb S with other genetic defects of haemoglobin

The commonest are S/β-thalassaemia, and sickle cell/C disease. In Hb S/β-thalassaemia, the MCV and MCH are lower than in homozygous Hb SS. The clinical picture is of sickle cell anaemia; splenomegaly is usual. Patients with sickle cell/C disease have a particular tendency to thrombosis and pulmonary embolism, especially in pregnancy. They also have a high incidence of retinal abnormalities. There is usually mild anaemia and splenomegaly. Diagnosis is made by haemoglobin electrophoresis, particularly with family studies.

Haemoglobin C disease

This genetic defect of haemoglobin is frequent in West Africa and is due to substitution of lysine for glutamic acid in the β-globin chain at the same point as the substitution in Hb S. Hb C tends to form rhomboidal crystals and in the homozygous state there is a mild haemolytic anaemia with marked target cell formation, cells with rhombodial shape and microspherocytes (see Fig. 6.20b). The spleen is enlarged. The carriers show a few target cells only.

Haemoglobin D disease

This is a group of variants all with the same electrophoretic mobility. Heterozygotes show no haematological abnormality while homozygotes have a mild haemolytic anaemia.

Haemoglobin E disease

This is the commonest haemoglobin variant in South East Asia. In the homozygous state, there is a mild microcytic, hypochromic anaemia. Haemoglobin E/β^0 thalassaemia, however, resembles homozygous β^0 thalassaemia both clinically and haematologically.

Prenatal diagnosis of genetic haemoglobin disorders

It is important to give genetic counselling to couples at risk of having a child with a major haemoglobin defect. If a pregnant woman is found to have a haemoglobin abnormality, her spouse should be tested to determine whether he also carries a defect. When both partners show an abnormality and there is a risk of a serious defect in the offspring, particularly β-thalassaemia major, it is important to offer antenatal diagnosis. Several techniques are available, the choice depending on the time in pregnancy and the potential nature of the defect.

Foetal blood sampling

This is performed in mid-second trimester on foetal blood obtained from the umbilical cord and is relatively safe. *In vitro* synthesis of individual globin chains is measured using incubation with a radioactive amino acid (leucine) to label the individual globin chains. At this stage normal β-chain production should be detected. The main disadvantage is the delay in making the diagnosis and, if necessary, performing abortion.

DNA diagnosis

Amniotic fluid cells can be obtained in the second trimester but trophoblast DNA may be obtained during the first trimester by chorionic villus biopsy using either a transcervical or transabdominal approach. The DNA is then analysed using one of the following methods.

Gene mapping
Where the mutation alters a restriction site to a particular enzyme, digestion will produce a different sized restriction fragment. This is best illustrated by Hb S in which the enzyme Mst II detects the A-T change (Fig. 6.21).

Restriction fragment length polymorphism (RFLP) linkage analysis
This technique is used widely to diagnose many genetic disorders. Scattered along each gene cluster are single base changes

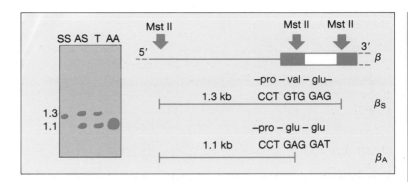

Fig. 6.21 Sickle cell anaemia: antenatal diagnosis. Direct DNA analysis. The DNA has been digested by the restriction enzyme Mst II. The replacement of an adenine base in the normal β-globin gene by thymine in the sickle cell gene removes a normal restriction site for Mst II, producing a larger 1.3 kb fragment than the normal 1.1 kb fragment to hybridize with the β-globin gene probe. In this case the trophoblast DNA (T) shows both normal (A) and sickle cell (S) restriction fragments and so is AS (sickle trait). (Courtesy of Dr J. Old and The Royal College of Obstetrics and Gynaecology.)

which may vary from one individual to the next i.e. are polymorphic. These changes give rise to sites recognized by restriction enzymes or remove sites previously identified so that the size of the DNA fragment produced by that restriction enzyme varies. A restriction site present is denoted as (+) and its absence as (−). The restriction fragment length polymorphisms (RFLPs) due to these sites are inherited in a Mendelian manner and can be used, provided they are sufficiently close to the gene of interest, as linkage markers to recognize a chromosome that carries a thalassaemia or other mutation (Fig. 6.22). The combination of various RFLPs along one chromosome is called the 'haplotype'. If two sites along a chromosome are found to occur together more frequently than by chance, this is known as linkage disequilibrium. Family studies are first needed to establish the linkage of normal and abnormal globin genes to particular haplotypes. The haplotypes of the foetal DNA are then analysed. This technique therefore requires a previous child or grandparents to be studied as well as parents, and the parents must not be homozygous. Rarely cross-over between the markers studied and the globin gene may lead to false results.

Oligonucleotide probes
These are short probes of about 17−19 nucleotides which can detect a single base change. Two are used, one to the normal, the other to the mutated sequence. Carriers have DNA that will hybridize with both probes. Normals or homozygous patients will hybridize with only one or other probe.

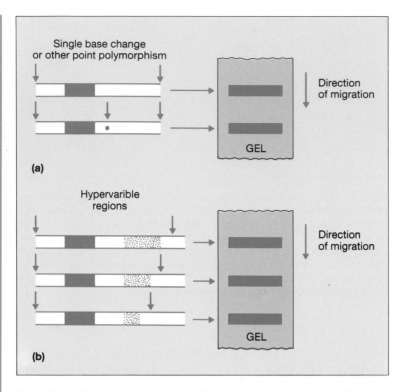

Fig. 6.22 (a) Restriction fragment length polymorphism analysis. A single point difference close to the gene to be studied (and for which a probe is available) produces a new restriction enzyme site so that the fragment of DNA hybridizing to the gene probe is smaller (and moves further in the gel).
(b) Hypervariable regions close to the gene to be studied (and for which a probe is available) result in different sizes of DNA fragments after restriction enzyme digestion. The different size of fragment is reflected in different mobility in the gel.

PCR gene amplification (Fig. 6.23)
A pair of DNA primers which flank the region to be studied and hybridize to opposite strands are chosen. The DNA is amplified by: (1) heat denaturation of the double-stranded DNA; (2) annealing the single stranded DNA to the pair of primers; (3) extension of the DNA from the primers with the Taq DNA polymerase which is heat insensitive; and (4) repeating this process through multiple cycles so that visible amounts of DNA can be synthesized. This can then be tested using direct restriction enzyme analysis, oligonucleotide probes or direct gene sequencing. A technique of 'mismatched PCR' *a*mplification *r*efractory *m*utation *s*ystem (ARMS) (Fig. 6.24) is now widely used. No gene product is obtained unless the primer matches the mutated gene to be amplified.

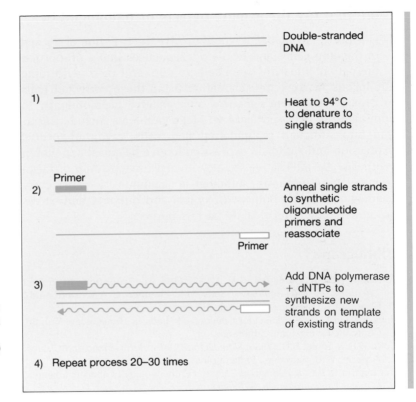

1) Heat to 94°C to denature to single strands — Double-stranded DNA

2) Primer — Anneal single strands to synthetic oligonucleotide primers and reassociate — Primer

3) Add DNA polymerase + dNTPs to synthesize new strands on template of existing strands

4) Repeat process 20–30 times

Fig. 6.23 Polymerase chain reaction. The primers are used, hybridizing to DNA on either side of the piece of DNA to be analysed. Repeated cycles of denaturation, association with the primers, incubation with a DNA polymerase and deoxyribonucleotides (dNTPs) results in amplification of the DNA over a million times within a few hours.

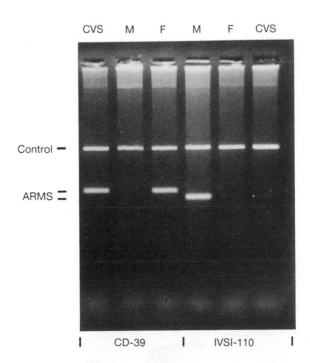

CVS M F M F CVS

Control —

ARMS =

CD-39   IVSI-110

Fig. 6.24 The rapid prenatal diagnosis of β-thalassaemia by ARMS. One parent has the common Mediterranean codon 39 (CD-39) mutation, the other the IVS1−110 G→A mutation. The foetus is heterozygous for the CD-39 mutation. CVS, foetal DNA from chorionic villus sampling; F, father, M, mother. (Courtesy of Dr J. Old and Professor D.J. Weatherall.)

Gene therapy for genetic defects of haemoglobin

This is not yet available. It would involve the insertion of normal
α- or β-globin genes and regulatory sequences into a proportion
of the patient's marrow stem cells *in vitro* and then performing
autologous marrow transplantation using these corrected cells
to reseed the patient's marrow after ablative chemotherapy to
eliminate the diseased marrow. Major problems include: insertion into sufficient repopulating stem cells, erythroid-specific
expression and sufficient expression to give balanced α/β-globin
synthesis. An alternative strategy involves reactivation of foetal
haemoglobin synthesis sufficient to maintain a satisfactory
haemoglobin level. Both hydroxyurea and butyrate derivatives
are undergoing clinical trials for this purpose.

Bibliography

Al-Refaie F.N. & Hoffbrand A.V. (1993) Oral iron chelation. In *Recent
Advances in Haematology*, 7 (eds M.K. Brenner & A.V. Hoffbrand).
Churchill Livingstone, Edinburgh, (in press).

Benz E.J. (ed.) (1989) *Molecular Genetics*. Methods in Hematology, Vol. 20.
Churchill Livingstone, Edinburgh.

Bunn H.F. & Forget B.G. (1985) *Hemoglobin: Molecular, Genetic and Clinical
Aspects*. W.B. Saunders, Philadelphia.

Gordon-Smith E.C. & Issaragrisil S. (1992) Epidemiology of aplastic anaemia.
Clinical Haematology, **5**, 475–491.

Hershko C. (ed.) (1989) Iron chelating therapy. *Clinical Haematology*, **2**,
195–496.

Hibbs J.R. & Young N.S. (1992) Viruses and the blood. *Clinical Haematology*,
5, 245–271.

Higgs D.R. & Weatherall D.J. (eds) (1993) Haemoglobinopathies. *Clinical
Haematology*, **6**, 1–331.

Hill A.V.S (1992) Molecular epidemiology of the thalassaemias (including
haemoglobulin E). *Clinical Haematology*, **5**, 209–238.

Kazazian H.H. (ed.) (1990) The thalassemia syndromes: molecular basis and
pre-natal diagnosis in 1990. *Seminars in Hematology*, **27**, 209–228.

Miller A.D. (1992) Human gene therapy comes of age. *Nature*, **357**, 455–460.

Nagel R.L. (ed.) (1991) Hemoglobinopathies. *Hematology/Oncology Clinics
of North America*, **5**, 375–596.

Old J.M., Thein S.L., Weatherall D.J., Cao A. & Loukopoulos D. (1989) Prenatal diagnosis of the major haemoglobin disorders. *Molecular Biology
and Medicine*, **6**, 55–63.

Powars D., Chan L.S. & Schroeder W.A. (1990) The variable expression of
sickle cell disease is genetically determined. *Seminars in Hematology*,
27, 360–376.

Sergeant G.R. (1992) *Sickle Cell Anaemia*, 2nd Edn. Oxford University
Press, Oxford.

Sullivan K.M. (ed.) (1991) Role of bone marrow transplantation in sickle cell
anemia. *Seminars in Hematology*, **28**, 177–267.

Weatherall D.J. & Clegg J.B. (1981) *The Thalassaemia Syndromes*, 3rd
Edition. Blackwell Scientific Publications, Edinburgh.

Weatherall D.J., Clegg J.B., Higgs D.R. & Wood W.G. (1988) The haemoglobinopathies. In *The Metabolic Basis of Inherited Disease*, 6th Edition
(eds C.R. Scryier, A.L. Beaudet, W.S. Sly & D. Valle). McGraw Hill, New
York, pp. 2281–2306.

Chapter 7
Aplastic Anaemia and Bone Marrow Transplantation

Aplastic anaemia

Aplastic (hypoplastic) anaemia is defined as pancytopenia (anaemia, leucopenia and thrombocytopenia) resulting from aplasia of the bone marrow. It is classified into primary types which include a congenital form (Fanconi anaemia) and an acquired form with no obvious precipitating cause. Secondary aplastic anaemia may result from a variety of industrial, iatrogenic and infectious causes (Table 7.1).

Pathogenesis

The underlying defect in all cases appears to be a substantial reduction in the number of haemopoietic pluripotential stem cells, and a fault in the remaining stem cells or an immune reaction against them, which makes them unable to divide and differentiate sufficiently to populate the bone marrow (Fig. 7.1). A primary fault in the marrow microenvironment has also been suggested but the success of bone marrow transplantation (BMT) shows this can only be a rare cause since normal donor stem cells are usually able to thrive in the recipient's marrow cavity.

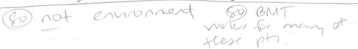
(handwritten) (so) not environment (so) BMT works for many of these pts.

Table 7.1 Causes of aplastic anaemia.

Primary	Secondary
Congenital (Fanconi and non-Fanconi types) *Idiopathic acquired*	*Ionizing radiations*: accidental exposure (radiotherapy, radioactive isotopes, nuclear power stations)
	Chemicals: benzene and other organic solvents, TNT, insecticides, hair dyes, chlordane, DDT
	Drugs Which regularly cause marrow depression (e.g. busulphan, cyclophosphamide, anthracyclines, nitrosoureas) Which occasionally or rarely cause marrow depression (e.g. chloramphenicol, sulphonamides, phenylbutazone, gold, and others)
	Infection: viral hepatitis (A or non-A, non-B)

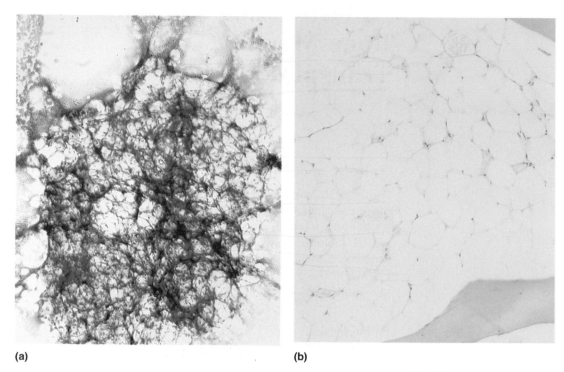

(a)   (b)

Fig. 7.1 Aplastic anaemia: low power views of bone marrow show severe reduction of haemopoietic cells with an increase in fat spaces. (a) Aspirated fragment. (b) Trephine biopsy.

Congenital

The Fanconi type has a recessive pattern of inheritance and is often associated with growth retardation and congenital defects of the skeleton (e.g. microcephaly, absent radii or thumbs), of the renal tract (e.g. pelvic or horseshoe kidney) or skin (areas of hyper- and hypopigmentation); sometimes there is mental retardation. There are chromosomal abnormalities (increased numbers of random breaks), best detected in peripheral blood lymphocytes. Some congenital cases do not show defects of other organs or chromosome changes; a few show an unusual sex-linked disorder with nail and skin atrophy (dyskeratosis congenita).

The usual age of presentation of Fanconi anaemia is 5–10 years. About 10% of cases develop acute myeloid leukaemia. Treatment is usually with androgens and/or BMT. The blood count usually improves with androgens but side effects, especially in children, are distressing (virilization) and liver abnormalities); remission rarely lasts more than 2 years. BMT may cure the patient but, because of the sensitivity of the patient's cells to alkylating agents (due to defective DNA repair), low-dose cyclophosphamide and low-dose total body irradiation (TBI) are usually combined as conditioning.

> hyperandrogenism in ♀ (androgen parts)

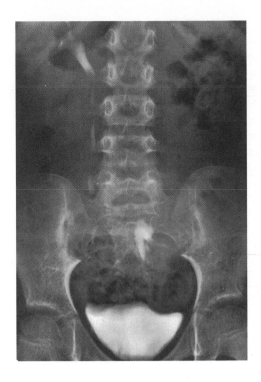

Fig. 7.2 Fanconi anaemia: intravenous pyelogram of a 9-year-old child showing a normal right kidney but a left kidney abnormally placed in the pelvis.

Idiopathic acquired

In most cases, an autoimmune mechanism in which the patient's T lymphocytes are thought to suppress haemopoietic stem cells seems likely on the basis of *in vitro* marrow culture experiments and clinical response to intense immunosuppression with, for example, anti-lymphocyte globulin (ALG), corticosteroids and cyclosporin. A defect of the marrow stem cells which limits their proliferative capacity seems likely in some instances. It may be that a structural defect of stem cells triggers a local cell-mediated autoimmune reaction against them.

Secondary

This is often due to direct damage to the haemopoietic marrow by radiation or cytotoxic drugs. The anti-metabolite drugs (e.g. methotrexate) and mitotic inhibitors (e.g. daunorubicin) cause only temporary aplasia but the alkylating agents, particularly busulphan, may cause chronic aplasia closely resembling the chronic idiopathic disease. In these cases, the drugs are known to be marrow depressants and often large doses have been given for prolonged periods. Some individuals develop aplastic anaemia, however, when exposed to drugs such as chloramphenicol or phenylbutazone (see Table 7.1) which are not

known to be cytotoxic, or they may develop the disease during
or within a few months of illness with viral hepatitis (hepatitis
A or non-A, non-B). Because the incidence of marrow toxicity
is particularly high for chloramphenicol, this drug should
be reserved for treatment of those infections which are life-
threatening (e.g. typhoid) and for which it is the optimum antibiotic. Chronic benzene exposure usually causes a hypercellular
dyserythropoietic marrow but may occasionally cause a true
aplastic anaemia. Rarely aplastic anaemia may be the presenting
feature of acute lymphoblastic or myeloid leukaemia, especially
in childhood. Myelodysplasia may also present with a hypoplastic marrow.

Clinical features

The onset is at any age with a peak incidence around 30 years
and a slight male predominance; it can be insidious or acute
with symptoms and signs resulting from anaemia, neutropenia
or thrombocytopenia. Infections, particularly of the mouth and
throat, are common and generalized infections are frequently
life-threatening; bruising, bleeding gums, epistaxes and menorrhagia are the most frequent haemorrhagic manifestations and
the usual presenting features, often with symptoms of anaemia.
The lymph nodes, liver and spleen are not enlarged.

Laboratory findings

1 Anaemia is normochromic, normocytic or macrocytic
(MCV often 95−110 fl). The reticulocyte count is reduced and
usually extremely low in relation to the degree of anaemia.
2 Leucopenia. There is a selective fall in granulocytes, usually
but not always to below $1.5 \times 10^9/l$. In severe cases, the lymphocyte count is also low. The neutrophils appear normal and their
alkaline phosphatase score is high.
3 Thrombocytopenia is always present and, in severe cases, is
less than $10 \times 10^9/l$.
4 There are no abnormal cells in the peripheral blood.
5 Bone marrow shows hypoplasia, with loss of haemopoietic
tissue and replacement by fat which comprises over 75% of the
marrow. Trephine biopsy is essential and may show patchy
cellular areas in a hypocellular background (Fig. 7.1). The main
cells present are lymphocytes and plasma cells; megakaryocytes
in particular are reduced or absent.

Diagnosis

The disease must be distinguished from other causes of pancytopenia (Table 7.2) and this is not usually difficult provided

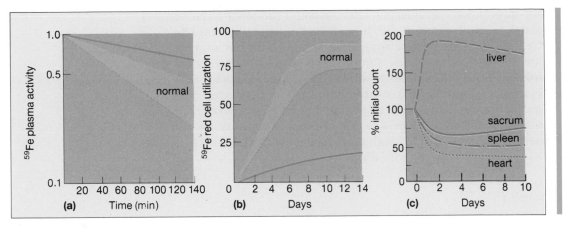

Fig. 7.3 ^{59}Fe ferrokinetic study of a plastic anaemia. (a) Slow clearance of ^{59}Fe. (b) Grossly reduced ^{59}Fe red cell utilization. (c) Surface counting evidence of liver uptake of ^{59}Fe and impaired bone marrow (sacral) uptake.

an adequate bone marrow sample is obtained. Ferrokinetic studies with labelled iron (^{59}Fe) are no longer performed routinely, but illustrate the marrow defect. They show slow clearance of iron from the bloodstream, poor uptake by the marrow, and subsequent inadequate incorporation into circulating red cells (Fig. 7.3). Most of the iron accumulates in the liver. If the reticulocyte count is raised, paroxysmal nocturnal haemoglobinuria must be excluded by examination of urine for haemosiderin and by the acid lysis test. In older patients, hypoplastic myelodysplasia may show similar appearances. Qualitative abnormalities of the cells and clonal cytogenetic changes suggest myelodysplasia rather than aplastic anaemia.

Treatment

General

The cause, if known, is removed, e.g. radiation or drug therapy is discontinued. Initial management consists largely of support care with blood transfusions, platelet concentrates and treatment

Table 7.2 Causes of pancytopenia.

1 Aplastic anaemia (including cytotoxic drug therapy)

2 Bone marrow infiltration (e.g. carcinoma, tuberculosis, lymphoma)

3 Leukaemia, some myelodysplastic syndromes, myeloma

4 Hypersplenism (e.g. portal hypertension, Felty's syndrome, storage diseases, e.g. Gaucher's disease)

5 Megaloblastic anaemia

6 Myelosclerosis (some cases)

7 Paroxysmal nocturnal haemoglobinuria (some cases)

and prevention of infection. In severely thrombocytopenic
(platelet count $<10 \times 10^9/l$) and neutropenic (neutrophils
$<0.5 \times 10^9/l$) patients, management is similar to the support
care of patients receiving intensive chemotherapy for acute
leukaemia. An anti-fibrinolytic agent (e.g. tranexamic acid) may
be used in patients with severe prolonged thrombocytopenia.
Oral antifungal agents (e.g. amphotericin and fluconazole) may
be given and oral quinolones, e.g. ciprofloxacin, and colistin are
used prophylactically in some units to reduce the incidence of
Gram-negative bacterial infections.

Specific

The choice of more specific therapy depends partly on correct
assessment of the patient's chance of spontaneous recovery.
In the most severe cases, assessed by reticulocyte, neutrophil
and platelet counts and degree of loss of haemopoietic marrow
tissue, the chance of survival beyond 6–12 months is less than
50%. Cases following viral hepatitis usually fall into this group.
Less severe cases may have an acute transient course, or a
chronic course with ultimate recovery, although the platelet
count often remains subnormal for many years. Relapses, sometimes severe and occasionally fatal, may also occur and, rarely,
the disease transforms into myelodysplasia, acute leukaemia or
paroxysmal nocturnal haemoglobinuria (p. 92).

The following 'specific' treatments are used with varying
success.

Anti-lymphocyte (thymocyte) globulin (ALG)

This is prepared in animals (e.g. horse or rabbit) and is of benefit
in about 50–60% of acquired cases (Fig. 7.4). The action may be
via elimination of suppressor killer T cells thought to be damaging
haemopoietic stem cells. It is given with immunosuppressive
corticosteroids which also reduce the side effects of ALG—fever,
rashes, hypotension or hypertension. Serum sickness with fever,
rash and joint pains may occur about 7 days after ALG administration and corticosteriod therapy is given to try to prevent this.
Cyclosporin therapy given with ALG and high doses of corticosteroids appears to be of additional benefit.

Patients who respond to the first course of ALG show an
improvement in blood counts within 4 months. Patients with
very severe disease (e.g. neutrophils $<0.2 \times 10^9/l$) respond less
well but age does not seem to be a factor. If there is no response
after 4 months, a second course of ALG prepared in a different
species may be tried. Overall, 50–60% of patients respond
to ALG, and up to 80% to combined ALG, steroids and cyclosporin (Fig. 7.4d).

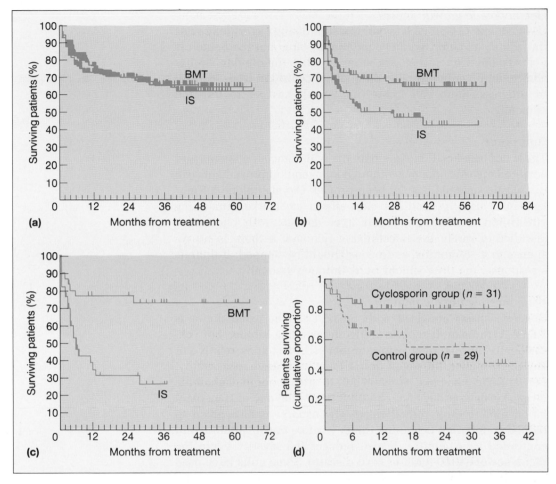

Fig. 7.4 (a) Comparison of bone marrow transplantation (BMT) with immunosuppression (IS) (ALG) in the treatment of aplastic anaemia. (b) Effect of low neutrophil count ($<0.2 \times 10^9/l$) on survival following BMT or IS ($p < 0.01$). (c) Survival of patients with aplastic anaemia who have $<0.2 \times 10^9/l$ neutrophils and are infected at time of treatment with either BMT or IS. (Data from cumulative European Bone Marrow Transplant Group, 1987.) (d) Survival of severe aplastic anaemia treated with ALG and high-dose steroids with or without (control group) cyclosporin. (From Frickhofen *et al.*, 1992.)

Cyclosporin
Alone, this is associated with an improvement in occasional patients. It had been reserved for cases not responding to ALG but recent studies suggest it should be given in combination with ALG and steroids.

High-dose methylprednisolone
High-dose methylprednisolone has been used as an alternative to ALG but side effects are major and it seems to have no advantage over ALG combined with cyclosporin and steroids.

Haemopoietic growth factors
GM-CSF and G-CSF (CSF = colony-stimulating factor) may raise
the white cell count while being administered but the benefit is
not sustained after they are stopped. IL-3 (interleukin 3) has
additional potential to raise the platelet count but trials are still
in progress. Stem cell factor (kit ligand) has yet to be tried
clinically.

Androgens
These are beneficial in some patients with Fanconi anaemia and
acquired aplastic anaemia although an overall improved survival
in aplastic anaemia has not been proved. Oxymetholone 2.5 mg/
kg/day is usually tried but side effects are marked including
virilization, salt retention and liver damage with cholestatic
jaundice or rarely hepatocellular carcinoma. If there is no response in 4–6 months, androgens should be stopped. If there is
a response, the drug should be withdrawn gradually.

Bone marrow transplantation
General aspects are dealt with on p. 130. The usual donor is
an HLA (human leucocyte antigen)-matching sibling but, occasionally, an identical twin, another HLA-matching relative or
an HLA-matched unrelated donor have been used successfully.
For aplastic anaemia, it is usual to give cyclophosphamide
50 mg/kg/day on days 5, 4, 3 and 2 before the day of transplantation and to omit radiotherapy. Cyclosporin is also given to
reduce graft failure beginning the day before transplantation and
continued for 6 months. It also reduces the severity if not the
incidence of GVHD (graft-vs-host disease). Some units have used
radiation, e.g. total lymphoid, or *in vivo* anti-thymocyte globulin
to reduce the risk of graft failure especially in multiply transfused
patients.
    BMT is indicated in younger patients (<20 years) with severe
aplastic anaemia (neutrophils <0.2 × 10^9/l) and if infections
have occurred, when the mortality without BMT is >50% in
some series (see Fig. 7.4). The overall success rate is about
60–70% long-term survival. In older subjects and those with
less severe disease, immunosuppression is usually tried first,
keeping BMT in reserve for failures, recognizing that the blood
and platelet support care needed may increase the risks associated
with BMT. The main causes of failure are graft rejection, GVHD
and cytomegalovirus infection.

Red cell aplasia

Chronic form

This is a rare syndrome characterized by anaemia with normal

Table 7.3 Classification of pure red cell aplasia.

Acute, transient	Chronic	
	Congenital	Acquired
Parvovirus infection	Diamond–Blackfan	Idiopathic
Infancy and childhood		Associated with thymoma, lymphoma, chronic T- or B-cell lymphocytic leukaemia
Drugs e.g. diphenylhydrantoin, azathioprine, co-trimoxazole		

leucocytes and platelets and grossly reduced or absent erythroblasts from the marrow. It may be congenital (Diamond–Blackfan syndrome) with recessive inheritance (Table 7.3). The acquired chronic form may occur with no obvious associated disease or precipitating factor (idiopathic), or in association with autoimmune diseases (especially SLE), with a thymoma or lymphoma. In some cases immunosuppression with, for example, corticosteroids or cyclosporin, is helpful. Androgens may also produce improvement in the congenital anaemia but the long-term effects on growth are a serious side effect of the prolonged use of steroids or androgens in infancy and childhood. If regular blood transfusions are needed iron chelation therapy will also be necessary. BMT has been carried out in some severe cases and stem cell factor is undergoing trials.

Transient form

Parvovirus infects red cell precursors and causes a transient red cell aplasia with the rapid onset of severe anaemia in patients with pre-existing shortened red cell survival, e.g. sickle cell disease or hereditary spherocytosis. Transient red cell aplasia with anaemia may also occur in association with drug therapy, and in normal infants or children, often with a history of a viral infection in the preceding 3 months. Recovery is usually within 1–2 months. Serum- or cell-mediated inhibition of erythropoiesis has been detected in some of these patients. Parvovirus may be the cause in some but not all of these cases.

Congenital dyserythropoietic anaemia

Congenital dyserythropoietic anaemias (CDAs) are a group of hereditary refractory anaemias characterized by ineffective erythropoiesis and erythroid multinuclearity. The white cell and platelet counts are normal. There is an increase in serum indirect bilirubin and absence of haptoglobins but the reticulocyte count is low for the degree of anaemia, despite increased marrow cellularity. The anaemia is of variable severity and usually first noted in infancy or childhood. Iron overload may develop

because of increased absorption and from transfusions; splenomegaly is common. The CDAs have been classified into four
types based on the degree to which megaloblastic changes, giant
erythroblasts and dyserythropoietic changes are present. Type II
is known as HEMPAS because there is *h*ereditary *e*rythroblast
*m*ultinuclearity with a *p*ositive *a*cidified *s*erum lysis test. The
basic lesion is a genetic defect in an enzyme *N*-acetylgluco-
saminyltransferase, which is concerned in glycosylation of several
red cell membrane proteins.

Bone marrow transplantation (BMT)

BMT involves eliminating an individual's bone marrow stem
cells and all the cells derived from them including the haemopoietic, lymphoid and histiocytic/macrophage systems. These
are replaced with bone marrow stem cells either from another
individual or with a previously harvested portion of the individual's own bone marrow cells. This portion has been protected
outside the body from the chemotherapy and/or radiotherapy
used *in vivo* to eliminate the patient's marrow. BMT may be
syngeneic (from an identical twin), *allogeneic* (from an HLA-
matched brother or sister, or from an HLA-matching close relative other than a sibling, or from an unrelated but HLA-matching
individual) or *autologous* (from the patient's own marrow)
(Table 7.4).

The principle diseases for which BMT has been performed are
listed in Table 7.5. Allogeneic BMT is most frequently performed
for patients with the malignant diseases acute leukaemia or
chronic myeloid leukaemia, for aplastic anaemia and for certain
genetic diseases, e.g. thalassaemia major. Autologous BMT is
frequently used for treatment of malignant lymphoma but is also
used in selected patients with other solid tumours, with acute
myeloid or lymphoblastic leukaemia or with multiple myeloma.

HLA matching

The HLA antigens are highly polymorphic cell surface molecules
encoded by a series of closely linked genes on chromosome 6
(see Fig. 21.7). They are clustered in three regions, class I, class

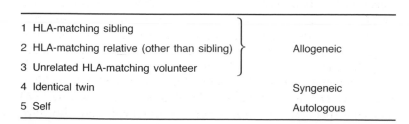

1 HLA-matching sibling	
2 HLA-matching relative (other than sibling)	Allogeneic
3 Unrelated HLA-matching volunteer	
4 Identical twin	Syngeneic
5 Self	Autologous

Table 7.4 Bone marrow transplantation: potential donors.

Table 7.5 Bone marrow transplantation: indications.

Allogeneic (or syngeneic)	Autologous
1 Severe aplastic anaemia	1 Malignant lymphoma usually post first relapse (Hodgkin's disease, non-Hodgkin's lymphoma)
2 Acute myeloid leukaemia	
3 Acute lymphoblastic leukaemia (usually in second remission or subsequently)	2 Other solid tumours, e.g. breast cancer
4 Chronic myeloid leukaemia	3 Acute leukaemia (in first or subsequent remission with or without 'purging of marrow')
5 Other malignant disorders of the marrow, e.g. myelodysplasia	4 Myeloma
6 Benign inherited disorders: thalassaemia major, severe combined immune deficiency, mucopolysaccharidoses, red cell aplasia, sickle cell anaemia, etc.	5 For 'gene therapy' of genetic disease, e.g. adenosine deaminase deficiency

II and class III. The class I genes encode the HLA-A, -B and -C antigens; and class II the HLA-D region (DR, DP and DQ genes). It is these class I and class II genes that function to restrict or direct T-cell responses. For BMT, matching of the class I and class II genes between recipient and donor is essential to prevent or reduce the allograft reactions of rejection and GVHD. The HLA specificities recognized by the World Health Organization (1992) are given in Appendix 1 (p. 416).

Class III antigens include various proteins, e.g. components of complement and tumour necrosis factor α and β, which are important in the immune system but not as major transplantation antigens. Beta$_2$-microglobulin is a non-polymorphic protein, encoded by chromosome 15 which binds non-covalently to class I molecules.

Identification of class I and class II antigens is usually performed by serological methods. Genetic differences in the class II HLA-D region molecules are the basis for proliferative responses in the mixed lymphocyte culture (MLC) assay. This is used for detecting possible differences in the HLA-D region between recipient and donor not detected by HLA-DR testing. Reaction of the donor's cells against recipient's cells suggests GVHD; recipient cell reaction against donor cells suggests graft rejection but this correlation is not established. HLA-DR, -DP and -DQ typing can also be carried out using molecular methods, e.g. restriction fragment length polymorphism analysis, employing oligonucleotide probes with polymerase chain reaction amplification.

The chance of a sibling being fully HLA matching with a patient with the same parents is theoretically 25% (Fig. 7.5) although because of cross-overs during meiosis, the true

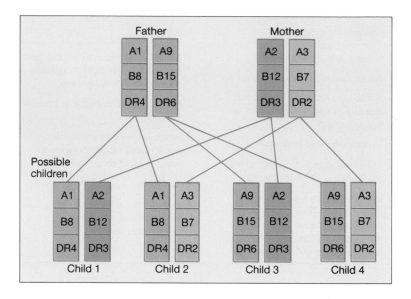

Fig. 7.5 An example of possible pattern inheritance of the A, B and DR series alleles of the HLA (human leucocyte antigen) complex.

incidence is slightly less. HLA matching is independent of sex or blood group. The chance of an unrelated potential donor matching is approximately 1:30 000, the incidence depending on the frequency of the patient's particular HLA types in the population from which the donor is selected.

The recipient

The patient is nursed in a protective environment with barrier nursing and is given high doses of chemotherapy with or without TBI in the days before the transplant (Fig. 7.6). This is aimed at eliminating the patient's bone marrow stem and progenitor cells and, if present, the bone marrow disease. Total body irradiation (TBI) is usually used in cases with malignant disease. It is administered as a single dose or in smaller doses over several days (fractionated). The 'conditioning' eliminates the patient's immune system and so reduces the risk (in allogeneic BMT) of failure of engraftment due to rejection of the donor stem cells by the recipient's immune cells. The drugs most commonly used are cyclophosphamide and busulphan but melphalan, cytosine arabinoside, etoposide or nitrosoureas are given in some protocols. Following the last dose of chemotherapy, at least 36 hours are allowed for the elimination of the drugs from the circulation before donor marrow cells are infused intravenously via an indwelling central venous catheter. The patient is given antiemetics and if high doses of cyclophosphamide are used, the drug mesna is given to reduce the risk of haemorrhagic cystitis caused by renal excretion of cyclophosphamide metabolites. Parenteral nutrition is usually needed and prophylactic oral antibiotics and antifungals are given.

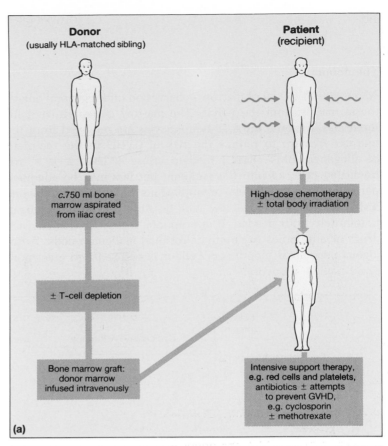

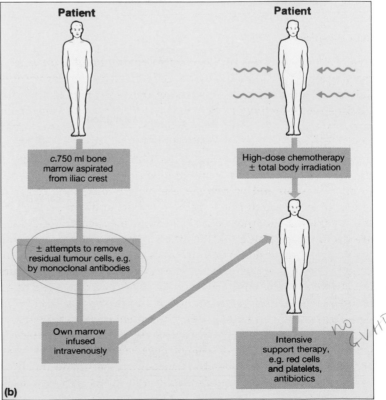

Fig. 7.6 Procedures for (a) allogeneic, and (b) autologous bone marrow transplantation.

The donor

About 500−1200 ml of marrow is harvested under general anaesthesia mainly from the pelvis. The marrow is heparinized, filtered and, in some units, T lymphocytes are removed from the
marrow *in vitro* to reduce the risk of GVHD in the recipient
of allogeneic BMT. It is hoped to infuse at least $2-4 \times 10^8$
nucleated cells/kg into the recipient but less may be adequate
particularly in syngeneic or autologous BMT. For autologous
BMT, the harvested marrow may be stored in liquid nitrogen
indefinitely until needed. If appropriate, it may be treated with
drugs or antibodies to eliminate residual malignant cells. Autologous peripheral blood stem cells may be used and give more
rapid platelet recovery.

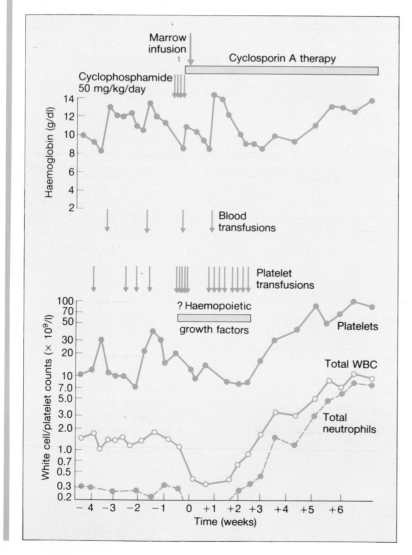

Fig. 7.7 Typical
haematological chart of a
patient undergoing allogeneic
marrow transplantation for
aplastic anaemia. WBC, white
blood cells.

Post-transplant course

After a period of about 2−3 weeks of severe pancytopenia, the first signs of successful engraftment are the appearance of monocytes followed by neutrophils in the blood with a subsequent increase in platelet count (Fig. 7.7). A reticulocytosis also begins in the second or third week and natural killer (NK) cells are among the earliest donor-derived cells to appear in the blood. The marrow cellularity gradually returns to normal but the marrow reserve remains impaired for 1−2 years. There is profound immune deficiency for 3−12 months. The immune system recovers slowly with a low level of CD4 helper and a raised CD8 : CD4 ratio for 6 months or more. Immune recovery is quicker after autologous and syngeneic BMT than following allogeneic BMT. Specific immunity can be enhanced post-BMT by immunizing both donor and recipient beforehand. The patient's blood group changes to that of the donor and antigen-specific immunity becomes that of the donor after about 60 days.

Complications (Table 7.6)

Infections

In the early post-transplant period bacterial or fungal infections are frequent. These may be reduced by reverse barrier nursing with laminar or positive pressure air flow, the use of skin and mouth antiseptics, oral antibiotics and antifungal therapy. If a fever or other evidence of an infection occurs, broad-spectrum i.v. antibiotics are commenced immediately after blood cultures and other appropriate microbiological specimens have been

Table 7.6 Complications of bone marrow transplantation.

Early (usually <100 days)	Late (usually >100 days)
Infections, especially bacterial, fungal, herpes simplex virus, CMV	Infections, especially varicella zoster, capsulate bacteria
Haemorrhage	Chronic GVHD (arthritis, malabsorption, hepatitis, scleroderma, sicca syndrome, lichen planus, pulmonary disease, serous effusions)
Acute GVHD (skin, liver, gut)	
Graft failure, especially aplastic anaemia	Chronic pulmonary disease
Haemorrhagic cystitis	Autoimmune disorders
Interstitial pneumonitis	Cataract
Others: veno-occlusive disease, cardiac failure	Infertility
	Second malignancies

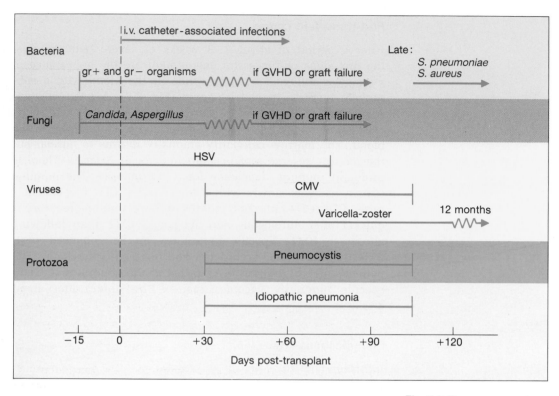

Fig. 7.8 Time sequence for development of different types of infection following allogeneic bone marrow transplantation. CMV, cytomegalovirus; gr+, gr−, Gram-positive or -negative; GVHD, graft-vs-host disease; HSV, herpes simplex virus.

taken. Failure of response to antibacterial agents is usually an indication to commence systemic antifungal therapy with amphotericin B. *Candida* species are the most frequent fungi involved. Viral infections, particularly with the herpes group of viruses, are frequent, with herpes simplex, cytomegalovirus (CMV) and varicella-zoster occurring at different peak intervals (Fig. 7.8).

Cytomegalovirus presents a particular threat since it is associated with a potentially fatal interstitial pneumonitis as well as with hepatitis and falling blood counts. The infection may be due to reactivation of CMV in the recipient or a new infection transmitted by the donor or by blood products. In CMV seronegative patients with CMV seronegative donors, CMV-negative blood products are given. CMV pneumonitis is particularly associated with GVHD and is rare in syngeneic or autologous BMT. The drug ganciclovir and CMV-immune globulin have been used in combination as therapy for established CMV infections. Ganciclovir may be useful prophylactically in reducing the incidence of CMV infection but is myelotoxic. Acyclovir has also been shown to be partly effective.

Pneumocystis carinii is another cause of pneumonitis; it may be prevented by prophylactic co-trimoxazole but if it does occur, treatment with co-trimoxazole in high doses is commenced with

additional benefit from corticosteroids. Varicella-zoster virus
(VZV) infection is also frequent post-BMT but occurs later with
a median onset at 4−5 months. Rarely disseminated VZV infection occurs. Intravenous acyclovir is indicated. Epstein−Barr
virus (EBV) infections are less frequent after BMT than after
solid organ transplants.

Haemopoietic growth factors especially GM-CSF, G-CSF and
IL-3 are now being used to accelerate recovery of haemopoiesis
and possibly enhance neutrophil and macrophage function post-
BMT. Immunoglobulin concentrates may also be given intravenously to reduce the consequences of post-transplant immune
deficiency.

Haemorrhage

Platelet concentrates are given to prevent haemorrhage until the
patient's platelet production is sufficient to maintain a count of
$20 \times 10^9/l$ or more. Platelets and blood transfusions given in the
post-transplant period are irradiated to kill lymphocytes which
possibly might cause GVHD. Trials of IL-3 therapy are in progress
to determine whether this will accelerate platelet recovery.

Graft-vs-host disease

This is caused by donor-derived immune cells, particularly T
lymphocytes, reacting against recipient tissues. It may occur
even when the MLC reaction between recipient and donor is
negative. Its incidence is increased with increasing age of donor
and recipient and if there is any degree of HLA mismatch between them. In acute GVHD, occurring in the first 100 days,
the skin, gastrointestinal tract or liver are affected (Table 7.7).
The skin rash typically affects the face, palms, soles and ears
but may in severe cases affect the whole body (Fig. 7.9). The
diagnosis is usually confirmed by skin biopsy which shows
initially single cell necrosis in the basal layer of the epidermis;
lymphocyte infiltration may be scanty. Typically the bilirubin
and alkaline phosphatase are raised but the other hepatic enzymes
are relatively normal.

Table 7.7 Acute graft-vs-host disease: clinical staging (Seattle system).

Stage	Skin	Liver (bilirubin mmol/l)	Gut (diarrhoea, l/day)
I	Rash <25%	20−35	0.5−1.0
II	Rash 25−50%	35−80	1.0−1.5
III	Erythroderma	80−150	1.5−2.5
IV	Bullae, desquamation	>150	>2.5 Severe pain, ileus

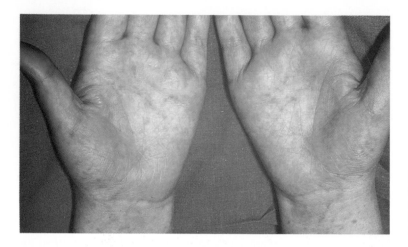

Fig. 7.9 Widespread erythematous skin rash in acute graft-vs-host disease following bone marrow transplantation.

In chronic GVHD, occurring after 100 days and usually evolving from acute GVHD, these tissues are involved but also the joints and other serosal surfaces, the oral mucosa and lacrimal glands. Features of scleroderma, Sjögren's syndrome and lichen planus may develop. The immune system is impaired (including hyposplenism) with risk of infection. Malabsorption and pulmonary abnormalities are frequent.

GVHD may be ameliorated or prevented by immunosuppressive drugs particularly cyclosporin and/or methotrexate and corticosteroids or by removing T lymphocytes from the donor marrow, e.g. with anti-T-cell monoclonal antibodies or by physical means. If GVHD does develop, it is usually treated with corticosteroids or ALG. Thalidomide and anti-T-cell monoclonal antibodies have also been tried.

Interstitial pneumonitis
This is one of the most frequent causes of death post-BMT (Fig. 7.10). CMV is a frequent agent but other herpes viruses and *Pneumocystis carinii* account for other cases; in many, no cause other than the previous radiation and chemotherapy can be implicated. Broncho-alveolar lavage or open lung biopsy may be needed to establish the diagnosis.

Graft failure
The risk of this is increased if the patient has aplastic anaemia or if T-cell depletion is used on donor marrow without compensation in the conditioning. This suggests that T cells are needed to overcome host resistance to engraftment of stem cells.

Haemorrhagic cystitis
This is usually due to the cyclophosphamide metabolite acrolein.

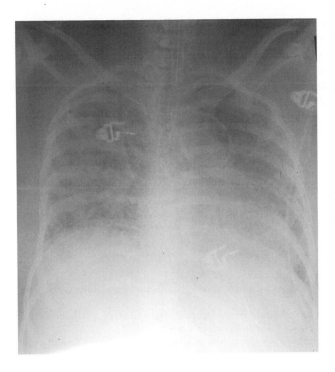

Fig. 7.10 Chest radiograph showing interstitial pneumonitis following bone marrow transplantation. Widespread diffuse mottling can be seen. The patient had received total body irradiation and had grade III graft-vs-host disease. No infective cause of the pneumonitis was identified. Possible causes include pneumocystis, cytomegalovirus, herpes, fungal infection, or a combination of these.

Mesna is given in an attempt to prevent this. Certain viruses, e.g. adeno or polyoma may also cause this complication.

Less frequent complications
These include veno-occlusive disease of the liver and cardiac failure due to the effect of the conditioning regimen (especially high doses of cyclophosphamide) and previous chemotherapy on the heart. Haemolysis due to ABO incompatibility between donor and recipient may cause problems in the first weeks.

Late complications
Relapse of the original disease, e.g. acute or chronic leukaemia, may occur; chronic GVHD, however, is associated with a reduction in leukaemic relapse. There are many other problems which may occur after the first 3 months, usually in patients with chronic GVHD. Infections are frequent, especially with Gram-negative or encapsulated organisms affecting the respiratory tract. The patients are functionally hyposplenic and penicillin prophylaxis is used. Varicella zoster and fungal infections are also frequent. The use of prophylactic co-trimoxazole and oral acyclovir for 3−6 months reduces the risk of pneumocystis and herpes infections respectively.

Delayed pulmonary complications include restrictive pneumonitis and bronchiolitis obliterans. Endocrine complications include hypothyroidism, growth failure with low growth

hormone levels in children, impaired sexual development and
infertility. These endocrine problems are more marked if TBI
has been used. Clinically apparent autoimmune disorders
are infrequent and include myasthenia, rheumatoid arthritis,
anaemia, thrombocytopenia or neutropenia. Autoantibodies are
frequently detected in the absence of symptoms. Second malignancies (especially non-Hodgkin's lymphoma) occur with a six
or sevenfold incidence compared with controls.

Other late complications include CNS disturbances, neuropathies and eye problems due to chronic GVHD (sicca syndrome)
or cataracts, radiation nephritis, and late bladder problems due
to previous haemorrhagic cystitis.

Bibliography

Burakoff S.J., Deeg H.J., Ferrara J. & Atkinson K. (1990) *Graft-vs-Host Disease*.
Marcel Dekker, New York.
Champlin R. (ed.) (1990) *Bone Marrow Transplantation*. Kluver Academic
Publishers, Boston.
Forman S.J. (ed.) (1990) Bone marrow transplantation. *Hematology/
Oncology Clinics of North America*, **4**, 507–710.
Frickhofen N., Kaltwasser J.P., Schrezenmeier H. *et al.* (1992) Treatment of
aplastic anemia with antilymphocyte globulin and methylprednisolone
with or without cyclosporine. (The German Aplastic Anemia Study
Group.) *New England Journal of Medicine*, **324**, 1358–1360.
Gordon-Smith E.C. (ed.) (1989) Aplastic anaemia. *Clinical Haematology*, **2**,
1–190.
Gordon-Smith E.C. & Rutherford T.R. (1991) Fanconi anaemia: constitutional
aplastic anemia. *Seminars in Hematology*, **28**, 104–112.
Prentice H.G., Kibbler C.C. & McWhinney P. (1992) Antimicrobial prophylaxis
and treatment after chemotherapy or marrow transplantation. In *Recent
Advances in Haematology*, Vol. 6 (eds A.V. Hoffbrand & M.K. Brenner).
Churchill Livingstone, Edinburgh, pp. 173–194.
Shahidi N.T. (1990) *Aplastic Anemia and Other Bone Marrow Failure
Syndromes*. Springer Verlag, Berlin.
Treleaven J. & Barrett J. (eds) (1992) *Bone Marrow Transplantation in
Practice*. Churchill Livingstone, Edinburgh.

Chapter 8
The White Cells 1: Granulocytes, Monocytes and their Benign Disorders

The white blood cells (leucocytes) may be divided into two broad groups—the phagocytes and the immunocytes. Granulocytes, which include three types of cell: neutrophils (polymorphs), eosinophils and basophils; together with monocytes comprise the phagocytes. Their normal development, function and benign disorders are dealt with in this chapter. Normally only mature phagocytic cells and lymphocytes are found in the peripheral blood (Table 8.1, Fig. 8.1). The lymphocytes, their precursor cells and plasma cells, which make up the immunocyte population, are considered in Chapter 9.

The function of phagocytes and immunocytes in protecting the body against infection is closely connected with two soluble protein systems of the body, immunoglobulins and complement. These proteins, which may also be involved in blood cell destruction in a number of diseases, are discussed together with the lymphocytes in Chapter 9.

Granulocytes

Neutrophil appearance

Neutrophil (polymorph)

This cell has a characteristic dense nucleus consisting of between two and five lobes and a pale cytoplasm with an irregular outline and containing many fine pink-blue (azurophilic) or grey-blue granules (Fig. 8.1a). The granules are divided into primary, which appear at the promyelocyte stage, and secondary (specific) which appear at the myelocyte stage and predominate in the mature neutrophil. Both types of granule are lysosomal in origin; the primary contains myeloperoxidase, acid phosphatase and other acid hydrolases, the secondary contains collagenase, lactoferrin and lysozyme (see Fig. 8.6). The lifespan of neutrophils in the blood is only about 10 hours.

Neutrophil precursors

These do not normally appear in normal peripheral blood but are present in the marrow (Fig. 8.2). The earliest recognizable

Table 8.1 White cells: normal blood counts.

Adults	Blood count	Children	Blood count
Total leucocytes	$4.00-11.0 \times 10^9/l$*	*Total leucocytes*	
Neutrophils	$2.50-7.5 \times 10^9/l$*	Neonates	$10.0-25.0 \times 10^9/l$
Eosinophils	$0.04-0.4 \times 10^9/l$	1 year	$6.0-18.0 \times 10^9/l$
Monocytes	$0.20-0.8 \times 10^9/l$	4$-$7 years	$6.0-15.0 \times 10^9/l$
Basophils	$0.01-0.1 \times 10^9/l$	8$-$12 years	$4.5-13.5 \times 10^9/l$
Lymphocytes	$1.50-3.5 \times 10^9/l$		

* Normal Black and Middle Eastern subjects may have lower counts due to an increased proportion of marginating neutrophils.

precursor is the myeloblast, a cell of variable size which has a large nucleus with fine chromatin and usually 2$-$5 nucleoli. The cytoplasm is basophilic and no cytoplasmic granules are present. The normal bone marrow contains up to 4% of myeloblasts. Myeloblasts give rise by cell division to promyelocytes which are slightly larger cells and have developed primary granules in the cytoplasm. These cells then produce myelocytes which have specific or secondary granules. The nuclear chromatin is now more condensed and nucleoli are not visible. Separate

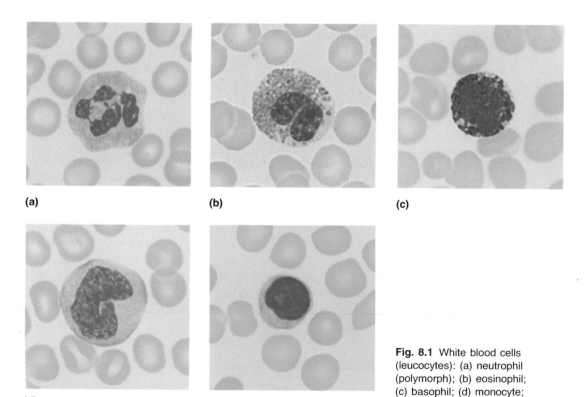

(a)   (b)   (c)

(d)   (e)

Fig. 8.1 White blood cells (leucocytes): (a) neutrophil (polymorph); (b) eosinophil; (c) basophil; (d) monocyte; (e) lymphocyte.

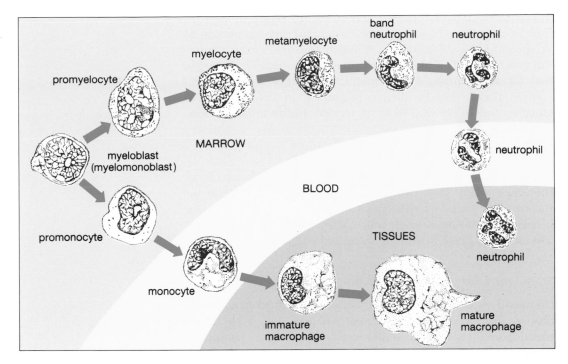

Fig. 8.2 The formation of the neutrophil and monocyte phagocytes. Eosinophils and basophils are also formed in the marrow in a process similar to that for neutrophils.

myelocytes of the neutrophil, eosinophil and basophil series can be indentified. The myelocytes give rise by cell division to metamyelocytes, non-dividing cells, which have an indented or horseshoe-shaped nucleus and a cytoplasm filled with primary and secondary granules. Neutrophil forms between the metamyelocyte and fully mature neutrophil are termed 'band', 'stab' or 'juvenile'. These cells may occur in normal peripheral blood. They do not contain the clear fine filamentous distinction between nuclear lobes which is seen in mature neutrophils.

Monocytes

These are usually larger than other peripheral blood leucocytes and possess a large central oval or indented nucleus with clumped chromatin (see Fig. 8.1d). The abundant cytoplasm stains blue and contains many fine vacuoles, giving a ground-glass appearance. Cytoplasmic granules are also often present. The monocyte precursors in the marrow (monoblasts and promonocytes) are difficult to distinguish from myeloblasts and monocytes.

Eosinophils

These cells are similar to neutrophils, except that the cytoplasmic granules are coarser and more deeply red staining (since they contain a basic protein) and there are rarely more than three nuclear lobes (see Fig. 8.1b). Eosinophil myelocytes can be recognized but earlier stages are indistinguishable from neutrophil precursors. The blood transit time for eosinophils is longer than for neutrophils. They enter inflammatory exudates and have a special role in allergic responses, in defence against parasites and in removal of fibrin formed during inflammation.

Basophils

These are only occasionally seen in normal peripheral blood. They have many dark cytoplasmic granules which overlie the nucleus and contain heparin and histamine (Fig. 8.1c). In the tissues they become mast cells. They have IgE attachment sites and their degranulation is associated with histamine release.

Granulocyte formation and kinetics

The blood granulocytes and monocytes are formed in the bone marrow from a common precursor cell (see Fig. 1.2). In the granulopoietic series progenitor cells, myeloblasts, promyelocytes and myelocytes form a proliferative or mitotic pool of cells while the metamyelocytes, band and segmented granulocytes make up a post-mitotic maturation compartment (Fig. 8.3). Large numbers of band and segmented neutrophils are held in the marrow as a 'reserve pool' or storage compartment. The bone marrow normally contains more myeloid cells than erythroid cells in the ratio of 2:1 to 12:1, the largest proportion being neutrophils and metamyelocytes. In the stable or normal state, the bone marrow storage compartment contains 10−15 times the number of granulocytes found in the peripheral blood. Following their release from the bone marrow, granulocytes spend 6−10 hours in the circulation before moving into the tissues where they perform their phagocytic function. In the bloodstream there are two pools usually of about equal size—the circulating pool (included in the blood count) and the marginating pool (not included in the blood count). It has been estimated that they spend on average 4−5 days in the tissues before they are destroyed during defensive action or as the result of senescence.

Control of granulopoiesis: myeloid growth factors

The granulocyte series arises from bone marrow progenitor cells which are increasingly specialized (see p. 1). Mixed myeloid precursors CFU_{GEMM} (see p. 2) arise from the pluripotential stem cells under the influence of growth factors IL (interleukin)-1, IL-3 and IL-6 which act synergistically and give rise to cells increasingly committed to red cell, neutrophil, eosinophil,

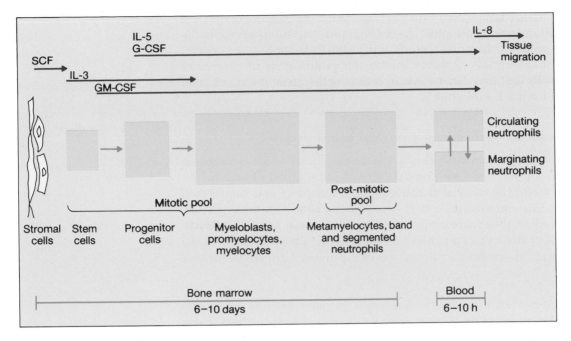

Fig. 8.3 Neutrophil kinetics. CSF, colony-stimulating factor; G, granulocyte; IL, interleukin; M, monocyte; SCF, stem cell factor.

basophil, monocyte or platelet production (Chapter 1). IL-1 has multiple actions concerned with the inflammatory response (see Fig. 8.7). GM-CSF increases commitment to granulocyte and monocyte production, G-CSF to neutrophils, IL-5 to eosinophils and M-CSF to monocytes (see Fig. 1.2). The growth factors not only stimulate proliferation of increasingly committed marrow precursors but also stimulate differentiation and affect the function of the mature cells on which they act (e.g. phagocytosis, superoxide generation and cytotoxicity in the case of neutrophils; phagocytosis, cytotoxicity and production of other cytokines by monocytes). They also affect the membrane integrity and surface adhesion properties of their target cells. GM-CSF tends to immobilize phagocytes causing their accumulation at local sites of inflammation.

The growth factors arise from stromal cells (endothelial cells, fibroblasts and macrophages) and from T lymphocytes and are responsible for basal production of phagocytes. Increased granulocyte and monocyte production in response to an infection is induced by increased production of growth factors from stromal cells and T lymphocytes, stimulated by endotoxin, IL-1 or tumour necrosis factor (TNF) (see Fig. 1.5). When there is an increase in their production, growth factors not normally found in plasma (e.g. GM-CSF) may appear there, e.g. during infection or during haemopoietic recovery following cytotoxic drug or radiation damage to the haemopoietic cells.

Other factors may play a role in controlling granulopoiesis. IL-8 stimulates neutrophil chemotaxis and migration across endo-thelial membranes. Transforming growth factor-β and a macro-phage inhibitory factor inhibit the proliferation of progenitor cells and may have a role in reversing the response to infection ('feedback inhibition').

Clinical applications of myeloid growth factors

Clinical administration of G-CSF intravenously or subcutaneously has been found to produce a rise of neutrophils, administration of GM-CSF a rise of neutrophils, eosinophils and monocytes, while administration of IL-3 produces a response similar to GM-CSF but the increase in granulocytes and monocytes is delayed; IL-3 also causes a rise in reticulocytes and platelets. Some of the indications for the clinical use of the myeloid growth factors are as follows.

Post-chemotherapy, radiotherapy or bone marrow transplan-tation. GM-CSF, G-CSF (Fig. 8.4) and IL-3 have been given to accelerate haemopoietic recovery, shortening the period of neutropenia, reducing the length of time in hospital, the need for antibiotics and the number of infections; hopefully, IL-3 will reduce platelet requirements and bleeding. It is expected, but not proven, that these effects will translate into an overall increase in patient survival and will enable more intensified chemo-therapy to be administered safely.

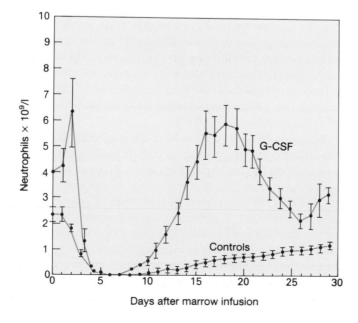

Fig. 8.4 Effect of G-CSF on recovery of neutrophils following autologous bone marrow transplantation (from Sheridan *et al.*, 1989).

AIDS. The myeloid growth factors may be given to improve granulocyte and monocyte numbers and function and reduce marrow toxicity of antiviral, antimicrobial and anti tumour therapy.

Myelodysplasia. GM-CSF and IL-3 have been given alone or in conjunction with chemotherapy in an attempt to improve bone marrow function, hopefully without accelerating leukaemic transformation.

Acute leukaemia. Trials are taking place of growth factors given immediately before, simultaneously with, or after chemo-therapy in an attempt to improve the killing of leukaemic cells by cytotoxics and to accelerate normal haemopoietic recovery. Uncontrolled acceleration of leukaemic cell proliferation must be avoided.

Aplastic anaemia. It is hoped that early acting factors (e.g. IL-3 or stem cell factor) with later acting factors (e.g. GM-CSF) may be of value but this has not been proven. GM-CSF although temporarily reducing neutropenia has not been found to have a long-term effect on neutrophil counts since these fall once GM-CSF therapy is discontinued.

Severe neutropenia. Both congenital and acquired neutropenia including cyclical and drug-induced neutropenia have been found to respond best to G-CSF.

Severe infection. GM-CSF and G-CSF have been used as adjuvants to antimicrobial therapy.

Peripheral blood stem cell transplants. GM-CSF or G-CSF increase the number of circulating multipotent progenitors, improving the harvest of sufficient peripheral blood stem cells for autotransplantation.

Phagocytic surface receptors

Three groups of receptors (adhesion molecules, receptors for immunoglobulin and complement components, and human leucocyte associated (HLA) antigens) occur on the surface of phagocytes.

Adhesion molecules

A large family of glycoprotein molecules termed adhesion molecules mediate the attachment of marrow precursors, leucocytes and platelets to various components of the extracellular matrix, to endothelium, to other surfaces and to each other. The adhesion

molecules on the surface of leucocytes are termed receptors
and these interact with molecules (termed ligands) on the surface
of potential target cells. Three main families exist.

1 *Immunoglobulin superfamily*. This includes receptors which
react with antigens (the T-cell receptors and the immunoglobulins) and antigen-independent surface adhesion molecules, e.g.
receptors for certain growth factors, e.g. c-*KIT* (the stem cell
factor receptor) and c-*FMS* (the M-CSF receptor) (see Chapter 1).

2 *Selectins*. These are mainly involved in leucocyte and platelet
adhesion to endothelium during inflammation and coagulation.

3 *Integrins*. These include three main subfamilies:

(a) *very late activation (VLA) antigens* which are involved in
cell adhesion to extracellular matrix, e.g. to collagen in wound
healing;

(b) *leucocyte cell adhesion molecules* (Leu-CAMs) which are
mainly involved in immune adherence; and

(c) *cytoadhesins*, e.g. platelet GPIIb/IIIa which are mainly
involved in platelet−vessel wall interaction.

The adhesion molecules are thus important in the development and maintainance of inflammatory and immune responses,
and in platelet−vessel wall and leucocyte−vessel wall interactions. Expression of adhesion molecules can be modified
by extracellular and intracellular factors and this alteration
of expression may be quantitative or functional. IL-1, TNF, γ-
interferon, T-cell activation, adhesion to extracellular proteins,
and viral infection may all up-regulate expression of these
molecules.

The pattern of expression of adhesion molecules on tumour
cells may determine their mode of spread and tissue localization,
e.g. the pattern of metastasis of carcinoma cells or of non-
Hodgkin's lymphoma cells into a follicular or diffuse pattern.
The adhesion molecules may also determine whether or not
cells circulate in the bloodstream or remain fixed in tissues.
They may also partly determine whether or not tumour cells are
susceptible to the body's defences, e.g. NK (natural killer) cell
activity. For example, infectious mononucleosis cells, which are
susceptible to NK activity, express adhesion molecules but these
molecules are absent from the surface of Burkitt lymphoma cells
which escape from immune destruction.

Fc and C3b receptors

Both monocytes and neutrophils have receptors on their surfaces
for the Fc portion of IgG (p. 167) and the C3b component
of complement (p. 172). These strengthen the binding of
the phagocytes to particles, whether bacteria or cellular
components, coated with IgG or C3. This results in activation of
phagocytosis.

Leucocyte antigens: HLA antigens, antigens recognized by cluster differentiation (CD) antibodies and neutrophil-specific antigens

Leucocytes exhibit two polymorphic sets of antigens (HLA class I and class II) coded for by the major histocompatibility complex (MHC) located on the short arm of chromosome 6 (see p. 411). Human leucocytes also carry surface antigens that are specific to certain subtypes but may also occur on non-haemopoeitic tissues. Monoclonal antibodies (termed cluster differentiation or CD) have been raised to these antigens and may be used to identify subgroups of normal and malignant haemopoietic cell populations, e.g. CD4 and CD8 T-lymphocyte subpopulations (see Appendix 2, p. 417, for full list). Neutrophils also express a number of specific antigens which may be the target for allo- or autoantibodies and have been termed NA, NB, etc.

Monocytes

Formation and kinetics

Monocytes spend only a short time in the marrow and, after circulating for 20–40 hours, leave the blood to enter the tissues where they mature and carry out their principle functions. Their extravascular lifespan after their transformation to macrophages may be as long as several months or even years. They may assume specific functions in different tissues, e.g. skin, gut, liver, etc. (Fig. 8.5). GM-CSF and M-CSF are involved in their production and activation.

Neutrophil and monocyte function

The normal function of neutrophils and monocytes may be divided into three phases.

Chemotaxis (cell mobilization and migration). The phagocyte is attracted to bacteria or the site of inflammation by chemotactic substances released from damaged tissues or by complement components and also by the interaction of leucocyte adhesion molecules with ligands on the damaged tissues.

Phagocytosis. The foreign material (bacteria, fungi, etc.) or dead or damaged cells of the host are phagocytosed (Fig. 8.6). Recognition of a foreign particle is aided by opsonization with immunoglobulin or complement since both neutrophils and monocytes have Fc and C3b receptors. Opsonization of normal body cells (e.g. red cells or platelets) also makes them liable to destruction by macrophages of the reticuloendothelial system,

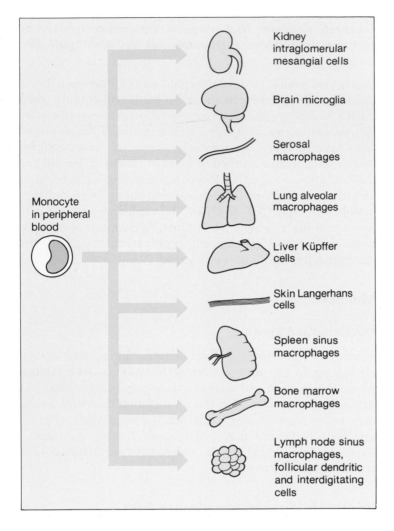

Kidney intraglomerular mesangial cells

Brain microglia

Serosal macrophages

Lung alveolar macrophages

Liver Küpffer cells

Skin Langerhans cells

Spleen sinus macrophages

Bone marrow macrophages

Lymph node sinus macrophages, follicular dendritic and interdigitating cells

Monocyte in peripheral blood

Fig. 8.5 Reticuloendothelial system: distribution of macrophages.

as in autoimmune haemolysis, idiopathic (autoimmune) thrombocytopenic purpura or many of the drug-induced cytopenias.

Macrophages also have a role in presenting foreign antigens to the immune system (see p. 164) and secrete a large number of growth factors (IL-1, TNF, IL-3, GM-CSF, G-CSF, M-CSF, IL-4 and IL-6). IL-1 has many biological effects in recruitment and activation of cells involved in the inflammatory response, in wound healing, in the immune response and in the early phases of haemopoiesis (see Fig. 8.7). IL-6 also has actions on a wide variety of haemopoietic and non-haemopoietic tissues.

Killing and digestion. This occurs by oxygen-dependent and oxygen-independent pathways (Fig. 8.6). In the oxygen-depen-

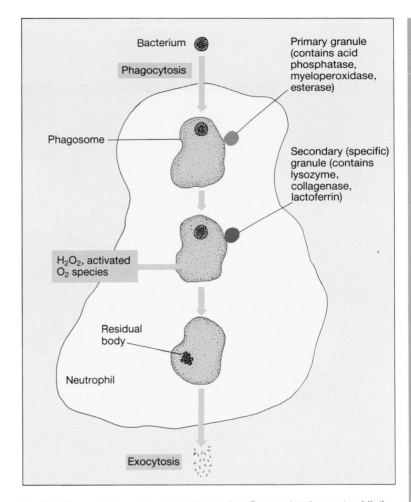

Fig. 8.6 Phagocytosis and bacterial destruction. On entering the neutrophil, the bacterium is surrounded by an invaginated surface membrane and fuses with a primary lysosome to form a phagosome. Enzymes from the lysosome attack the bacterium. Secondary granules also fuse with the phagosomes, and new enzymes from these granules and lactoferrin attack the organism. Various types of activated oxygen, generated by glucose metabolism, also help to kill bacteria. Undigested residual bacterial products are excreted by exocytosis.

dent reactions, superoxide (O_2^-), hydrogen peroxide (H_2O_2) and other activated oxygen (O_2) species, are generated from O_2 and NADPH. In neutrophils, H_2O_2 reacts with myeloperoxidase and intracellular halide to kill bacteria; activated oxygen may also be involved. The non-oxidative microbicidal mechanism involves a fall in pH within phagocytic vacuoles into which lysosomal enzymes are released. An additional factor, lactoferrin — an iron-binding protein present in neutrophil granules — is bacteriostatic by depriving bacteria of iron.

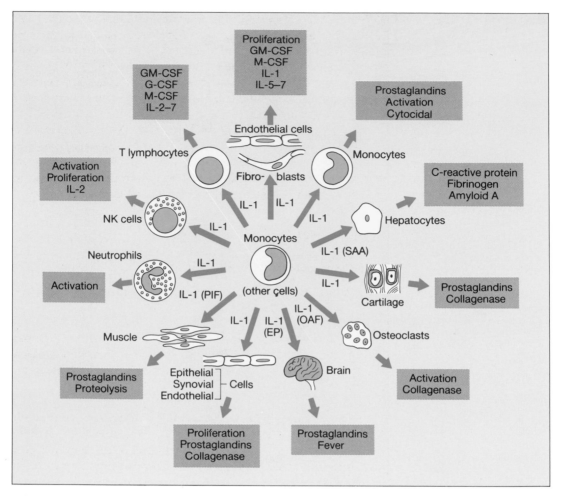

Fig. 8.7 Some of the effects of interleukin (IL)-1 on target cells and tissues. (From Oppenheim *et al.*, 1986.) CSF, colony-stimulating factor; EP, endogenous pyrogen; G, granulocyte; M, monocyte; NK, natural killer; OAF, osteoclast-activating factor (this may be TNFα, induced by IL-1); PIF, proteolysis-inducing factor; SAA, serum amyloid A.

Defects of phagocytic cell function

Chemotaxis. These defects occur in rare congenital abnormalities (e.g. 'lazy leucocyte' syndrome, complement abnormalities) and in more common acquired abnormalities either of the environment, e.g. corticosteroid therapy, hypophosphataemia, aspirin, alcohol, high plasma osmolarity (as in diabetes), or of the leucocytes themselves, e.g. in acute or chronic myeloid leukaemia, myelodysplasia and the myeloproliferative syndromes.

Phagocytosis. These defects usually arise because of a lack of opsonization which may be due to congenital or acquired causes of hypogammaglobulinaemia, to lack of complement components or to a lack of a serum factor which stimulates phagocytosis ('tufsin') following splenectomy or splenic infarction, e.g. in sickle cell disease.

Killing. This abnormality is clearly illustrated by the rare X-linked or autosomal recessive chronic granulomatous disease which results from abnormal leucocyte oxidative metabolism. There is an abnormality affecting different elements of the respiratory burst oxidase or its activating mechanism. The patients have recurring infections, usually bacterial but sometimes fungal, which present in infancy or early childhood in most cases.

Other rare congenital abnormalities may also result in defects of bacterial killing, e.g. myeloperoxidase deficiency and the Chédiak–Higashi syndrome (see below). Acute or chronic myeloid leukaemia and myelodysplastic syndromes may also be associated with defective killing of ingested microorganisms.

Benign disorders

Variations in neutrophil morphology

A number of the hereditary conditions may give rise to changes in granulocyte morphology.

Pelger–Huët anomaly. In this uncommon condition bilobed neutrophils are found in the peripheral blood. Occasional unsegmented neutrophils are also seen. Inheritance is autosomal dominant.

May–Hegglin anomaly. In this rare condition the neutrophils contain basophilic inclusions of RNA (resembling Döhle bodies) in the cytoplasm. There is an associated mild thrombocytopenia with giant platelets. Inheritance is autosomal dominant.

Alder's (Alder–Reilly) anomaly. In this rare anomaly deep purple granules are found in granulocytes, monocytes and lymphocytes. Inheritance is autosomal recessive.

Other rare disorders. In contrast to these three relatively benign anomalies which are not associated with major clinical problems, other rare congenital leucocyte disorders may be associated with severe disease. The Chédiak–Higashi syndrome is inherited in an autosomal recessive manner, there are giant granules in neutrophils, eosinophils, monocytes and lymphocytes accompanied by neutropenia, thrombocytopenia, marked hepatosplenomegaly and often partial albinism. Affected children usually die from infection or haemorrhage. Abnormal leucocyte granulation or vacuolation is also seen in patients with rare mucopolysaccharide disorders, e.g. Hurler's syndrome.

Common morphological abnormalities. Figure 8.8 shows some of the more common abnormalities of neutrophil morphology

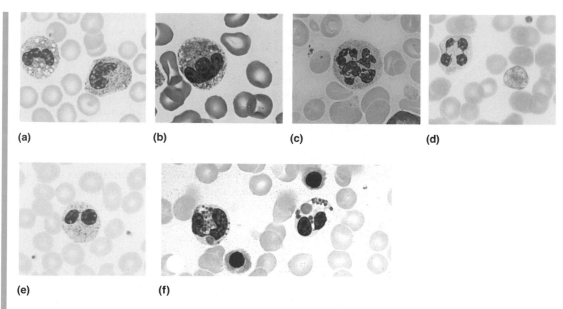

(a)   (b)   (c)   (d)

(e)   (f)

Fig. 8.8 Abnormal white blood cells. (a) Neutrophil leucocytosis: toxic changes shown by the presence of red-purple granules in the band-form neutrophils. (b) Neutrophil leucocytosis: a Döhle body can be seen in the cytoplasm of the neutrophil. (c) Megaloblastic anaemia: hypersegmented oversized neutrophil in peripheral blood. (d) May–Hegglin anomaly: the neutrophils contain basophilic inclusions 2–5 μm in diameter; there is an associated mild thrombocytopenia with giant platelets. (e) Pelger–Huët anomaly: coarse clumping of the chromatin in pince-nez configurations. (f) Chédiak–Higashi syndrome: bizarre giant granules in the cytoplasm of neutrophils.

which can be seen in the peripheral blood. Hypersegmented forms occur in megaloblastic anaemia, Döhle bodies and toxic changes in infection. The 'drumstick' appears on the nucleus of a proportion of the neutrophils in normal females and is due to the presence of two X chromosomes. Pelger cells are seen in the benign congenital abnormality but also in patients with acute myeloid leukaemia or myelodysplasia.

Neutrophil leucocytosis

An increase in circulating neutrophils to levels greater than $7.5 \times 10^9/l$ is one of the most frequently observed blood count changes. The causes of neutrophil leucocytosis are given in Table 8.2. Neutrophil leucocytosis is sometimes accompanied by fever due to the release of leucocyte pyrogens. Other characteristic features of reactive neutrophilia (Table 8.2, 1–5) include: (a) a 'shift to the left' in the peripheral blood differential white cell count, i.e. an increase in the number of band forms and the occasional presence of more primitive cells such as metamyelocytes and myelocytes; (b) the presence of cytoplasmic toxic granulation and Döhle bodies (Fig. 8.8a, b); and (c) an elevated neutrophil alkaline phosphatase score. For this the strength of the staining of each of 100 neutrophils is scored between 0 and 4. The maximum score is therefore 400; a normal score is between 20 and 100.

The leukaemoid reaction

The leukaemoid reaction is a reactive and excessive leucocytosis usually characterized by the presence of immature cells (e.g. myeloblasts, promyelocytes and myelocytes) in the peripheral blood. Occasionally lymphocytic reactions occur. Associated disorders include severe or chronic infections, severe haemolysis or metastatic cancer. Leukaemoid reactions are often particularly marked in children. Granulocyte changes such as toxic granulation and Döhle bodies and a high neutrophil alkaline phosphatase score help to differentiate the leukaemoid reaction from chronic myeloid leukaemia. The presence of a large proportion of myelocytes, a low neutrophil alkaline phosphatase score and the Philadelphia chromosome help to confirm chronic myeloid leukaemia.

Eosinophilic leucocytosis (eosinophilia)

The causes of an increase in blood eosinophils above $0.4 \times 10^9/l$ are listed in Table 8.3.

Basophil leucocytosis (basophilia)

An increase in blood basophils above $0.1 \times 10^9/l$ is uncommon. The usual cause is a myeloproliferative disorder such as chronic myeloid leukaemia or polycythaemia vera. Reactive basophil increases are sometimes seen in myxoedema, during smallpox or chickenpox infection, and in ulcerative colitis.

Table 8.2 Causes of neutrophil leucocytosis.

1 Bacterial infections (especially pyogenic bacterial, localized or generalized)
2 Inflammation and tissue necrosis, e.g. myositis, vasculitis, cardiac infarct, trauma
3 Metabolic disorders, e.g. uraemia, eclampsia, acidosis, gout
4 Neoplasms of all types, e.g. carcinoma, lymphoma, melanoma
5 Acute haemorrhage or haemolysis
6 Corticosteroid therapy (inhibits margination)
7 Myeloproliferative disease, e.g. chronic myeloid leukaemia, polycythaemia vera, myelosclerosis
8 Treatment with myeloid growth factors, e.g. G-CSF, GM-CSF

Table 8.3 Causes of eosinophilia.

1 Allergic diseases, especially hypersensitivity of the atopic type, e.g. bronchial asthma, hay fever, urticaria and food sensitivity
2 Parasitic diseases, e.g. amoebiasis, hookworm, ascariasis, tapeworm infestation, filariasis, schistosomiasis and trichinosis
3 Recovery from acute infection
4 Certain skin diseases, e.g. psoriasis, pemphigus and dermatitis herpetiformis
5 Pulmonary eosinophilia and the hypereosinophilic syndrome
6 Drug sensitivity
7 Polyarteritis nodosa
8 Hodgkin's disease and some other tumours
9 Eosinophilic leukaemia (rare)
10 Treatment with GM-CSF

Table 8.3 Causes of eosinophilia.

Monocytosis

A rise in blood monocyte count above $0.8 \times 10^9/l$ is infrequent. The conditions listed in Table 8.4 may be responsible.

Neutropenia

The lower limit of the normal neutrophil count is $2.5 \times 10^9/l$ except in Blacks and the Middle East where $1.5 \times 10^9/l$ is normal. When the absolute neutrophil level falls below $0.5 \times 10^9/l$ the patient is likely to have recurrent infections and when the count falls to less than $0.2 \times 10^9/l$ the risks are very serious particularly if there is also a functional defect. Neutropenia may be selective or part of a general pancytopenia (Table 8.5). The possible mechanisms are illustrated in Fig. 8.9.

Congenital
Kostmann's syndrome is an autosomal recessive disease presenting in the first year of life with life-threatening infections. G-CSF produces a clinical response.

Drug-induced neutropenia
Selective neutropenia due to the patient's individual susceptibility may follow therapy with a large number of drugs (Table 8.5). Although, in the majority, the drug damages the marrow

1 Chronic bacterial infections: tuberculosis, brucellosis, bacterial endocarditis, typhoid
2 Protozoan infections
3 Chronic neutropenia
4 Hodgkin's disease
5 Myelodysplasia (especially chronic myelomonocytic leukaemia)
6 Treatment with GM-CSF or M-CSF

Table 8.4 Causes of monocytosis.

Table 8.5 Causes of neutropenia.

SELECTIVE NEUTROPENIA

Congenital
- Kostmann's syndrome

Acquired

Drug-induced
- Anti-inflammatory drugs (aminopyrine, phenylbutazone)
- Antibacterial drugs (chloramphenicol, co-trimoxazole, sulphasalazine)
- Anticonvulsants (phenytoin)
- Anti-thyroids (carbimazole)
- Hypoglycaemics (tolbutamide)
- Phenothiazines (chlorpromazine thioridazine)
- Psychotropics and antidepressants (clozapine mianserin, imipramine)
- Miscellaneous (gold, penicillamine, mepacrine, amodiaquine, etc.)

Benign (racial or familial)

Cyclical

Immune
- Autoimmune
- Systemic lupus erythematosus (SLE)
- Felty's syndrome
- Hypersensitivity and anaphylaxis

Infections
- Viral, e.g. hepatitis, influenza, HIV
- Fulminant bacterial infection, e.g. typhoid, miliary tuberculosis

PART OF GENERAL PANCYTOPENIA (see Table 7.2)

Bone marrow failure

Splenomegaly

---

precursor cell (a toxic mechanism), in others an immune mechanism is present which in some cases only damages neutrophils but in others also affects marrow precursors. A drug–hapten mechanism affecting circulating neutrophils may be responsible in some cases, e.g. aminopyrine. In this, an antibody is formed

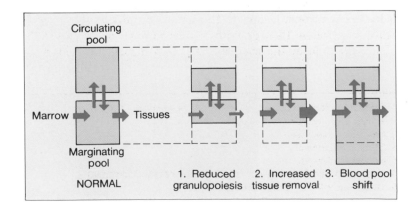

Fig. 8.9 Different kinetic mechanisms of neutropenia (from Boggs & Winkelstein, 1978).

to a drug–protein complex acting as an antigen. Complement is bound to the complex and deposited on the neutrophil surface. The immune complex and complement-coated neutrophils are rapidly removed from the circulation by reticuloendothelial (RE) macrophages. In other cases, the drug acts as a hapten on the cell surface or rarely the drug may stimulate an autoimmune reaction directed against neutrophils in the absence of the drug.

Cyclical neutropenia
This is a rare syndrome with 3–4-week periodicity. Severe but temporary neutropenia occurs. Monocytes tend to rise as the neutrophils fall.

Autoimmune neutropenia
In some cases of chronic neutropenia an autoimmune mechanism can be demonstrated. The antibody may be directed against one of the neutrophil specific antigens (NA, NB, etc).

Idiopathic benign neutropenia
An increase in the marginating fraction of blood neutrophils and a corresponding reduction in the circulating fraction occurs in many normal Africans and in other races and also, rarely, as a familial abnormality. Despite their low peripheral blood neutrophil count, these subjects have no increased susceptibility to infection and their bone marrow appears normal.

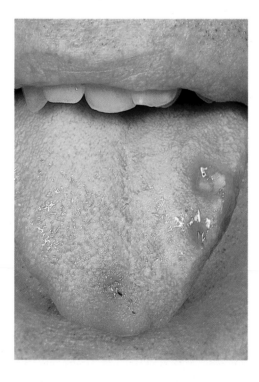

Fig. 8.10 Ulceration of the tongue in severe neutropenia.

Clinical features

Severe neutropenia is particularly associated with infections of the mouth and throat. Painful and often intractable ulceration may occur at these sites (Fig. 8.10), on the skin or at the anus. Septicaemia rapidly supervenes. Organisms carried as commensals by normal individuals may become pathogens. Other features of infections associated with severe neutropenia are described on p. 220.

Diagnosis

Bone marrow examination is useful in determining the level of damage in granulopoiesis, i.e. whether there is reduction in early precursors or whether there is reduction only of circulating and marrow neutrophils with late precursors remaining in the marrow. This situation has erroneously been referred to as 'maturation arrest'. Marrow aspiration and trephine biopsy may also provide evidence of leukaemia, myelodysplasia or other infiltration.

Management

The treatment of patients with acute severe neutropenia is described on p. 221. In many patients with drug-induced neutropenia spontaneous recovery occurs within 1 or 2 weeks after stopping the drug. Patients with chronic neutropenia have recurrent infections which are mainly bacterial in origin although fungal and viral infections (especially herpes) also occur. Early recognition and vigorous treatment with antibiotics, antifungal or antiviral agents, as appropriate, is essential. Prophylactic antibacterial agents, e.g. oral co-trimoxazole or ciprofloxacin and colistin, and antifungal agents, e.g. oral amphotericin and fluconazole, may be of value in reducing the incidence and severity of infections due to severe neutropenia. The haemopoietic growth factor G-CSF may be used to stimulate neutrophil production and is effective in a variety of benign chronic neutropenic states. Corticosteroid therapy or splenectomy has been associated with good results in some patients with autoimmune neutropenia. On the other hand, corticosteroids impair neutrophil function and should not be used indiscriminately in patients with neutropenia.

Bibliography

Boggs D.R. & Winkelstein A. (1978) *White Cell Manual*, 3rd Edition. F.A. Davis, Philadelphia.
Bronchud M.H. & Dexter T.M. (1989) Clinical use of haematopoietic growth

factors. *Blood Reviews*, **3**, 66–70.

Engelfriet P.C. & von dem Borne A.E.G.Kr. (1987) Immune cytopenias. *Clinical Immunology and Allergy*, **1**, 2.

Jasmin C. (ed.) (1990) Growth and differentiation factors in hematology. *Leukaemia Research*, **14**, 675–733.

Leader (1990) Adhesion molecules in diagnosis and treatment of inflammatory diseases. *Lancet*, **ii**, 1351–1352.

Mertelsman R. & Hermann F. (eds) (1990) *Haematopoietic Growth Factors: Clinical Applications*. Marcel Dekker, New York.

Metcalfe D. (1990) The colony-stimulating factors. *Cancer*, **65**, 2185–2195.

Morstyn G. (1990) The impact of colony-stimulating factors as cancer chemotherapy. *British Journal of Haematology*, **75**, 303–307.

Oppenheim J.J., Kovacs E.J., Matsushima M. & Durum S.K. (1986) There is more than one interleukin 1. *Immunology Today* **7**, 45–56.

Patarroyo M. & Makgoba M.W. (1989) Leucocyte adhesion to cells in immune and inflammatory responses. *Lancet*, **ii**, 1139–1142.

Sachs L. (1990) The control of growth and differentiation in normal and leukaemic blood cells. *Cancer*, **65**, 2196–2206.

Yong K. & Khawaja A. (1990) Leucocyte adhesion molecules. *Blood Reviews*, **4**, 211–225.

Chapter 9
The White Cells 2: Lymphocytes and their Benign Disorders

Lymphocytes are the immunologically competent cells which assist the phagocytes in the defence of the body against infection and other foreign invasion and add specificity to the attack. A complete description of the functions of these cells is beyond the scope of this book, but information essential to an understanding of the diseases of the lymphoid system, and of the role of lymphocytes in haematological diseases is included here.

Lymphocytes (Fig. 9.1)

Primary lymphocyte formation

In postnatal life the bone marrow and thymus are the primary lymphopoietic organs (Fig. 9.2) in which lymphocytic stem cells undergo division not dependent upon antigenic stimulation although driven by non-specific cytokines (see Fig. 9.4). In the

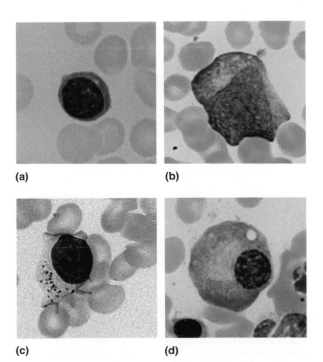

(a)   (b)

Fig. 9.1 Lymphocytes:
(a) small lymphocyte;
(b) activated lymphocyte;
(c) large granular
lymphocyte; (d) plasma cell.

(c)   (d)

foetus, the yolk sac, liver and spleen are also primary lymphopoietic. The secondary or reactive lymphoid tissue is found in
the lymph nodes and the spleen together with the organized and
diffuse lymphoid tissues of the alimentary and respiratory tracts
and the circulating lymphocytes in the blood and tissue spaces.

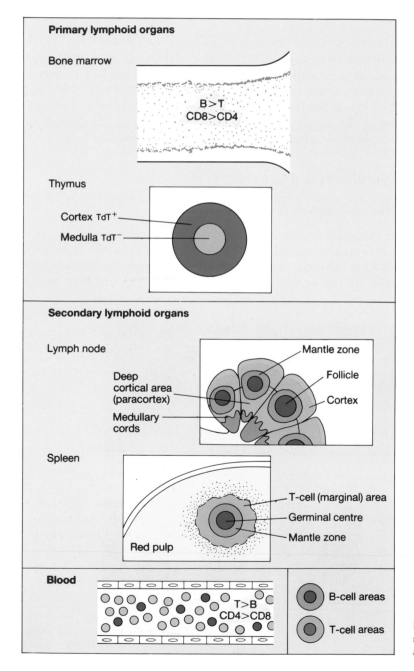

Fig. 9.2 Primary and
secondary lymphoid organs
and blood.

Table 9.1 Functional aspects of T and B cells.

	T cells	B cells
Origin	Thymus	Bone marrow
Distribution	Parafollicular areas of cortex in nodes, periarteriolar in spleen	Germinal centres of lymph nodes, spleen, gut, respiratory tract; also subcapsular and medullary cords of lymph nodes
Blood	80% of lymphocytes; CD4 > CD8	20% of lymphocytes
Membrane receptors	For phytohaemagglutin, for T-cell growth factors, for antigens	For Fc portion of IgG, immune complexes and C3, for B-cell growth factors, for antigens
Bone marrow	CD8 > CD4	
Function	Cell-mediated immunity, e.g. against intracellular organisms including bacteria, viruses, protozoa and fungi; also against transplanted organs	Humoral immunity, e.g. against bacteria
Surface markers	CD1 CD2 CD3 CD4 or 8 CD5 CD6 CD7 MHC class I and II	CD19 CD20 CD22 CD9 (pre B-cells) CD10 Ig receptors for Fc, C3 MHC class I and II
Genes rearranged	TCR α, β, γ, δ	IgH, Igκ, Igλ
Growth and differentiation factors	IL-1, IL-2, IL-3, IL-4, IL-6, IL-7, IL-9	TNF, IL-1, IL-4, IL-6, IL-7, IL-10, also IL-2, γIFN

C, complement; H, heavy; IFN, interferon; Ig, immunoglobulin; IL, interleukin; κ, kappa; λ, lambda; MHC, major histocompatibility complex; TCR, T-cell receptor; TNF, tumour necrosis factor.

Functional aspects of lymphocytes — T and B cells

The immune response depends upon two types of lymphocytes, B and T cells (Table 9.1). In man, B cells are derived from the bone marrow stem cells. Whether any of the cells are processed outside the bone marrow to become mature B lymphocytes is uncertain. In birds, this process takes place in the bursa of Fabricius but an equivalent organ has not been identified in man.

T cells also derive from bone marrow stem cells but undergo processing in the thymus where self-reacting T cells are eliminated by contact with epithelial and dendritic cells. The earliest cell, a prothymocyte which is surface CD7+, probably comes from the bone marrow and populates the subcapsular cortex.

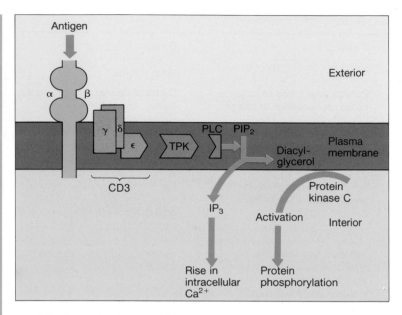

Fig. 9.3 The mechanism by which antigen binding to the T-cell antigen receptor–CD3 complex activates an associated tyrosine protein kinase (TPK) which then activates phospholipase C (PLC). The consequent hydrolysis of an inositol lipid (PIP_2) results in the generation of the second messengers inositol trisphosphate (IP_3) and diacylglycerol, which stimulate a rise in intracellular calcium ions and protein phosphorylation, respectively. (From Brenner & Holtbrand, 1989.)

The mature helper cells express CD4 and suppressor cells express CD8 antigen as well as CD2 (the sheep red cell receptor), CD3 and other T-cell antigens (Table 9.1). The cells also express one of two T-cell antigen receptors, $\alpha\beta$ or $\gamma\delta$. Binding of antigen produces signals which activate the cell and lead to cell division (Fig. 9.3).

The immune response

One of the most striking features of the immune system is its capacity to produce a highly specific response. For both T and B cells this specificity is achieved by the presence of a particular receptor on the lymphocyte surface. The immune system contains many clones of lymphocytes. Each of these clones has a receptor which shows minor differences in structure from that of any other clone, and consequently will only bind to a restricted number of antigens. The B-cell receptor is essentially identical to the immunoglobulin it will secrete. The T-cell receptor (TCR) is more complex. The portion that recognizes antigen is structurally analogous to immunoglobulin, and has either α and β, or in a small minority, γ and δ chains. Variability is produced during B- or T-cell development by rearrangement of the genes coding for immunoglobulins in B cells or for the TCR in T cells (see p. 169). When an antigen is encountered only those clones to which the antigen binds are induced to proliferate and mature into effector cells—the phenomenon of clonal selection.

After activation by certain antigens, particularly polysaccharides, B cells recognizing that antigen proliferate and mature into plasma cells which secrete specific immunoglobulin antibodies. Specialized macrophages (antigen-presenting cells, APCs) play a role in processing many antigens before presenting them to B and T lymphocytes which will respond (Fig. 9.4a).

T cells are unable to bind antigen free in solution and require it to be made available on APCs found particularly in lymphoid tissues. Antigen on APCs is presented as a peptide in association with molecules of the major histocompatibility complex (MHC) which is called HLA (Fig. 9.4). T cells therefore must recognize not only the antigen, but also 'self' MHC molecules. The CD4 molecule in helper cells recognizes class II (HLA-DP, -DQ and -DR) molecules, and the CD8 molecule in suppressor cells recognizes class I (HLA-A, -B and -C) molecules and cross-stabilizes the APC/T-cell links. The antigen recognition site of the TCR is joined to the CD3 molecule which has several sub-units and acts to transduce the signal to proliferate to the T-cell interior (see Fig. 9.3). Adhesion molecules (see p. 147) are also important in binding T or B cells to APCs (Fig. 9.4).

Although the primary interaction between T cells, B cells and APCs is dependent on the presence of the appropriate antigen, the cells so activated then release amplification factors (cytokines), IL-1, IL-2 and other T- and B-cell growth and differentiation factors (Table 9.1) which induce proliferation and differentiation of the activated clone (Fig. 9.4c).

The cytokines, IL-7 and IL-10, act as early B-cell growth factors while IL-2, IL-4, IL-6 and tumour necrosis factor (TNF) act later to cause proliferation and differentiation. For T cells, IL-2 is the main growth factor but IL-3, IL-4, IL-6 and IL-7 also act as early factors.

Immunoglobulins

These are a heterogenous group of proteins produced by plasma cells and B lymphocytes which react with particular antigens. They are divided into five subclasses or isotypes: IgG, IgA, IgM, IgD and IgE. IgG, the most common, contributes about 80% of normal serum immunoglobulin (Ig), and is further subdivided into four subclasses: IgG_1, IgG_2, IgG_3 and IgG_4. IgA is subdivided into two. IgM is usually produced first in response to antigen, IgG subsequently and for a more prolonged period. The same cell can switch from IgM to IgG, IgA or IgE synthesis. IgA is the main Ig in secretions, particularly of the gastrointestinal tract.

IgD and IgE (involved in delayed hypersensitivity reactions)
are minor fractions. Some important biochemical and biological
properties of the three main Ig subclasses are summarized in
Table 9.2.

The immunoglobulins are all made up of the same basic structure (Fig. 9.5) consisting of two heavy chains which are called
gamma (γ) in IgG, alpha (α) in IgA, mu (μ) in IgM, delta (δ) in

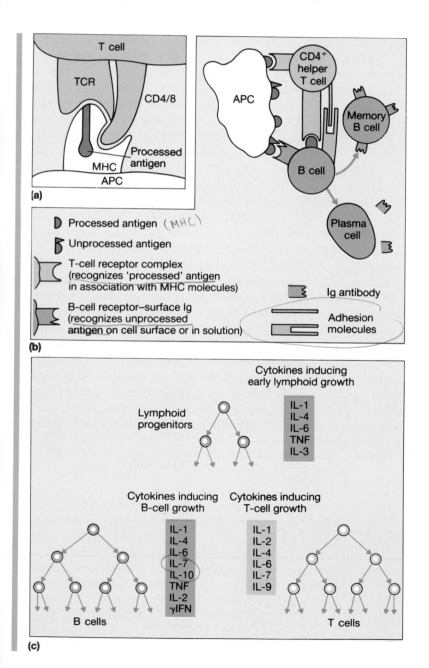

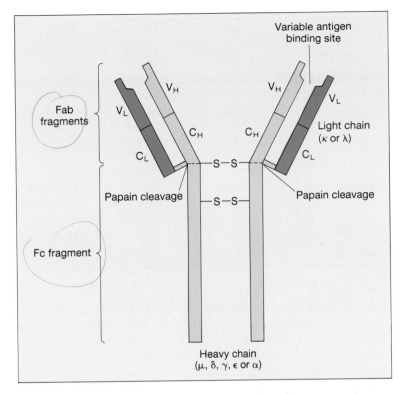

Fig. 9.5 Basic structure of an immunoglobulin molecule. Each molecule is made up of two light (κ or λ) (dark blue areas) and two heavy (light blue areas) chains, and each chain is made up of variable (V) and constant (C) portions, the V portions including the antigen-binding site. The heavy chain (μ, δ, γ, ϵ or α) varies according to the immunoglobulin class. IgA molecules form dimers, while IgM forms a ring of five molecules. Papain cleaves the molecules into an Fc fragment and two Fab fragments.

Fig. 9.4 (*Opposite*) (a) T lymphocytes recognize antigens after they have been processed intracellularly to peptides and have become associated with newly formed MHC molecules. The T-cell receptor (TCR) complex recognizes this combination of antigen and MHC (class I for cytotoxic T cells, class II for helper T cells) and the interaction is stabilized by the CD4 or CD8 molecules.
(b) Production of an antibody response requires cellular interaction between antigen-specific helper T cells and B lymphocytes and antigen-presenting cells (APCs). The mechanism underlying these interactions are incompletely understood. One model is shown. Helper T cells recognize processed antigen in association with MHC class II molecules on the APC surface. They form a bridge with B lymphocytes which recognize the same antigen in the unprocessed form on the APC. B cells *may* also present the processed antigen to the T cell. The bridging between helper T cells and B cells is cemented by antigen-independent receptor−ligand (adhesion molecule) interaction, on the B cell. CD40/CD40 ligand binding is needed for IgM to IgG class switch.
(c) Cytokines involved in early lymphoid cell growth and in the proliferation of more mature B cells and T cells, e.g. in cell amplification in the immune response. IFN, interferon; Ig, immunoglobin; IL, interleukin; MHC, major histocompatibility complex; TNF, tumour necrosis factor.

	IgG	IgA	IgM
Molecular weight	140 000	140 000	900 000
Sedimentation constant	7S	7S	19S
Normal serum level (g/l)	6.0–16.0	1.5–4.5	0.5–1.5
Present in	Serum and extracellular fluid	Serum and other body fluids, e.g. of bronchi and gut	Serum only
Complement fixation	Usual	Yes (alternative pathway)	Usual and very efficient
Placental transfer	Yes	No	No
Heavy chain	(γ_{1-4})	α (α_1 or α_2)	μ

Table 9.2 Some properties of the three main classes of immunoglobulin.

IgD and epsilon (ε) in IgE and two light chains — kappa (κ) or lambda (λ) — which are common to all five immunoglobulins. The heavy and light chains each have highly variable regions which give the immunoglobulin specificity, and constant regions in which there is virtual complete correspondence in amino acid sequence in all antibodies of a given isotype or isotype subclass. In the variable regions of both the heavy and light chains there are hypervariable or complement-determining regions and frame-work regions with less variability. They can be broken into a constant Fc fragment and two highly variable Fab fragments. IgM molecules are much larger because they consist of five subunits.

The main role of immunoglobulins is defence of the body against foreign organisms. However, they also play a vital role in the pathogenesis of a number of haematological disorders. Secretion of a specific immunoglobulin from a monoclonal population of lymphocytes or plasma cells occurs in macro-globulinaemia, most cases of multiple myeloma and in other disorders (p. 272). Bence-Jones protein found in the urine in some cases of myeloma consists of a monoclonal secretion of light chains or light chain fragments (either κ or λ). Immuno-globulins may coat blood cells in a variety of immune or auto-immune haematological disorders and cause:

1 agglutination (e.g. in cold agglutinin disease, p. 89);

2 destruction by macrophages of the RE (reticuloendothelial) system which have receptors for the Fc portion of the immuno-globulin (as in warm type autoimmune haemolytic anaemia, immune thrombocytopenia or rhesus disease of the newborn); or

3 complement coating of the cells which, in turn, may lead either to RE system macrophage destruction (via C3 receptors)

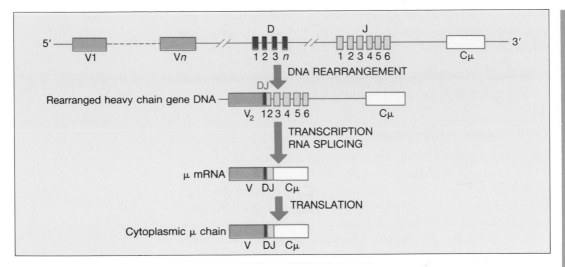

Fig. 9.6 Rearrangement of a heavy-chain immunoglobulin gene. One of the V segments is brought into contact with a D, a J and a C (in this case Cμ) segment, forming an active transcriptional gene from which the corresponding mRNA is produced. The DJ rearrangement precedes VDJ joining.

(as in many drug-induced immune disorders of blood cells) or to direct lysis if the complement sequence goes to completion (as in ABO incompatible blood transfusion).

Immunoglobulin gene rearrangements

The immunoglobulin heavy-chain and κ and λ light-chain genes occur on chromosomes 14, 2 and 22 respectively in man. In the embryonic germ-line state the heavy-chain genes occur as segments for variable (V), diversity (D), joining (J) and constant (C) regions. Each of the V, D and J segments contain a number (n) of different gene segments (Fig. 9.6). In cells not committed to immunoglobulin synthesis, these gene segments remain in their separate germ-line state. During early differentiation of B cells, there is rearrangement of heavy-chain genes so that one of the variable heavy-chain segments combines with one of the D segments and one of the J region segments and its adjacent C region. They thus form a transcriptionally active gene for the heavy chain. The protein-coding segments of the C region mRNA are joined after splicing out intervening RNA. The class of immunoglobulin secreted depends on which of the 9 (4γ, 2α, 1μ, 1δ, 1ε) constant regions is used. Diversity is introduced by the variability of which V segment joins with which D and with which J segment. Additional diversity is generated in B (and T) cells by the enzyme terminal deoxynucleotidyl transferase (TdT) which inserts a variable number of new bases into the DNA of the D region at the time of gene rearrangement. In the arbitrary example shown in Fig. 9.6, V_2 joins with D_1 and J_2. For the light chains similar rearrangements occurs within the light-chain gene segments. Enzymes called recombinases are needed both in B and T cells to join up the adjacent pieces of DNA after excision of intervening sequences. These recognize certain heptamer- and nonamer-conserved sequences flanking the various gene segments. Rearrangement occurs during the ontogeny of B cells in the sequence heavy, κ and λ genes (Fig. 9.7). Mistakes in recombinase activity play an important role in the chromosome translocations of B- or T-cell malignancy.

T-cell receptor rearrangements

The vast majority of T cells contain a TCR composed of a heterodimer of α and β chain. In a minority of T cells, the TCR is composed of γ and δ chains. The α, β, γ and δ genes of the TCRs each include V, D, J and C regions. During T-cell ontogeny, rearrangements of these gene segments occur in an analogous fashion to those for immunoglobulin genes in developing B cells, so creating T cells expressing a wide variety (10^{12} or more) of TCR structures (Fig. 9.8). TdT is involved in creating additional diversity and the same recombinase enzymes used in B cells are involved in joining up TCR gene segments.

Complement

This consists of a series of plasma proteins constituting an amplification enzyme system which is capable of lysis of bacteria

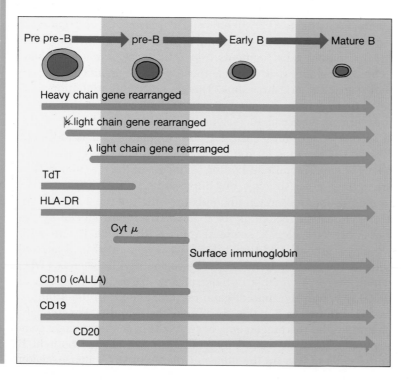

Fig. 9.7 The sequence of immunoglobulin gene rearrangement, antigen and immunoglobulin expression during early B-cell development. Intracytoplasmic CD22 is also a feature of very early B cells.

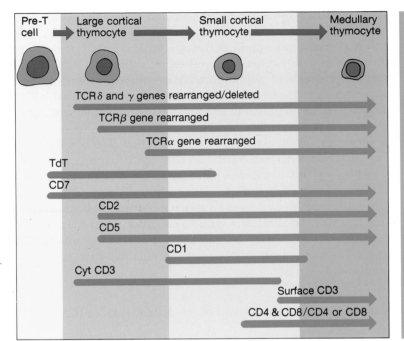

Fig. 9.8 The sequence of events during early T-cell development. The earliest events appear to be the expression of surface CD7, intranuclear TdT and intracytoplasmic CD3 followed by T-cell receptor (TCR) gene rearrangement. Early medullary thymocytes may express both CD4 and CD8, but they then lose one or other of these structures.

or of blood cells or can 'opsonize' (coat) bacteria or cells so that they are phagocytosed. The complement sequence consists of nine major components — C1, C2, etc. — which are activated in turn (denoted thus $\overline{C1}$) and form a cascade, resembling the coagulation sequence (Fig. 9.9). The most abundant and pivotal protein is C3 which is present in plasma at a level of about 1.2 g/l. The early (opsonizing) stages leading to coating the cells with C3b can occur by two different pathways:

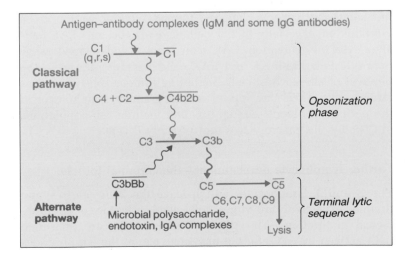

Fig. 9.9 The complement (C) sequence. The activated factors are denoted by a bar over the number. Both pathways generate a C3 convertase. In the classical pathway, the convertase is the major (b) component of C4 and C2 (C4b2b). In the alternate pathway, it is the combination of C3b and the major fragment (b) of factor B (C3bBb).

1 the classical pathway usually activated by IgG or IgM coating of cells; or
2 the alternate, more rapid, pathway activated by IgA, endotoxin (from Gram-negative bacteria) and other factors (Fig. 9.9).

Macrophages and neutrophils have C3b receptors and they phagocytose C3b-coated cells. C3b is degraded to C3d which is detected in the antiglobulin test using an anti-complement agent (p. 396). If the complement sequence goes to completion, there is generation of an active phospholipase that punches holes in the cell membrane (e.g. of the red cell or bacterium), causing direct lysis. The complement pathway also generates biologically active fragments C3a and C5a which act directly on phagocytes, especially neutrophils, to stimulate the respiratory burst associated with production of oxygen metabolites. Both may trigger anaphylaxis by release of mediators from tissue mast cells and basophils which may cause vasodilation and increased permeability.

Natural killer (NK) and lymphokine-activated killer (LAK) cells

NK refers to a function rather than a specific cell type. NK cells can kill cells which they recognize as foreign. They lack antigen-specific receptors but recognize other target structures on the target cell. They do this by two mechanisms:
1 direct; and
2 antibody-dependent cell-mediated cytotoxicity (ADCC). In this, antibody binds to antigen on the cell surface; NK cells then bind to the Fc portion of the bound antibody and kill the target cell.
In either case, adhesion molecules on the NK cell bind to ligands on the target cell. NK cells are activated by γ-interferon and IL-2. LAK also refers to a function rather than a specific cell type. LAK cells may be derived from NK cells and kill by the same mechanisms, but are formed after activation by a lymphokine, especially IL-2. T cells may also become LAK cells after cytokine activation. LAK cells have a wider target range than NK cells. Both NK and LAK cells may have a role in the removal of altered host cells, including tumour cells as well as foreign cells. They may appear as large granular lymphocytes in the peripheral blood (see Fig. 9.1) and include sub-populations of CD8 T cells, macrophages and possibly B cells.

Further lymphocyte development — the germinal follicle

The B and T lymphocytes which leave the bone marrow and thymus respectively are 'virgin' cells, at an early stage of immunological maturation. When these T and B cells are presented with antigen by APCs for the first time, e.g. in the lymph nodes

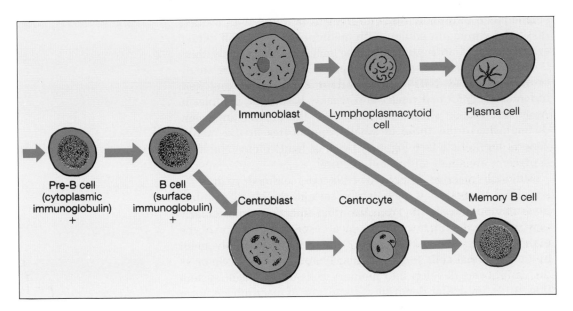

Fig. 9.10 Suggested maturation of B lymphocytes after leaving the marrow. The bone marrow stages of B-cell development are illustrated in Fig. 9.7. Centroblasts and centrocytes are the follicle centre cells.

or spleen, they transform into T or B immunoblasts (Fig. 9.10).

Immunoblasts are the largest lymphoid cells. They have a light nucleus with fine chromatin pattern with very large nucleoli which are often solitary and found in the middle of the nucleus or at an indentation of the nuclear membrane. They have a broad rim of strongly basophilic cytoplasm. The T immunoblasts either carry out their primary T-cell function and die or they become 'memory' T lymphocytes. These latter cells react more intensely and quickly during subsequent stimulation by the same antigen. B immunoblasts give rise to plasma cells (see Fig. 9.10). Initially, these are small cells with features intermediate between those of small lymphocytes and mature plasma cells (plasmacytoid lymphocytes) and they secrete chiefly IgM. With further development they enlarge and become typical plasma cells which are responsible for the production of immunoglobulins.

Plasma cells are larger than lymphocytes. Typically, they have an eccentric round nucleus with a 'clock-face' chromatin pattern. With the exception of a perinuclear light-staining Golgi body, the cytoplasm is strongly basophilic (see Fig. 9.1). During the primary immune response plasmacytoid lymphocytes predominate and the associated immunoglobulin production is small.

In the lymph nodes and other collections of lymphoid tissue, germinal centres arise as a result of continuing response to antigenic stimulation. The typical dividing cells, known as centroblasts, arise from small B lymphocytes; their progeny are known as centrocytes. These two types of lymphocyte are also known as follicle centre cells. *Centroblasts* vary in size but are usually smaller than immunoblasts. The nucleus is round with a finely dispersed chromatin pattern with medium-sized nucleoli, which are often found at the inner nuclear membrane. Typically there is a rim of strongly basophilic cytoplasm. *Centrocytes* are small- or medium-sized cells with round or conspicuous, notched, indented or deformed nuclei and weakly basophilic cytoplasm. Apart from their shape, the nuclei of these cells are easily distinguished from those of small lymphocytes in the mantle zone of the follicle (see Fig. 9.2) by their light colour. Nucleoli, if present, are small and usually central.

Although reactive lymphoid cells are confined mainly to lymphoid tissues, they may also be seen in the blood in infectious mononucleosis (p. 176) and other infections (particularly viral) and during other immunological responses. In some of the malignant lymphomas (Chapter 13) there is blood involvement by the abnormal cells (e.g. 'follicular lymphoma' cells). Some of the centrocytes develop into memory cells of the B-cell system (Fig. 9.10). Follicular dendritic cells, a type of macrophage, form a framework to which the follicle centre B lymphocytes adhere; a few T cells, mainly of the CD4 type also enter the germinal follicle. *Lymphoblasts* are seen in the tissue or blood in lymphoblastic lymphoma or lymphoblastic leukaemia and cannot be distinguished by conventional microscopy from other early blast cells (e.g. in a normal marrow). They are not identified in normal germinal follicles. Special staining or immunophenotyping is needed to identify them (p. 216).

Lymphocyte circulation

Lymphocytes in the peripheral blood migrate through post-capillary venules into the substance of the lymph nodes or into the spleen. T cells home to the perifollicular zones of the cortical areas of lymph nodes (paracortical areas) (see Fig. 9.2) and to the peri-arteriolar sheaths surrounding the central arterioles of the spleen. B cells selectively accumulate in germinal follicles of the lymph nodes and spleen and also at the subcapsular periphery of the cortex and in the medullary cords of the lymph nodes. Lymphocytes return to the peripheral blood via the efferent lymphatic stream and the thoracic duct. The majority of the recirculating cells (e.g. in the thoracic duct or peripheral blood) are T cells with median duration of a complete circulation of about 10 hours (see Table 9.1). In normal peripheral blood and germinal centres CD4 helper cells predominate, but in the marrow and gut the major T-cell subpopulation is CD8 positive. T cells expressing the γδ receptor home particularly to the lungs, skin and gut. The majority of B cells are more sessile and spend long periods in the spleen and lymph nodes.

Benign disorders

Lymphocytosis

Lymphocytosis often occurs in infants and young children in response to infections which produce a neutrophil reaction in adults. Conditions particularly associated with lymphocytosis are listed in Table 9.3.

Infectious mononucleosis

Infectious mononucleosis (glandular fever) is a disease character-ized by fever, sore throat, lymphadenopathy and atypical lymph-ocytes in the blood. These are T cells reacting against B lymphocytes infected with Epstein–Barr virus (EBV). The condition is associated with a rising titre of antibody against the EBV. Individuals without antibody to this virus are prone to the infection. As many people have antibodies without having had the obvious features of the disease, it appears that subclinical infection is common. There is a low infectivity rate. Sporadic groups of cases occur, particularly in young people living together in boarding schools, colleges and military institutions. The dis-ease is associated with a high titre of heterophile (reacting with cells of another species) antibody which reacts with sheep, horse or beef red cells. A similar clinical syndrome without heterophile antibodies may occur in young adults with toxoplasmosis or cytomegalovirus and other viral infections.

Clinical features

The majority of patients are between the ages of 15 and 40 years. A prodromal period of a few days occurs with lethargy, malaise, headaches, stiff neck and a dry cough. In established disease the following features may be found.

Table 9.3 Causes of lymphocytosis.

1 Infections
- Acute: infectious mononucleosis, rubella, pertussis, mumps, acute infectious lymphocytosis, infectious hepatitis, cytomegalovirus, HIV, herpes simplex or zoster
- Chronic: tuberculosis, toxoplasmosis, brucellosis, syphilis

2 Thyrotoxicosis

3 Chronic lymphocytic leukaemia and polymphocytic leukaemia (B- and T-cell types)

4 Acute lymphoblastic leukaemia

5 Non-Hodgkin's lymphoma (some)

6 Hairy cell leukaemia

1 Bilateral cervical lymphadenopathy is present in 75% of cases. Symmetrical generalized lymphadenopathy occurs in 50% of cases. The nodes are discrete and may be tender.

2 Over half of patients have a sore throat with inflamed oral and pharyngeal surfaces. Follicular tonsillitis is frequently seen.

3 Fever may be mild or severe.

4 A morbilliform rash, severe headache and eye signs, e.g. photophobia, conjunctivitis and periorbital oedema are not uncommon.

5 Palpable splenomegaly occurs in over half the patients and hepatomegaly in about 15%.

6 About 5% of patients are jaundiced.

7 Occasionally, in the most severely affected patients, there is widespread mucosal bleeding with epistaxis, tachycardia with ECG (electrocardiograph) abnormalities, or evidence of nervous system disease, e.g. convulsions, coma, stupor, various pareses or palsies involving cranial nerves or lower motor neurones. Involvement of mesenteric nodes may produce a clinical picture similar to that of acute appendicitis.

8 Immunosuppressed patients, e.g. following renal, bone marrow or cardiac transplantation or with AIDS (acquired immune deficiency syndrome) who are carriers of EBV, may develop lymphoma-like proliferations of B lymphocytes which carry the EBV genome. The proliferation usually resolves if the immunosuppression can be discontinued. In some patients, however, a monoclonal malignant lymphoma develops.

Diagnosis

1 Pleomorphic atypical lymphocytosis. A moderate rise in white cell count (e.g. $10-20 \times 10^9/l$) with an absolute lymphocytosis is usual, and some patients have even higher counts. Large numbers of atypical lymphocytes are seen in the peripheral blood film (Fig. 9.11). These cells are variable in appearance but most have nuclear and cytoplasmic features similar to those seen during reactive lymphocyte transformation. The greatest

Fig. 9.11 Infectious mononucleosis: representative 'reactive' lymphocytes in the peripheral blood film of a 21-year-old man (see also Fig. 9.1b).

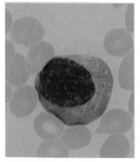 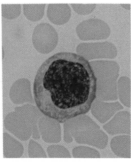 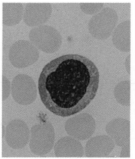 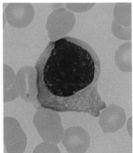

(a)   (b)   (c)   (d)

number of atypical lymphocytes are usually found between the seventh and 10th day of the illness and these cells may persist in the blood for 1 or 2 months.

2 Heterophile antibodies. Heterophile antibodies against sheep red cells may be found in the serum at high titres. Similar antibodies are occasionally found in normal people and were often seen in the past in patients suffering from serum sickness. Differential absorption studies before titration against sheep red cells allow distinction between these heterophile antibodies (the Paul—Bunnell test). Antibodies present in normal people and those suffering from serum sickness are absorbed by a suspension of guinea-pig kidney which is rich in Forsmann antigen. The antibody in infectious mononucleosis is not absorbed by guinea-pig kidney but is absorbed by antigens on the membrane of ox red cells. Modern slide screening tests in kit form (the monospot test) substitute more sensitive formalized horse red cells for the sheep cells used in the Paul—Bunnell test. Highest titres occur during the second and third week and the antibody persists in most patients for 6 weeks.

3 EBV antibody. If viral diagnostic facilities are available a rise in the titre of antibody against the EBV capsid antigen may be demonstrated during the first 2—3 weeks. Specific antibody to the EBV nuclear antigen develops later but persists for life.

4 Haematological abnormalities other than the atypical lymphocytosis are frequent. Occasional patients develop an autoimmune haemolytic anaemia. The IgM autoantibody is typically of the 'cold' type and usually shows 'i' blood group specificity. Thrombocytopenia is frequent and an autoimmune thrombocytopenic purpura occurs in a smaller number of patients.

5 Patients with infectious mononucleosis may have false-positive serology for syphilis or rheumatoid arthritis or a positive antinuclear factor test.

Differential diagnosis

The differential diagnosis of infectious mononucleosis includes a large number of conditions with similar clinical findings or blood film appearance. Apart from acute leukaemia, cytomegalovirus infection and toxoplasmosis, influenza, rubella, infectious hepatitis, follicular tonsillitis or agranulocytosis are most likely to create initial diagnostic confusion. Initial infection with HIV (human immunodeficiency virus) may also cause a similar syndrome. In the rare condition of childhood known as acute infective lymphocytosis the fever is mild and there is no lymphadenopathy, splenomegaly or heterophile antibody.

Treatment

In the great majority of patients only symptomatic treatment is required. There is no evidence to suggest that either antibiotics or corticosteroids influence the course of the disease. Patients tend to develop an erythematous rash if given ampicillin therapy.

Course and prognosis

Most patients recover fully 4–6 weeks after initial symptoms. However, convalescence may be slow and associated with severe malaise and lethargy. Relapse occurs in about 6% of cases but almost all patients eventually recover. Isolated fatalities have resulted from encephalitis, oedema of the glottis, severe hepatic necrosis or splenic rupture. Some individuals develop a chronic fatigue syndrome and persistent high titres of EBV antibody.

Lymphopenia

Lymphopenia may occur in severe bone marrow failure, with corticosteroid and other immunosuppressive therapy, in Hodgkin's disease and with widespread irradiation. It also occurs in a variety of immune deficiency syndromes the most important of which is AIDS (see p. 179).

Immune deficiencies

A large number of inherited or acquired deficits in any of the

Table 9.4 Classification of immune deficiencies.

Primary	B cell (antibody deficiency)	X-linked agammaglobulinaemia, acquired common variable hypogammaglobulinaemia, selective IgA or IgG subclass deficiencies
	T cell	Thymic aplasia, purine nucleoside phosphorylase (PNP) deficiency
	Mixed B and T cell	Severe combined immune deficiency (due to adenosine deaminase deficiency (ADA) or other causes) Bloom's syndrome Ataxia-telangiectasia Wiskott–Aldrich syndrome
Secondary	B cell (antibody deficiency)	Myeloma Nephrotic syndrome, protein losing enteropathy
	T cell	AIDS Hodgkin's disease, non-Hodgkin's lymphoma Drugs: steroids, cyclosporine, azathioprine, etc.
	T and B cell	Chronic lymphocytic leukaemia, post-bone marrow transplantation and post-chemotherapy/radiotherapy

components of the immune system may cause an impaired immune response with increased susceptibility to infection (Table 9.4). A primary lack of T cells (as in AIDS) leads not only to bacterial infections but also to viral, protozoal, fungal and mycobacterial infections. In some cases, however, lack of specific subsets of T cells which control B-cell maturation may lead to a secondary lack of B-cell function as in many cases of common variable immune deficiency which may develop in children or adults of either sex. In others, a primary defect of B cells or APCs is present. X-linked agammaglobulinaemia is due to a failure of B-cell development. Pyogenic bacterial infections dominate the clinical course. Rare syndromes include aplasia of the thymus, severe combined (T and B) immune deficiency due to adenosine deaminase deficiency and selective deficiencies of IgA or IgM. Acquired immune deficiency occurs after cytotoxic chemotherapy or radiotherapy and is particularly pronounced after bone marrow transplantation where dysregulation of the immune system persists for 2 years or more and is responsible for a high incidence of serious viral infections, e.g. with cytomegalovirus or herpes zoster. Immune deficiency is also frequently associated with tumours of the lymphoid system including chronic lymphocytic leukaemia, Hodgkin's disease and myeloma. A major cause of acquired immunodeficiency is HIV infection and the clinical and haematological aspects of this disease are considered next.

Acquired immune deficiency syndrome

Aetiology

This syndrome is caused by infection with HIV, a retrovirus of the lentivirus subgroup. The usual cause is the HIV-1 virus (Fig. 9.12). A second retrovirus, HIV-2, has also been associated with AIDS in Africa and Europe. The geographical origin of the HIV virus is still unclear, but some evidence suggests it was present in Africa a decade before its appearance in the USA and Europe.

Following the initial recognition of cases in the USA in 1979, the epidemic has expanded rapidly. The World Health Organization has estimated that by the year 2000 there may be 15–20 million people infected with HIV, with 5–6 million cases of AIDS.

Virus structure

The virus contains RNA encoding three groups of structural genes encoding virion proteins and other genes which code for proteins which regulate viral replication. The three groups of structural genes are:

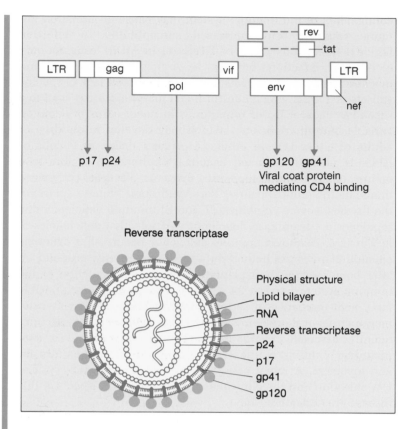

Fig. 9.12 The structure of the HIV genome and virus. gp, glycoprotein; p, protein; numbers are molecular weight (kDa).

1 gag (group-specific antigen) coding for proteins within the viral particle, e.g. p24, which can be detected in serum of some patients with HIV infection;
2 pol coding for reverse transcriptase which converts the RNA to DNA in the host cell and for other enzymes;
3 env which codes for envelope proteins.

Epidemiology

The virus is transmitted in semen, blood and other body fluids. Most infection occurs during intimate sexual contact or from blood or blood products. Homosexual activity and unprotected anal intercourse are dominant risk factors. AIDS is also seen frequently in intravenous drug abusers, haemophiliacs, thalassaemics and other patients who have been transfused with HIV-infected blood or blood products and in the heterosexual partners of those infected with HIV.

Pathogenesis

HIV produces its predominant effects through infection of T-helper (CD4) cells. Some CD4 cells are lysed directly by replicating HIV, but the virus remains latent in most host cells unrecognized by the patient's immune system. When such latently infected T cells are activated, the virus replicates and cell death follows. Activation may be due to other viruses, cytokines released from B cells or by antigen presented by APCs. The CD4 antigen appears to be the main receptor for HIV, and CD4+ APCs are also an important site for viral replication. Direct infection by the virus of other cells, e.g. brain cells or bone marrow cells, may also account for some of the pathology of the disease. The consequences of helper T-cell depletion on cell-mediated immune responses leave the HIV patient open to infections.

Clinical features

The clinical outcome of HIV infection has been classified into four stages or groups (Table 9.5). The factors which determine the progression from one stage to another remain uncertain. A prodromal period of about 6 weeks follows initial infection. Symptoms resembling infectious mononucleosis with transient lymphadenopathy may then occur. A proportion of patients pass through the asymptomatic (possibly with alteration in blood cell composition) and persistent lymphadenopathy stages (Table 9.5) to the AIDS-related conditions and to fully developed AIDS. The AIDS-related conditions or complex comprise a variety of manifestations including generalized lymphadenopathy with

Table 9.5 Classification of HIV infection.

Group I	*Initial infection* Symptomatic (e.g. mononucleosis-like syndrome, mild meningoencephalitis) or asymptomatic seroconversion
Group II	*Chronic asymptomatic infection* Normal tests but may have anaemia, neutropenia, thrombocytopenia, low CD4 lymphocytes and lymphopenia, hypergammaglobulinaemia
Group III	*Persistent generalized lymphadenopathy* Laboratory test abnormalities as in group II may or may not be present
Group IV	*Other diseases* (a) Constitutional disease — fever, weight loss, diarrhoea (b) Neurological disease — either central (e.g. dementia or myelopathy) or peripheral neuropathies (c) Secondary infectious disease — e.g. *Pneumocystis carinii*, toxoplasmosis, *Cryptococcus*, cryptosporidiosis, atypical *Mycobacteria*, herpes simplex or zoster, oral hairy leucoplakia, histoplasmosis, candidiasis, cytomegalovirus, *Salmonella* (d) Secondary cancers — e.g. Kaposi's sarcoma, non-Hodgkin's lymphoma, squamous carcinoma of the mouth or rectum (e) Other conditions — clinical problems related to HIV and decreased cellular immunity not included above

persistent fever, weight loss, unexplained diarrhoea, CNS manifestations and haematologic abnormalities including thrombocytopenia, leucopenia and anaemia. Fully developed AIDS is
associated with a wide spectrum of opportunistic infections
including *Pneumocystis carinii* (Fig. 9.13) and others listed in
Table 9.5.

A proportion of patients develop Kaposi's sarcoma, a vascular
skin tumour of endothelial cell origin (Fig. 9.14), while others
have developed non-Hodgkin's lymphoma.

Diagnosis

1 The blood count reveals a progressive lymphopenia. The
depletion of helper T cells results in a fall of the CD4:CD8
(helper:suppressor) ratio from the normal value of $1.5-2.5:1$ to
less than $1:1$. An absolute CD4 count of less than $0.2 \times 10^9/l$ is
usually associated with clinical disease and a bad prognosis.
2 A polyclonal rise in serum immunoglobulin is often found. A
paraprotein occurs in serum of about 10% of AIDS patients.
3 HIV infection is confirmed by serological detection of antibodies to one of the HIV antigens by enzyme-linked immunoabsorbent assay (ELIZA) or by immunoblotting (western blot
assay). Confirmation may also be provided by detection of HIV
antigen in the blood or positive culture of the virus. The lag
period between infection and a positive antibody test is usually
several months.
4 AIDS patients show depressed delayed-type skin reactivity
to common antigens.

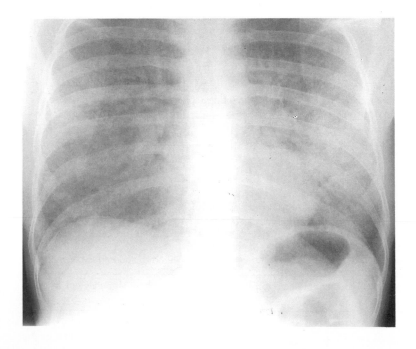

Fig. 9.13 *Pneumocystitis
carinii* infection: a chest
radiograph showing the typical
'bat wing' shadowing of both
lung fields.

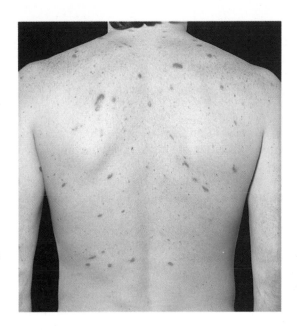

Fig. 9.14 Kaposi's sarcoma in AIDS: a vascular tumour of endothelial origin in a homosexual male (HIV antigen-positive).

5 Examination of the lymph nodes reveal a spectrum of changes. In the type I pattern there is follicular and paracortical hyperplasia with attenuation of mantle zones. In type II there is a loss of germinal centres but diffuse lymphoid hyperplasia and in type III, an end stage, lymphocyte depletion predominates.

Haematological aspects

The most frequent abnormalities in the blood cells are anaemia, thrombocytopenia and neutropenia either individually or combined, and lymphopenia with a reduced number of CD4 lymphocytes. The bone marrow may be hypercellular (with an increase of plasma cells and lymphocytes), normocellular or hypocellular. The cells may be dysplastic and fibrosis may occur. Marrow examination can be used to diagnose opportunistic infections, e.g. tuberculosis, cryptococcus, histoplasmosis.

The mechanism for the cytopenias include infections, autoimmune reactions and impaired marrow production either due to HIV infection of progenitors or lack of growth factors perhaps due to HIV infection of accessory cells. The drugs used in therapy, especially azidothymidine (AZT) but also ganciclovir, pentamidine and trimethoprim may also cause cytopenias, especially if the patient is folate-deficient. Serum B_{12} levels tend to be low in AIDS probably due to intestinal B_{12} malabsorption, but megaloblastic anaemia due to B_{12} deficiency is unusual. Therapy of the cytopenias is difficult. Haemopoietic growth factors (e.g. erythropoietin, G-CSF, GM-CSF) have been tried. Corticosteroids, intravenous γ-globulin or even splenectomy have been used in severe cases of thrombocytopenia.

This may also respond to AZT (zidovudine) therapy. Lymphomas
are treated in the usual way, although these tend to be high
grade and if the patient already has AIDS, the prognosis is
extremely bad.

Treatment

Much of the therapy is aimed at preventing or treating infections,
e.g. with prophylactic antibiotics or antifungals and inhalation
of pentamidine.

AZT has been successful in improving both morbidity and
mortality. Acyclovir may be of benefit by inhibiting the replication of herpes viruses which may otherwise accelerate the
disease process. Present treatment strategies attempt to combine
antiretroviral drugs with lymphokines to suppress HIV with
concurrent stimulation of lymphoid and myeloid cell proliferation. Drugs such as suramin and ribavarin have been developed
to inhibit viral reverse transcriptase. Trials are underway in
chimpanzees to stimulate antibodies against the virus using
recombinant envelope antigens as immunogen. Synthetic peptides corresponding to virus envelope sequences and anti-
idiotypes are also being explored as vaccines. Soluble CD4
receptor is also in trial. The success of future vaccines may
depend on their ability to neutralize a number of HIV variants
which mutate in the envelope gene of the virus allowing for
different serotypes.

Differential diagnosis of lymphadenopathy

The principal causes of lymphadenopathy are listed in Table 9.6.
The clinical history and examination give essential information. The age of the patient, length of history, associated
symptoms of possible infectious or malignant disease, whether
the nodes are painful or tender, consistency of the nodes and
whether there is generalized or local lymphadenopathy, are all
important. The size of the liver and spleen are assessed. In the
case of local node enlargement, inflammatory or malignant disease
in the associated lymphatic drainage area are particularly
considered.

Further investigations will depend on the initial clinical diagnosis but it is usual to include a full blood count, blood film
and ESR (erythrocyte sedimentation rate). Chest X-ray, monospot
test, *Toxoplasma* titres and anti-HIV and Mantoux tests are
frequently needed. In many cases, it will be essential to make a
histological diagnosis by node biopsy but a fine needle aspirate
may sometimes avoid the need for this. CT (computerized
tomography) scanning is valuable in determining the presence

THE WHITE CELLS 2: LYMPHOCYTES

185

Table 9.6 Causes of lymphadenopathy.

Localized	Generalized
Local infection • pyogenic infection (e.g. pharyngitis, dental abscess, otitis media), actinomyces • viral infection (e.g. cat scratch fever, lymphogranuloma venereum) • tuberculosis	**Infections** • viral (e.g. infectious mononucleosis, measles, rubella, viral hepatitis), HIV • bacterial (e.g. brucellosis, syphilis, tuberculosis, *Salmonella*, bacterial endocarditis) • fungal (e.g. histoplasmosis) • protozoal (e.g. toxoplasmosis)
Lymphoma • Hodgkin's disease • non-Hodgkin's lymphoma	Non-infectious inflammatory diseases (e.g. sarcoidosis, rheumatoid arthritis, SLE, other connective tissue diseases, serum sickness)
Carcinoma (secondary)	Leukaemias, especially CLL, ALL
	Lymphoma: non-Hodgkin's lymphoma, Hodgkin's disease
	Waldenström's macroglobulinaemia
	Rarely secondary carcinoma
	Angioimmunoblastic lymphadenopathy
	Sinus histocytosis with massive lymphadenopathy
	Reaction to drugs and chemicals (e.g. hydantoins and related chemicals, beryllium)
	Hyperthyroidism

and extent of deep node enlargement. Subsequent investigations will depend on the diagnosis made and the patient's particular features. In some cases of deep node enlargement, where enlarged superficial nodes are not available for biopsy, bone marrow or liver biopsies may be needed in an attempt to reach a histological diagnosis and avoid the need for a diagnostic laparotomy.

Bibliography

Anon. (1991) The biology of complement. *Immunology Today*, **12**, 291–342.
Brenner M.K. & Hoffbrand A.V. (1989) Lymphocytes and their benign disorders. In *Postgraduate Haematology*, 3rd Edition (eds A.V. Hoffbrand & S.M. Lewis). Heinemann Medical, Oxford, pp. 325–358.
Brostoff J., Scadding G.K., Male D. & Roitt I.M. (eds) *Clinical Immunology*. Gower Medical, London.
Costello C. (ed.) (1990) Haematology in HIV disease. *Clinical Haematology*, **3**, 1–213.
Hirano T., Akira S., Taga T. & Kishimoto T. (1990) Biological and clinical aspects of interleukin-6. *Immunology Today*, **11**, 443–449.
Mitsuyasu R.T. & Golde D.W. (eds) (1991) Hematologic and oncologic aspects of HIV disease. *Hematology/Oncology Clinics of North America*, **5**, 195–370.
Roitt I.M. (1991) *Essential Immunology*, 7th Edition. Blackwell Scientific Publications, Oxford.
Roitt I.M., Brostoff J. & Male D.K. (1990) *Immunology*, 2nd Edition. Gower Medical, London.

Chapter 10
Haematological Malignancies: General Aspects

This chapter summarizes current knowledge on the mechanisms by which normal haemopoietic cells become malignant. Chromosomal abnormalities are frequent in these tumours and are often of value in diagnosis and classification and provide a sensitive test for minimal residual disease (disease still present when the patient appears to be in full remission). The chapter begins with a summary of the terms used for these chromosomal changes. The different techniques used to show that the haemopoietic neoplasms are monoclonal (i.e. arise by mitotic division from a single somatic cell) are described. The normal bone marrow stem or progenitor cell or early lymphoid cell from which each of the tumours is postulated to arise is then detailed.

Malignant transformation is now known to be associated with changes in the function of various cellular genes called oncogenes (proto-oncogenes) and tumour-suppressor genes (anti-oncogenes). These genes code for proteins which are normally involved in cell proliferation and differentiation. How these genes may be activated or inactivated in the tumour cells is discussed. A final section summarizes the practical applications of some of the techniques described in the diagnosis and management of malignant haematological diseases.

Chromosome nomenclature

The normal somatic cell has 46 chromosomes and is called diploid; ova or sperm have 23 chromosomes and are called haploid. The chromosomes occur in pairs and are numbered 1 to 22 in decreasing size order; there are two sex chromosomes, XX in females, XY in males. Karyotype is the term used to describe the chromosomes derived from a mitotic cell which have been set out in numerical order. A somatic cell with more or less than 46 chromosomes is termed aneuploid; more than 46 is hyperdiploid, less than 46 hypodiploid; 46 but with chromosome rearrangements, pseudodiploid.

Each chromosome has two arms, the shorter called 'p', the longer called 'q'. These meet at the centromere. On staining each arm divides into regions numbered outwards from the centromere and each region divides into bands (Fig. 10.1). When a whole chromosome is lost or gained, a − or + is put

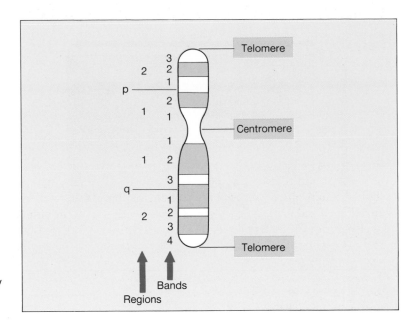

Fig. 10.1 A schematic representation of a chromosome. The bands may be divided into sub-bands according to staining pattern.

in front of the chromosome number; if part of the chromosome is lost or gained, the + or − is put after the chromosome number. Chromosome translocations are denoted by 't', the two chromosomes involved placed in brackets, the lower numbered chromosome first. Inversion implies part of the chromosome runs in the opposite direction to normal and isochrome is the term used when a chromosome divides horizontally at its centromere, rather than vertically which is normal.

Establishment of clonality

The leukaemias, lymphomas and myeloma are thought to arise by genetic alteration within a single cell in the marrow or peripheral lymphoid tissue (Fig. 10.2). Mitotic division in successive generations of cells derived from the original abnormal cell gives rise to a 'clonal' population which, when sufficiently large, causes clinically apparent disease. The evidence for the clonal origin of these tumours is based on a number of techniques most of which are used only for research (Table 10.1).

G6PD isoenzyme analysis

The G6PD (glucose-6-phosphate dehydrogenase) gene is situated on the X chromosome. Two different forms of the enzyme, A and B, exist and can be distinguished by electrophoresis. Females who have two X chromosomes may, therefore, be heterozygous for the two forms (G6PD A/G6PD B). According to the Lyon

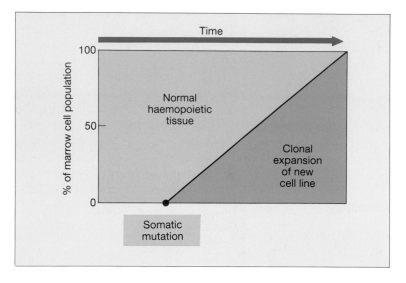

Fig. 10.2 Theoretical graph to show the replacement of normal marrow cells by a clonal population of malignant cells arising from a single cell with an acquired genetic alteration ('somatic mutation').

hypothesis, one of the two X chromosomes in each female cell becomes inactivated. This inactivation remains fixed. In the case of a female heterozygous for G6PD, the somatic cells will be a mosaic, some cells expressing G6PD A and others G6PD B. All the cells in a clone of cells derived from one cell in such an individual, however, will express either G6PD A or G6PD B but not both.

X-linked RFLP

Restriction fragment length polymorphism (RFLP) indicates the variation in the size of a DNA fragment, detectable with a given probe, after digestion with a restriction enzyme (see p. 117). Differences in size of the RFLP detected can be due to a point mutation in a restriction site, or to a shift in the position of the

Table 10.1 Establishment of clonality.

G6PD isoenzyme analysis	Applicable to 'informative' females only
X-linked RFLP analysis	
Light chain restriction	Applicable to B-lymphoid tumours only
Immunoglobulin and TCR gene rearrangements	Applicable to lymphoid malignancies
Cytogenetics	
Chromosomal translocational analysis	
Point mutations	

G6PD, glucose-6-phosphate dehydrogenase; RFLP, restriction fragment length polymorphism; TCR, T-cell receptor.

restriction site due to deletion or duplication of neighbouring DNA. In females, the two X chromosomes can be informative by having different RFLP haplotypes (see p. 117). In a clone of cells, only one of the X chromosomes will be active (see Lyon hypothesis above). DNA active in transcription is usually hypomethylated whereas resting DNA is methylated. Since the DNA of the active X chromosomes will be hypomethylated the use of a second restriction enzyme (e.g. Hpa I) sensitive to the methylation status of the DNA, followed by Southern blotting using a single X chromosome probe, will be informative of whether only one (as in a monoclonal tumour) or both (as in a polyclonal proliferation) X chromosomes are active in the tissue examined.

Light chain restriction

This method is only applicable to B-lymphoid tumours. A mature B lymphocyte expresses a surface immunoglobulin which is characteristic of the individual cell in terms of light and heavy chain usage. A polyclonal population of B cells express a wide variety of different immunoglobulin molecules on the surfaces of the cells; the individual immunoglobulin molecules of each cell will contain either κ or λ light chains but not both. If there is a monoclonal population derived from a single cell only one immunoglobulin and therefore only one type of light chain, either κ or λ, will be expressed. Analysis of surface light chain expression is appropriate to determine monoclonality of proliferations of relatively mature surface immunoglobulin-expressing B-cell tumours (e.g. B-cell chronic lymphocytic leukaemia (B-CLL) or B-cell lymphoma) and this technique is widely used, e.g. to distinguish B-CLL from a benign polyclonal lymphocytosis.

Immunoglobulin and T-cell receptor gene rearrangements

During normal B-lymphocyte development (ontogeny), the cells sequentially rearrange their genes coding for the heavy and light (κ and λ) chains of the immunoglobulins (see p. 169). The patterns of rearrangements are different for different B cells according to the immunoglobulin they are destined to secrete. During T-lymphocyte ontogeny, rearrangement of the genes for the α, β, γ and δ chains of the T-cell antigen receptor occurs. The diversity of these rearrangements accounts for the diversity of the T cells formed (see p. 170). In a clonal population of B or T cells, the immunoglobulin or T-cell receptor (TCR) genes, respectively, will be clonally rearranged. This clonal rearrangement can be detected by Southern blot or PCR analysis. Gene rearrangement analysis has the advantage of detecting commit-

ment to B- or T-cell development at a very early stage of B- or
T-cell development, before surface immunoglobulin or T-cell
antigen expression occurs, e.g. in precursor B-ALL or T-ALL (B-
or T-acute lymphoblastic leukaemia) blast cells.

Cytogenetics

A chromosome abnormality characteristic of a particular tumour
acts as a clonal marker and helps define the various cell lineages
which are part of the clone. For example, the Philadelphia (Ph)
chromosome, found in myeloid cells of chronic myeloid
leukaemia (CML), has now been identified in this disease in
the erythroid and megakaryocytic cells as well as in B and
T lymphocytes and their precursors. Thus, the tumour is established as clonal and is presumed to arise from a multipotent
bone marrow stem cell which can give rise to all these different
cell types.

Chromosomal translocation analysis

If the tumour cells contain a chromosomal translocation, certain
genetic elements which have been exchanged will give different
restriction fragment lengths detected by Southern blotting, compared with normal cells in which the genetic elements are in the
normal non-translocated state. Restriction enzyme digestion and
a probe to the particular DNA sequence (e.g. an oncogene) which
has been translocated are needed. Alternatively, PCR techniques
can be used.

Point mutations

Certain tumours show particular mutations in their DNA compared with the original tissue, e.g. point mutations in the *RAS*
or *FMS* oncogenes in myelodysplasia or acute leukaemia. These
may be detected by RFLP analysis, by oligonucleotide probes or
by PCR (polymerase chain reaction) techniques (see p. 118). The
presence of the same mutation throughout the tumour tissue
indicates clonality.

Clonal progression

Some of the chromosomal translocations commonly associated
with different types of leukaemia and lymphoma are listed in
Table 10.2. In many cases of leukaemia and other tumours, the
disease develops new characteristics during its clinical course.
This may be accompanied by new chromosome changes. This is
illustrated by CML in which the clone present in the chronic
phase is replaced by a new clone when the disease enters the

Table 10.2 Some of the more frequent chromosomal abnormalities in leukaemia and lymphoma.

Disease	Chromosomal abnormality*	Oncogene(s) involved
Myeloid		
AML M$_2$	t(8;21)	AML1 (*CBFα*), *MTGA*
	t(6;9)	*DEK, CAN*
AML M$_3$	t(15;17)	*RARA, PML*
AML M$_4$	inv(16), del(16q)	*CBFβ, MYH*11
AML M$_5$	del(11q); t(9;11); t(11;19)	
AML M$_6$	+8	*MYC*
MDS	−5/del(5q)	*FMS* (in some), *IRF*
	−7/del(7q)	
CML	t(9;22)	*ABL, BCR*
Lymphoid		
	⎰ t(4;11)	*AF4 (FELL), MLL (ALL1, HRX)*
	⎪ t(9;22)	*ABL, BCR*
Precursor	⎨ t(1;19)	*PBX-1, E2A*
B lineage	⎪ Hyperdiploidy	
	⎱ Hypodiploidy	
Burkitt lymphoma,	⎰ t(8;14)†	*MYC*
B-ALL	⎨ t(2;8)	*MYC*
	⎱ t(8;22)	*MYC*
T-ALL	t(8;14)†	*MYC*
	t(11;14)	*RBTN-1* or *RBTN-2*
	t(10;14)	*HOX-11 (TCL3)*
	t(1;14)	*TAL-1*
	t(7;9)	*TAL-2*
	t(7;19)	*LYL-1*
Follicular	t(14;18)	*BCL-2*
lymphoma		
B lymphoma	t(11;14)†	*BCL-1*
B-CLL	t(14;19)	*BCL-3*
T-CLL	inv(14q) or t(14q)	

* Other chromosomal abnormalities may occur in many of the conditions listed.
† The breakpoints on chromosome 14 are in different positions in T-ALL, B-CLL and B-ALL or Burkitt's lymphoma. ALL, acute lymphoblastic leukaemia; AML, acute myeloid leukaemia; CLL, chronic lymphocytic leukaemia; CML, chronic myeloid leukaemia; *HOX*, homeobox; MDS, myelodysplasia; *PBX*-1, pre B-cell leukaemia transcription factor-1; *RARA*, retinoic acid receptor; *RBTN*, rhombotin gene; *TAL*, T-ALL oncogene; *MYH*, myosin heavy chain.

acute phase. In 70% of cases new chromosome changes are superimposed on the original Ph chromosome. Selection of sub-clones may occur during treatment, e.g. multi-drug-resistant clones or clones with other more malignant characteristics which may survive and proliferate prefentially in later stages of the disease.

Cells of origin of the leukaemias, lymphomas, myeloproliferative diseases and myeloma

There is now considerable evidence based on similarities of surface, intracytoplasmic and intranuclear antigens, biochemical

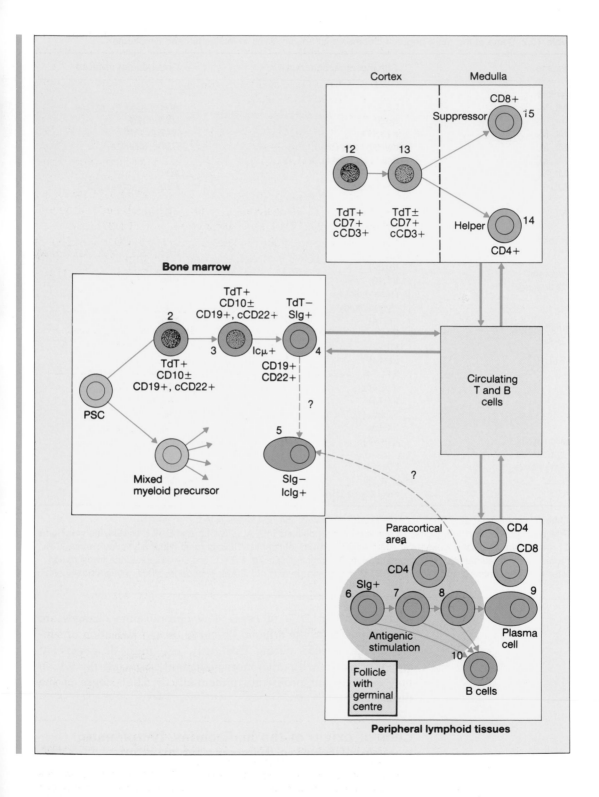

characteristics and on immunoglobulin and TCR gene rearrangement studies that the leukaemias, lymphomas, myeloproliferative diseases and multiple myeloma arise by clonal expansion of one or other particular cell in the marrow, thymus or peripheral lymphoid tissue (Fig. 10.3).

The acute leukaemias are associated with a predominance of lymphoblasts or myeloblasts in the marrow (see Chapter 11). *Acute lymphoblastic leukaemia* (ALL) is thought to arise from early cells in the lymphoid series. The most common form, precursor B-ALL, appears to arise from a population of very early B-lymphoid progenitors which have nuclear TdT (terminal deoxynucleotidyl transferase), show early B-cell antigenic markers (surface CD19 and intracytoplasmic CD22) and have rearranged immunoglobulin genes. If surface CD10 antigen is present, the disease has been termed common ALL. In some cases, the precursor B-ALL blasts (either CD10+ or CD10−)

Fig. 10.3 (*Opposite*) Diagram showing possible normal cells of origin in the bone marrow, peripheral lymphoid tissues and thymus of the leukaemias, lymphomas and myeloma.

Normal cell	Suggested derived tumour
Bone marrow	
1 PSC	Chronic myeloid leukaemia
2 Lymphoid progenitor	C-ALL*
3 Pre-B cell	Pre-B-ALL
4 B cell	B-ALL
5 Plasma cell	Multiple myeloma
11 Mixed myeloid precursors	AML
Peripheral lymphoid tissues	
6 'Virgin' peripheral B cells	} CLL, B-cell lymphomas
7 Follicular peripheral B cells (centrocytic, centroblastic, etc.)	
8 Lymphoplasmacytoid cells	Macroglobulinaemia
9 Peripheral plasma cell	Peripheral plasmacytoma
10 Coronal lymphocyte	B-prolymphocytic leukaemia
Thymus	
12 Large thymic cortical blast	} Thy-All, some T lymphomas
13 Thymic cortical cell	
14 T4+ cell	} Some T lymphomas, mycosis fungoides, T-prolymphocytic leukaemia and T-CLL (these probably arise in T cells in peripheral lymphoid tissues)
15 T8+ cell	

* Antigen present on surface of non-T, non-B lymphoid stem cells.
ALL, acute lymphoblastic leukaemia; c, cytoplasmic; CD, human cell surface markers; CLL, chronic lymphocytic leukaemia; IcIg, intracytoplasmic immunoglobulin; Icμ, intracytoplasmic μ heavy chain; PSC, pluripotential stem cell; SIg, surface immunoglobulin; TdT, terminal deoxynucleotidyl transferase.

have intracytoplasmic immunoglobulin and the disease is then termed pre-B-ALL. More mature ALL-expressing surface immunoglobulin is rare and termed B-ALL. About 10–20% of cases of ALL, termed T-ALL, arise from early cortical thymocytes. The blasts contain nuclear TdT, but in addition express the T antigens' surface CD7 and intracytoplasmic CD3 and have rearrangement of the TCR genes δ, γ and β.

Acute myeloid (myeloblastic) leukaemia (AML) probably arises from a pluripotent stem cell or myeloid progenitor, committed in varying degrees to the erythroid, granulocytic– monocytic and megakaryocytic lines. Typically, AML blasts express the surface antigens CD13 and CD33, are negative for nuclear TdT and have both the immunoglobulin and TCR receptor genes in the germ-line (unrearranged) configuration.

Chronic myeloid leukaemia (CML) probably derives from a stem cell, capable of entering both the myeloid or lymphoid lineages and, indeed, the disease may transform into either acute myeloid or acute lymphoblastic leukaemia. The other myeloproliferative diseases, *polycythaemia rubra vera*, myelo- fibrosis and *essential thrombocythaemia* and the myelodys- plastic syndromes also seem to be stem cell disorders based on G6PD isoenzyme, cytogenetic and X-linked RFLP analysis of the different cell lineages.

B-cell chronic lymphocytic leukaemia (CLL), the B-cell lymphomas, some cases of macroglobulinaemia and peripheral plasmacytomas are thought to arise from more mature cells in the bone marrow or peripheral lymphoid organs. The origin of myeloma is more controversial. A bone marrow origin in an early B-lymphoid cell has been postulated but recent evidence suggests an origin in a post-germinal centre B cell of the peri- pheral lymphoid tissues, the tumour cells then homing to the marrow, the main site of the disease. Certain unusual T-cell disorders, Sézary's syndrome, mycosis fungoides, some T-cell lymphomas and the rare T-CLL, appear to arise from more mature T cells, either in the thymus or in the peripheral lymphoid tissues. Current evidence suggests that the malignant cell in Hodgkin's disease arises in peripheral lymphoid tissue from an early lymphoid cell genotypically either B or T, although, as in the other neoplasms, the predominant malignant cells have more mature features than the presumed cell of origin of the clone.

The reason why particular cells of the marrow or lymphoid tissue are prone to malignant transformation is unclear. Cells of the lymphoid system appear to be particularly liable to transform at the stage of their development when gene rearrangements are occurring. Why the malignant clones escape partly or completely from normal physiological control factors is also uncertain. Loss of adhesion molecules (see p. 148) from the cell surface may allow them to enter the peripheral blood at an immature stage and also to escape normal surveillance, e.g. by natural killer cells. It is an intriguing observation that different leukaemias (or lymphomas) are prone to occur at different ages, e.g. CD10+ precursor B-ALL is most common in children aged about 4 years, AML occurs at any age with almost equal incidence, CML occurs particularly in young- and middle-aged adults, while myelodysplasia, myeloma, polycythaemia rubra vera and CLL are diseases predominantly of older people.

Malignant transformation

Much is now known about the molecular changes in haemopoietic cells associated with malignant transformation, and general aspects of this with specific examples in individual haemopoietic neoplasms are discussed next.

Oncogenes

Changes in the function of certain normal genes known as cellular oncogenes (or proto-oncogenes, now commonly called oncogenes) may lead to malignant transformation of the normal cells. These genes are part of the normal genetic make up and code for proteins involved in cell proliferation, survival or differentiation (Fig. 10.4). Oncogenes were first discovered as the transforming (from normal to malignant) elements (v-oncs) of acutely transforming retroviruses (see p. 205). These viruses cause tumours in animals but have not been described to cause tumours in humans. v-oncs were subsequently shown to have been 'transduced' by the viruses from oncogenes of normal mammalian DNA. Oncogenes are generally named after the mammalian species in which virus-induced tumours were first reported (Table 10.3).

Table 10.3 Cellular oncogenes and tumour-suppressor genes implicated in human leukaemias and lymphomas.

Extracellular growth factor	*SIS*
Membrane-associated tyrosine kinases (including growth factor receptors)	*FMS, KIT, ERB*-B
Intracellular signal transducers	
GTP-binding	H-*RAS*, K-*RAS*, N-*RAS*
Serine–threonine kinases	*MOS, PIM, RAF*
Nuclear	
Transcription factors	*JUN, FOS, MYC, MYB, ETS, TAL*-1, *TAL*-2, *PBX*
Hormone receptor	*ERB*-A
Tyrosine kinase	*ABL**
Tumour suppressor (recessive)	p53, Rb
Mitochondrial (inhibits apoptosis)	*BCL*-2
Unknown	*BCL*-1

* The *BCR–ABL* fusion protein found in CML is cytoplasmic.

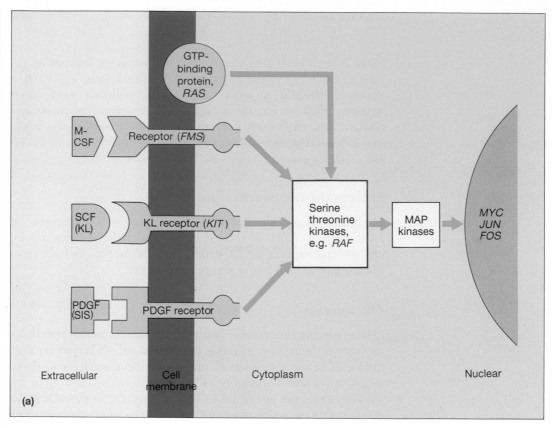

(a)

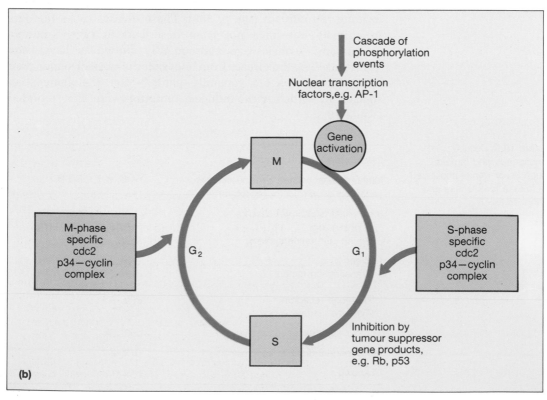

(b)

Classification

Oncogenes are highly conserved genes which have been found in many species ranging from yeasts through fruit flies and primates, to man. Oncogenes are widely distributed among human chromosomes. They may be classified according to the function or presumed function of the protein for which they code (see Table 10.3). The products of tumour-suppressor genes or anti-oncogenes tend to inhibit the process of cell division and proliferation (see below).

Function of protein products

Extracellular growth factors

The best example of this is c-*SIS* which codes for the β chain of platelet-derived growth factor (PDGF). PDGF stimulates mitogenesis and growth of a variety of cells mainly of connective tissue origin.

Membrane-associated tyrosine kinases (including growth factor receptors)

These growth factor receptors are composed of three domains: an extracellular ligand-binding portion, a transmembrane portion and a cytoplasmic portion which, in response to ligand binding, induces phosphorylation of various proteins, including the receptor itself (see Fig. 1.8, p. 9). This phosphorylation occurs specifically on tyrosine residues. *FMS* and *KIT*, which code for the receptors for monocyte colony-stimulating factor (M-CSF) and stem cell factor (SCF or kit ligand) respectively, are typical oncogenes coding for growth factor receptors.

Intracellular signal transducers

These proteins regulate the levels of intracellular second messengers normally in response to the binding of growth factors to their receptors. They include:
1 *RAS proteins.* N-*RAS*, H-*RAS* and K-*RAS* encode proteins of 21 000 MW (p21 *RAS*) which are weakly homologous to classical G proteins. The *RAS* proteins bind GTP (guanosine triphosphate) which is hydrolysed to GDP (guanosine diphosphate) by

Fig. 10.4 (*Opposite*) (a) Examples of oncogene products which act at different stages of the pathways by which growth signals are transduced through the cell membrane into the nucleus. The signal may activate the cell into cycle (as in this figure) or cause functional activation or differentiation. (b) A simplified diagram of the cell cycle to show the involvement of nuclear transcription factors, the cdc2 p34−cyclin complex and tumour-suppressor genes. GTP, guanosine triphosphate; KL, kit ligand; M, mitosis; MAP, mitogen-activated protein; M-CSF, monocyte colony-stimulating factor; PDGF, platelet-derived growth factor; S, DNA synthetic phase; SCF, stem cell factor.

an intrinsic GTPase activity of the molecule. When *RAS* is bound to GTP, the protein is 'active' and stimulates cell division. A second protein, GAP (GTPase-activating protein), binds to the *RAS* protein and stimulates the intrinsic rate of GTP hydrolysis.

2 *Serine—threonine kinases.* These phosphorylate proteins on serine or threonine residues rather than on tyrosine.

Nuclear oncogenes

These can be classified into three groups:

1 *Transcription factors*: The protein products of these factors bind to DNA at the promoter sequences of a variety of genes and regulate their transcription (see Fig. 10.4b). The transcription factors involved in human leukaemia/lymphoma largely fall into five families: helix-loop-helix, homeobox, zinc finger, LIM and REL.

2 Certain hormone receptors also function as transcriptional regulators in a like manner. These include receptors for various steroids including the oestrogen and glucocorticoid receptors.

3 The protein coded for by *ABL*, a tyrosine kinase, appears to be normally localized to the nucleus. Its function is unknown. When it is translocated to the *BCR* region on chromosome 22 in the Philadelphia translocation, the resulting *BCR—ABL* fusion protein is localized to the cytoplasm.

Tumour-suppressor genes (recessive oncogenes, anti-oncogenes)

Although the exact normal function of the tumour-suppressor genes (e.g. p53, Rb) is unclear, in general they appear to act as components of feedback control mechanisms which regulate entry of the cell from the G_1 phase of the cell cycle into the S phase and passage through the S phase to G_2 and mitosis (see Fig. 10.4b). Their protein products are often located in the nucleus. Loss of function of these tumour-suppressor genes by deletion or mutational 'inactivation' may be one event in a multi-step process in tumour development. Homozygous loss or inactivation is found in many tumours and is particularly associated with progression of a tumour to a more malignant phenotype. Loss of one tumour-suppressor gene allele may be inherited and so predisposes to the development of tumours if the second allele becomes mutated or deleted. This underlies the frequency of some tumours, e.g. retinoblastoma, in certain families.

Prevention of cell death

The oncogene *BCL*-2 codes for a protein which inhibits cell death by apoptosis.

Table 10.4 Mechanism of activation of proto-oncogenes in human leukaemias.

Chromosome translocations and rearrangements

Point mutations

Inactivation

Amplification

Activation of oncogenes in haematological malignancies

There is an obvious link between the activation of oncogenes or loss of function of tumour-suppressor genes and the disturbed balance between cell proliferation and differentiation which is a characteristic of malignancy. One activation event is often insufficient to cause malignant transformation. Multiple alterations within one oncogene or changes in two or more oncogenes or tumour-suppressor genes appear to be necessary for the cell to reach a fully malignant phenotype. The mechanisms by which the normal cellular oncogenes may be activated are listed in Table 10.4 and include the following.

Translocation and rearrangements

These are the best studied mechanisms and frequently occur in leukaemias and lymphomas (see Table 10.2). Aberrant activity of the recombinase enzyme which is involved in immunoglobulin or T-cell receptor gene rearrangement in immature B or T cells is important in generating translocations in lymphoid malignancies. DNA sequences involved in normal VDJ rearrangements (see p. 169) are often found at translocation breakpoints. Some translocations fuse parts of two genes. The resulting chimeric gene encodes a fusion protein, e.g. *BCR-ABL* in t(9;22) in CML (see Fig. 10.6b), *RARA-PML* in t(15;17) in AML M_3 or *E2A-PBX*-1 in t(1;19) in pre-B-ALL. Translocations involving oncogenes which occur in the myeloid and lymphoid malignancies are illustrated by those involving the oncogenes *RARA*, *MYC*, *ABL* and *BCL*-2 and are discussed next.

Retinoic acid receptor (RARA)

In the 15;17 translocation associated with AML M_3 in the FAB classification (see p. 210), the *RARA* is translocated from chromosome 17 to chromosome 15. A chimeric gene is created between *RARA* and a locus, termed *PML* (promyelocytic) leukaemia. The *PML-RARA* chimeric gene produces a fusion protein which localizes to the nucleus. How it disturbs cell proliferation and differentiation is unclear. The disease responds to treatment with high doses of *trans*-retinoic acid which causes differentiation of the abnormal promyelocytes (see p. 229).

MYC

In Burkitt's lymphoma and B-ALL, one of three translocations is found (most frequently t(8;14)) all of which bring the *MYC* oncogene into close proximity with one of the immunoglobulin

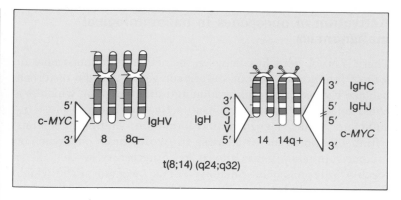

Fig. 10.5 Diagram to show the genetic events in one of the three translocations found in Burkitt's lymphoma and B-acute lymphoblastic leukaemia. The oncogene c-*MYC* is normally located on the long arm (q) of chromosome 8. In the 8;14 translocation, c-*MYC* is translocated into close proximity to the immunoglobulin heavy chain gene on the long arm of chromosome 14. Part of the heavy chain gene (the V region) is reciprocally translocated to chromosome 8. C, constant region; IgH, immunoglobulin heavy chain gene; J, joining region; V, variable region.

genes (Fig. 10.5). Immunoglobulin genes normally rearrange during B-cell development and it is at this point in development that they may be prone to this pathological translocation. As a result, expression of the *MYC* gene is deregulated and the gene is expressed in parts of the cell cycle during which it should normally be switched off.

ABL

In the Ph translocation 5′ exons of *BCR* are fused to the 3′ exons of *ABL* (Fig. 10.6). The resulting chimeric *BCR-ABL* gene codes for a fusion protein of size 210 kDa (p210). This has tyrosine kinase activity in excess of the normal 145 kDa *ABL* product.

The Ph translocation is observed in CML and in a minority of cases of ALL, and rarely in AML. The same molecular defect has also been found in a proportion of patients with otherwise undistinguishable CML who did not show the Ph chromosome by conventional light microscopy (Fig. 10.7).

In some cases of Ph+ ALL, the breakpoint in *BCR* occurs in the same region as in CML. In other cases of Ph+ ALL, however, the breakpoint in *BCR* is further upstream, in the intron between the first and second exons, leaving only the first *BCR* exon intact. This chimeric *BCR-ABL* gene is expressed as a p190 protein which like p210 has enhanced tyrosine kinase activity. There is speculation that patients with ALL expressing p190 are truly *de novo* cases of ALL, whereas patients with ALL expressing p210 are really cases of CML, transformed into lymphoid blast crisis with no detectable previous chronic phase, but there is no clinical evidence for this.

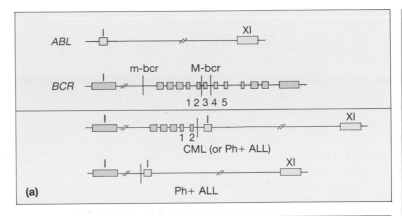

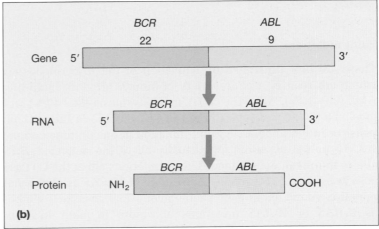

Fig. 10.6 (a) Schematic representation of the *BCR* and *ABL* genes showing known exons (indicated as boxes); introns are shown as lines. The arabic numerals below the *BCR* genes identify the exons within the major (M-bcr) breakpoint cluster region. Representative positions for the breakpoints in CML and Ph+ ALL are shown as vertical lines. The region of the first intron on the *BCR* gene involved in some cases of Ph+ ALL is known as the minor *BCR* (m-bcr) region. (b) The fusion gene gives rise to a chimeric protein. The fusion gene in M-bcr gives rise to a protein of MW 210 000 (p210) whereas the fusion gene in m-bcr gives rise to a protein of MW 190 000 (p190) (see Fig. 10.7).

BCL-2

This oncogene is translocated from chromosome 18 to chromosome 14 in the (14;18) translocation found in about 85% of cases of follicular lymphoma and in some cases of diffuse lymphoma and B-CLL.

The translocation *BCL*-2 gene is over-expressed. The *BCL*-2 protein is localized to the inner mitochondrial membrane and prevents programmed cell death (apoptosis) of the tumour cells.

Normal	Ph−, bcr − → p145	
CML	Ph+, bcr + → p210	
	Ph−, bcr + → p210	
	Ph−, bcr − → p145	(atypical cases; ?myelodysplasia)
ALL	Ph+, bcr + → p210	(?blast transformation of CML)
	Ph+, bcr − → p190	(?*de novo* ALL)
	Ph−, bcr − → p145	(*de novo* ALL)

Fig. 10.7 Patterns of involvement of the Philadelphia chromosome, the major bcr (5.8 kb) region and *ABL* tyrosine protein kinase in CML (chronic myeloid leukaemia) and ALL (acute lymphoblastic leukaemia). bcr+ is the rearrangement within the major bcr region; p is the molecular weight of tyrosine kinase.

Point mutations

These are best illustrated by activation of the *RAS* oncogenes which are seen in a wide variety of human tumours including AML (20−30%), ALL (15−20%), myelodysplasia (20−40%) and myeloma (20%), but typically not in CLL or CML in the chronic phase or in lymphomas. A point mutation in one of three codons (12, 13 or 61) accounts for virtually all of the activated *RAS* alleles in human malignancy. These mutations affect the GTPase activity of the p21 protein. Activation of N-*RAS* is the usual mutation found in human haemopoietic malignancies, whereas K-*RAS* or H-*RAS* mutations are more frequent in non-haemopoietic tumours. *RAS* mutations may occur in *de novo* cases of myelodysplasia or AML and disappear in later phases of the disease, or they may appear in later stages suggesting they can be an early or late event in the multistep process of tumour development.

Point mutations have also been described in the *FMS* oncogene in cases of myelodysplasia and AML. Exactly how these affect the function of the product, the M-CSF receptor, is still unclear, but constitutive (in the absence of M-CSF binding) activation of the M-CSF receptor tyrosine kinase activity seems likely.

Inactivation

Biallelic loss or functional inactivation of tumour-suppressor genes may lead to tumour development. This is best documented for the retinoblastoma gene both in the development of retinoblastomas in families where loss of one allele is inherited and in AML where loss or mutation of both alleles is acquired.

Biallelic inactivation has also been described for the p53 gene in patients with CML in blast transformation, *de novo* AML or myelodysplasia. Alteration of one allele may, however, also have a dominant effect if the mutated protein product interferes with the function of the product of the normal allele.

Amplification

Although this is a well-documented mechanism of oncogene overexpression in animal and some human tumours, its role in human haemopoietic neoplasms is probably minor. Oncogene amplification may be a feature of tumour progression and duplication of the Ph chromosome is one of the features of progression of CML from chronic to an accelerated or acute phase, but whether this acceleration is caused by increased expression of the *BCR−ABL* fusion protein is unknown.

Gains or losses of all or parts of the chromosomes are common in the leukaemias and myelodysplasias. Gains are common in chromosomes 8, 12, 19, 21 and Y; losses most commonly affect chromosomes 5, 6, 7, 11, 20 and Y. Some of these numerical abnormalities result in extra copies of oncogenes (e.g. of *MYC* and *MOS* in +8) or loss of one allele (e.g. of *FMS* in −5q). It is likely that expression of the corresponding oncogene is altered.

Retroviral infection as a cause of haematological malignancy

Retroviruses are RNA viruses which contain the enzyme reverse transcriptase which converts viral RNA into DNA which then integrates with host cell DNA (Fig. 10.8). Human immuno-deficiency virus (HIV) which causes the disease AIDS (acquired immune deficiency syndrome) is a retrovirus (see Fig. 9.12). HTLV-1 (human T-cell lymphotrophic virus) is believed to cause the disease adult T-cell leukaemia/lymphoma (ATLL) (see p. 270) but the exact mechanism is uncertain. HTLV-1 lacks an oncogene and the DNA from the virus does not integrate into host DNA close to a known oncogene and the integration site is different in different patients.

Inherited and acquired predisposition to leukaemia and lymphoma

The evidence that activated oncogenes are involved in leukaemo-genesis is generally indirect but it has been possible to reproduce some leukaemias resembling those in humans in transgenic mice, in which activated oncogenes are introduced into the germ-line, e.g. a CML-like disease may be produced in mice by the *BCR−ABL* fusion gene producing p210 while an ALL-like disease is caused by introduction of the p190 fusion gene. Nevertheless, in human leukaemias, a similar oncogene abnormality may be associated with different types of disease,

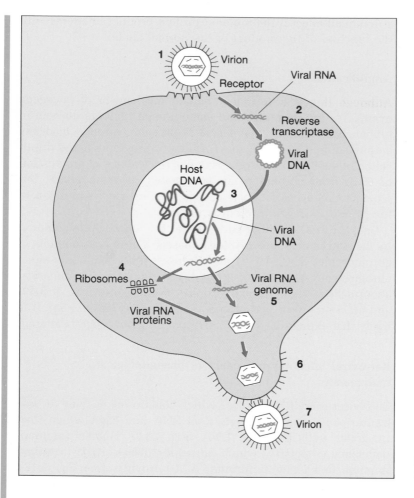

Fig. 10.8 The life cycle of a retrovirus.

e.g. *BCR−ABL* rearrangement with p210 expression in both chronic phase CML and in ALL.

How the translocations, mutations and other changes in oncogenes listed above are brought about in the development of human leukaemias (and other tumours) is largely obscure. Certain constitutional and acquired disorders predispose to leukaemia but it is difficult in each case to relate the DNA abnormalities in these disorders to changes in function of known oncogenes. It seems that several factors including host susceptibility, and chemical, physical and radiation damage to chromosomes may all be involved in oncogene activation (Fig. 10.9).

1 *Hereditary*. There is a greatly increased incidence of leukaemia in some hereditary diseases, particularly Down's syndrome (where ALL, or less frequently AML, occurs with a 20−30-fold increased frequency), Bloom's syndrome, Fanconi anaemia, ataxia−telangiectasia, Klinefelter's syndrome, osteogenesis imperfecta and Wiskott−Aldrich syndrome. There is also an

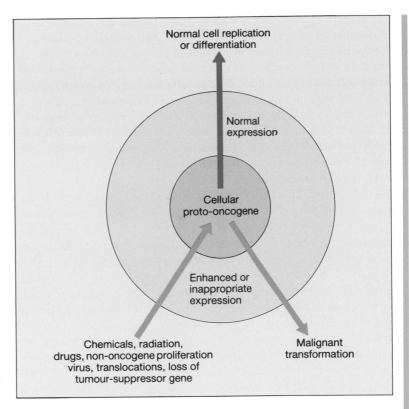

Normal cell replication
or differentiation

Normal
expression

Cellular
proto-oncogene

Enhanced or
inappropriate
expression

Chemicals, radiation,
drugs, non-oncogene proliferation
virus, translocations, loss of
tumour-suppressor gene

Malignant
transformation

Fig. 10.9 Possible
mechanisms of oncogenesis
due to enhanced or
inappropriate expression of an
oncogene.

increased risk if a sibling has acute leukaemia and this risk is
substantially greater in the case of identical twins and in certain
high-risk families. The explanations for these findings are largely
unknown. Inherited lack of one allele for a tumour-suppressor
gene occurs in some cancer-prone families. The somatic cells of
patients with Fanconi anaemia and Bloom's syndrome which
show multiple chromosome breaks are more susceptible to
oncogenic viral transformation *in vitro*.

2 *Chemicals.* Chronic exposure to benzene may cause bone
marrow hypoplasia, dysplasia and chromosome abnormalities
and is an unusual cause of myelodysplasia or AML. Other
industrial solvents and chemicals may less commonly cause
leukaemia.

The alkylating agents, e.g. chlorambucil, mustine, melphelan,
procarbazine and nitrosoureas (e.g. BCNU, CCNU) predispose to
AML especially if combined with radiotherapy or if used to treat
patients with lymphocytic or plasmacytic disorders. Direct
damage to DNA and/or immunosuppression causing reduction
of host resistance to neoplasms are likely mechanisms.

3 *Radiation*, especially to the marrow, is leukaemogenic. This
is illustrated by survivors of the atom bomb explosions in Japan
who were irradiated and by patients with ankylosing spondylitis.

The effects of radiation are also shown by the increased risk of leukaemia in children born to mothers who received abdominal X-rays during pregnancy or, in one as yet unconfirmed study, in children of fathers who work in nuclear reprocessing plants, and by patients given extended field irradiation (e.g. for lymphomas). Some population studies have shown an increased incidence of leukaemia in families living close to electrical pylons or exposed to high levels of radioactive radon gas. Exactly how radiation predisposes to leukaemia is unknown. Chromosomal breaks and recombinations and activation of oncogenes by point mutations are potential mechanisms.

4 *Predisposing haematological diseases.* AML occurs with an increased incidence in patients with CML, myeloproliferative diseases (polycythaemia vera, myelofibrosis and essential thrombocythaemia), myelodysplasia, paroxysmal nocturnal haemoglobinuria, aplastic anaemia, multiple myeloma and Hodgkin's disease. This seems to be due to clonal progression often with new chromosomal abnormalities in a disease of stem or very early progenitor cells. The nature of the precipitating factor for this 'second event' is unclear.

5 *Viruses.* These seem more important in the aetiology of leukaemia in animals and birds than in humans. As mentioned on p. 270 a viral aetiology is established in ATLL. HTLV-1 has been demonstrated by electron microscopy and by cell culture in the cells of patients with this disease. However, many people infected with this virus (and so anti-HTLV-1 positive) do not develop the tumour.

Epstein—Barr virus (EBV) DNA has been found integrated into the genome of endemic (African) Burkitt lymphoma cells but not into the genome of sporadic Burkitt lymphoma cells. The EBV genome is also present in the tumour cells of patients developing lymphomas who were receiving immunosuppressive therapy after solid organ (e.g. kidney or heart) transplantation, in many AIDS patients developing lymphomas, and has also been detected in the cells of a proportion of patients with Hodgkin's disease. All these patients have disturbed T-cell immunity (e.g. due to chronic malaria in the case of endemic Burkitt lymphoma). Correction of this by discontinuation of immunosuppressive therapy post-transplantation may result in spontaneous resolution of the tumour.

Indirect evidence for a virus aetiology is the rare occurrence of leukaemia in cells of donor origin in patients following bone marrow transplantation for acute leukaemia. Nevertheless, numerous attempts to identify viruses in patients with AML, ALL, CML or CLL have been unsuccessful.

Chromosome, gene rearrangement and oncogene studies in diagnosis and disease monitoring

The detection of chromosome or oncogene abnormalities (e.g. the Ph translocation or *BCR−ABL* fusion gene or the *BCL*-2 translocation or of clonal immunoglobulin or TCR gene rearrangement by Southern blotting or by the PCR technique) may be important in several aspects of the management of patients with leukaemia or lymphoma.

1 *For initial diagnosis* of the type of leukaemia, lymphoma or myeloproliferative disorder. A clonal immunoglobulin gene rearrangement occurs in a B-cell tumour and a clonal T-cell receptor rearrangement in a T-cell tumour. Cross-lineage gene rearrangements occasionally occur, however (e.g. of the T-cell

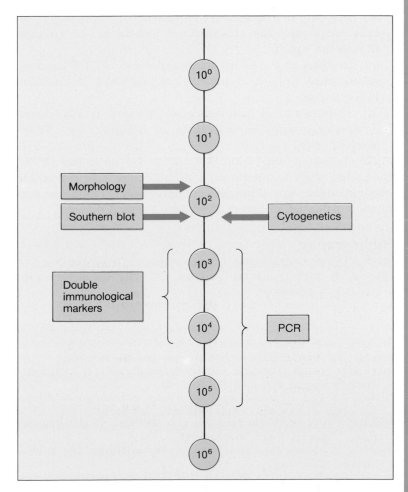

Fig. 10.10 Sensitivity of detection of leukaemic cells in bone marrow using five different techniques. $10^1 - 10^6 = 1$ cell in 10 to 1 cell in 10^6 detected.

receptor in precursor B-ALL or of the immunoglobulin genes in T-ALL), so the analysis must be interpreted with caution.

2 *For establishing prognosis*, e.g. in ALL where cytogenetic findings may give independent prediction of the possibility for cure by chemotherapy/radiotherapy alone. For instance, Ph+ ALL has a particularly poor prognosis, whereas hyperdiploidy in ALL is a favourable finding.

3 *Monitoring the response to therapy* (Fig. 10.10). The detection of minimal residual disease (disease which cannot be seen by conventional staining and microscopy of the blood or bone marrow) in AML, ALL or CML after chemotherapy or bone marrow transplantation is possible using:

(a) cytogenetic analysis (which will detect residual leukaemic cells only if they are dividing so making chromosome analysis possible); *in situ* hybridization techniques can be used, however, to detect, e.g. monosomy and trisomy of interphase cells;

(b) detection of translocated or mutated oncogenes by the PCR technique. The abnormalities present in the original disease are sought;

(c) detection of the clonal immunoglobulin or TCR gene re-arrangement present in the original leukaemic clone using PCR analysis;

(d) combination of immunological markers which detect 'leukaemia-specific' combinations of antigens, e.g. TdT+ myeloid cells.

The molecular tests using PCR may detect up to one in 10^5 cells. They must be interpreted with caution because of possible changes in genotype of the cells with progression of disease, and possible patchy distribution of minimal residual disease.

Bibliography

Bishop J.M. (1991) Molecular themes in oncogenes. *Cell*, **64**, 235−248.

Catovsky D. (ed.) (1991) *The Leukemic Cell*, 2nd Edition. Churchill Livingstone, Edinburgh.

Glover D.M. & Haines B.D. (eds) (1989) *Oncogenes*. Oxford University Press, Oxford.

Green A.R. (1992) Transcription factors, translocations and haematological malignancies. *Blood Reviews*, **6**, 118−124.

Marshall C.J. (1991) Tumour suppressor genes. *Cell*, **64**, 313−326.

Potter M.N. (1992) Detection of minimal residual disease in acute lympho-blastic leukaemia. *Blood Reviews*, **6**, 68−82.

Rabbitts T.H. (1991) Translocations, master genes, and differences between the origins of acute and chronic leukaemias. *Cell*, **67**, 641−644.

Rowley J.D. (1990) Molecular cytogenetics: Rosetta Stone for understanding cancer. *Cancer Research*, **50**, 3816−3825.

Sandberg A. (1990) *The Chromosomes in Human Cancer*, 2nd Edition. Elsevier, Amsterdam.

Sawyers C.L., Denny C.T. & Witte O.N. (1991) Leukaemia and the disruption of normal haematopoiesis. *Cell*, **64**, 337−350.

Wiernik P.H., Canellos G.P., Kyle R.A. & Schiffer C.A. (eds) (1991) *Neo-plastic Diseases of the Blood*, 2nd Edition. Churchill Livingstone, Edinburgh.

Chapter 11
Acute Leukaemias

The leukaemias are a group of disorders characterized by the accumulation of abnormal white cells in the bone marrow. These abnormal cells may cause bone marrow failure, a raised circulating white cell count and infiltrate organs. Thus common but not essential features include abnormal white cells in the peripheral blood, a raised total white cell count, evidence of bone marrow failure (i.e. anaemia, neutropenia, thrombocytopenia) in the acute leukaemias, and involvement of other organs (e.g. liver, spleen, lymph nodes, meninges, brain, skin or testes).

Classification of leukaemia

The main classification is into acute and chronic leukaemia (Table 11.1). Acute leukaemia, in which there are over 50% myeloblasts or lymphoblasts in the bone marrow at clinical presentation, is further subdivided into acute myeloid (myeloblastic) leukaemia (AML) and acute lymphoblastic leukaemia (ALL) on the basis of morphology and cytochemistry. AML is further subdivided into eight variants on a morphological basis according to the French–American–British (FAB) scheme (Table 11.2). ALL is subdivided on a morphological basis according to the FAB classification into L_1, L_2 and L_3 types. Immunophenotyping, chromosome and gene rearrangement studies are also used to distinguish AML from ALL and to subclassify them.

The chronic leukaemias comprise two main types, chronic myeloid leukaemia (CML) and chronic lymphocytic (lymphatic) leukaemia (CLL). Other chronic types include hairy cell leukaemia, prolymphocytic leukaemia and various leukaemia/lymphoma syndromes. In addition, there are a variety of myelodysplastic syndromes, some of which are regarded as chronic or 'smouldering' forms of leukaemia and others as 'pre-leukaemia' (see Chapter 12).

The acute leukaemias

Pathogenesis

The leukaemic cell population in ALL and AML probably result from clonal proliferation by successive divisions from a single

Acute (see Table 11.2)
- Acute myeloid (myeloblastic) leukaemia (AML): M_0-M_7
- Acute lymphoblastic leukaemia (ALL): L_1, L_2, L_3, precursor B-ALL, B-ALL, T-ALL

Chronic (see Table 12.1)
- Chronic myeloid (granulocytic) leukaemia (CML/CGL)
- Chronic lymphocytic (lymphatic) leukaemia (CLL)
- Other chronic lymphoid leukaemias, e.g. hairy cell, prolymphocytic, lymphoma/leukaemia syndromes

Myelodysplastic syndromes (see Table 12.6)

Table 11.1 Classification of leukaemias.

AML	ALL
M_0 undifferentiated	L_1 blast cells small, uniform high nuclear to cytoplasmic ratio
M_1 without maturation	
M_2 with granulocytic maturation	L_2 blast cells larger, heterogenous, lower nuclear to cytoplasmic ratio
M_3 acute promyelocytic	
M_4 granulocytic and monocytic maturation	L_3 vacuolated blasts, basophilic cytoplasm (usually B-ALL)
M_5 monoblastic or monocytic	*NB* Both L_1 and L_2 include cases of c-ALL, pre-B-ALL, null-ALL and T-ALL (see Table 11.4), which are indistinguishable on conventional (Romanowsky) morphology
M_6 erythroleukaemia	
M_7 megakaryoblastic	

ALL, acute lymphoblastic leukaemia; AML, acute myeloid leukaemia.

Table 11.2 Classification of acute leukaemia according to the French–American–British (FAB) group.

abnormal stem or progenitor cell (see p. 187). The possible mechanisms of leukaemic transformation, abnormalities of the leukaemic cell and the conditions that predispose to leukaemic transformation have been discussed in Chapter 10. In acute leukaemia the blast cells fail to differentiate normally but are capable of further divisions. Their accumulation results in replacement of the normal haemopoietic precursor cells of the bone marrow by myeloblasts or lymphoblasts and, ultimately, in bone marrow failure. The clinical condition of the patient can be correlated with the total number of leukaemic cells in the body (see Fig. 11.9). When the abnormal cell number approaches 10^{12} the patient is usually gravely ill with severe bone marrow failure. Peripheral blood involvement by the leukaemic cells and infiltration of organs such as the spleen, liver and lymph nodes may not occur until the leukaemic cell population comprises 60% or more of the marrow cell total.

The disease may be recognized by conventional morphology only when blast cells in the marrow exceed 5% of the cell total (unless the blast cells have some particular abnormal feature, e.g. Auer rods in AML). This corresponds to a total cell count in excess of 10^8. The term 'relapse' is applied to this detectable state after a complete remission has been induced by treatment. When the number of leukaemic cells is 5% or less in the bone marrow, the leukaemia is usually undetectable by conventional morphology and termed in 'complete remission' if the blood count is also normal and the patient clinically well with no other symptoms of the disease. Using modern sensitive cyto-genetic, molecular biological or immunological techniques 'minimal residual disease' may, however, be detectable although the blood and marrow appear normal.

The clinical presentation and mortality in acute leukaemia arises mainly from neutropenia, thrombocytopenia and anaemia because of bone marrow failure and, less commonly, from organ infiltration, e.g. of the meninges or testes.

Incidence

The acute leukaemias comprise over half of the leukaemias seen in clinical practice. ALL is the common form in children; its incidence is highest at 3−4 years, falling off by 10 years. The common (CD10+) precursor B type which is most usual in children has an equal sex incidence; however, there is a male predominance for T-ALL which, like null (CD10−)-ALL, has a later peak age incidence. There is a lower frequency of ALL after 10 years of age with a secondary rise after the age of 40. AML occurs in all age groups. It is the common form of acute leukaemia in adults, including the elderly, and is the usual type to complicate myelodysplasia (see p. 245) and other haematological diseases. AML forms only a minor fraction (10−15%) of the leukaemias in childhood.

Clinical features

Due to bone marrow failure
1 Pallor, lethargy and dyspnoea from anaemia.
2 Fever, malaise, features of mouth, throat, skin, respiratory, perianal or other infections (Fig. 11.1), including septicaemia, are common. The organisms involved are considered in detail below (see p. 220).
3 Spontaneous bruises, purpura, bleeding gums, menorrhagia and bleeding from venepuncture sites because of thrombo-cytopenia are common (Fig. 11.2). Occasionally there is a major internal haemorrhage. A bleeding tendency due to thrombo-cytopenia and disseminated intravascular coagulation (DIC) is characteristic of the promyelocytic variant of AML, AML M_3.

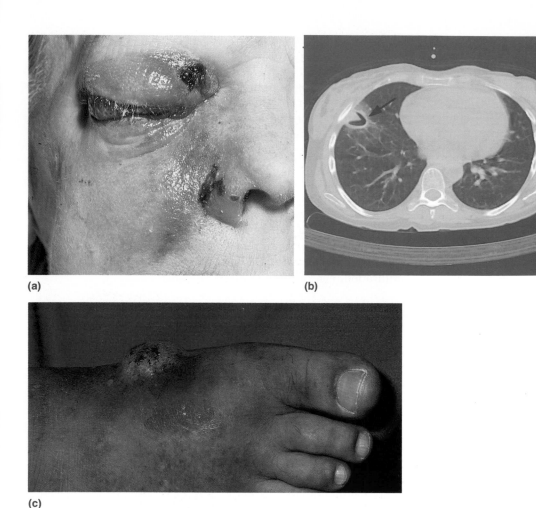

(a)   (b)

(c)

Fig. 11.1 (a) An orbital infection in a female patient (aged 68 years) with acute myeloblastic leukaemia and severe neutropenia (haemoglobin 8.3 g/dl, white cells 15.3 × 10⁹/l, blasts 96%, neutrophils 1%, platelets 30 × 10⁹/l). (b) CT scan of a chest showing cavitating mass (arrowed) in the periphery of the right upper lobe which at operation (lobectomy) proved to be an aspergilloma. (c) Skin infection (*Pseudomonas aeruginosa*) in a female patient (aged 33 years) with acute lymphoblastic leukaemia receiving chemotherapy and with severe neutropenia (haemoglobin 10.1 g/dl, white cells 0.7 × 10⁹/l, neutrophils < 0.1 × 10⁹/l, lymphocytes 0.6 × 10⁹/l, platelets 20 × 10⁹/l).

Due to organ infiltration
1 Tender bones, especially in children.
2 Superficial lymphadenopathy in ALL (Fig. 11.3).
3 Moderate splenomegaly, hepatomegaly especially in ALL.
4 Gum hypertrophy and infiltration (Fig. 11.4), skin involvement, particularly in the myelomonocytic (M_4) and monocytic (M_5) types. Lysosyme released by the blast cells may cause renal damage with potassium leakage and hypokalaemia in AML M_5.
5 Meningeal syndrome, particularly in ALL and more rarely

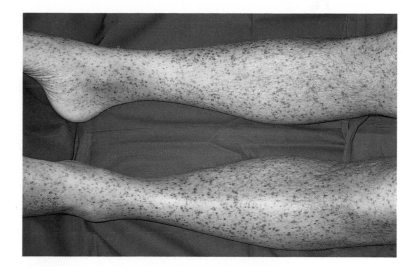

Fig. 11.2 Purpura over the lower limbs in a male patient (aged 53 years) with acute myeloblastic leukaemia (haemoglobin 6.1 g/dl, white cells 20×10^9/l with 90% blasts, platelets 5×10^9/l).

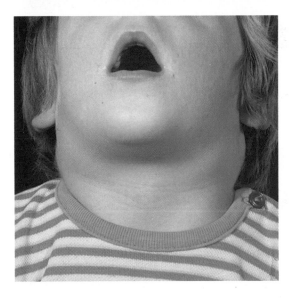

Fig. 11.3 Acute lymphoblastic leukaemia: marked cervical lymphadenopathy in a boy. (Courtesy of Professor J.M. Chessels.)

AML especially M_4, M_5 subtypes—headache, nausea and vomiting, blurring of vision and diplopia. Fundal examination may reveal papilloedema and sometimes haemorrhage.

6 Other occasional manifestations of organ infiltration include testicular swelling in ALL or signs of mediastinal compression in T-ALL (Fig. 11.5).

Laboratory findings

Haematological investigations may reveal the following:

1 A normochromic normocytic anaemia.

2 The total white cell count may be decreased, normal or increased up to 200×10^9/l or more.

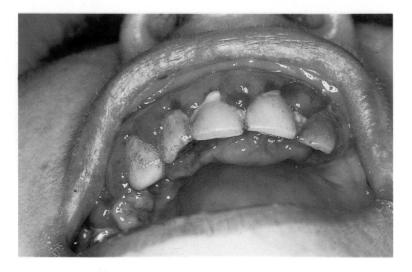

Fig. 11.4 Acute myeloid
leukaemia FAB type M$_5$
(monocytic): the gums are
swollen and haemorrhagic
due to infiltration by leukaemic
cells.

3 Thrombocytopenia in most cases, often extreme in AML.
4 Blood film examination typically shows variable numbers of
blast cells. In AML, the blasts may contain Auer rods (Fig. 11.6)
and other abnormal cells may be present, e.g. promyelocytes,
myelocytes, agranular neutrophils, pseudo-Pelger cells or myelomonocytic cells. In AML M$_6$ (erythroleukaemia) many erythro-

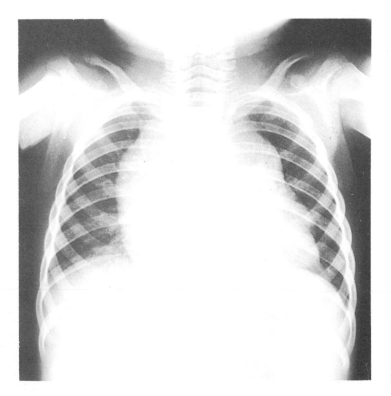

Fig. 11.5 Chest X-ray of a
boy aged 6 years with Thy-
ALL. There is a large
mediastinal mass due to
thymic enlargement.

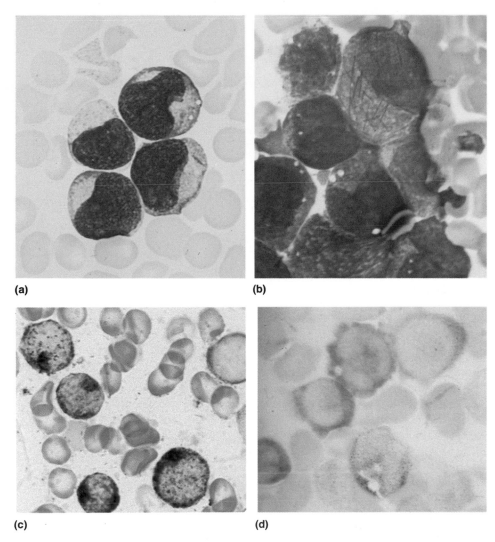

(a)   (b)

(c)   (d)

Fig. 11.6 Acute myeloblastic leukaemia. (a) M_2: the blast cells show cytoplasmic granules and Auer rods. (b) M_3: the blast cells show multiple Auer rods. Special stains: (c) Sudan black B shows black staining in the cytoplasm; (d) M_4 (myelomonocytic): non-specific esterase/chloracetate staining shows orange-staining monoblast cytoplasm and blue-staining (myeloblast) cytoplasm.

blasts may be found and these may also be seen in smaller numbers in other forms. ALL (Fig. 11.7) must be differentiated from infectious mononucleosis and other causes of lymphocytosis. **5** The bone marrow is hypercellular with a marked proliferation of leukaemic blast cells which amount to over 50% and typically over 75% of the marrow cell total. In ALL the marrow may be difficult to aspirate because of increased reticulin fibre. In AML M_7 the patient typically has an acute onset of pancytopenia with marrow fibrosis.

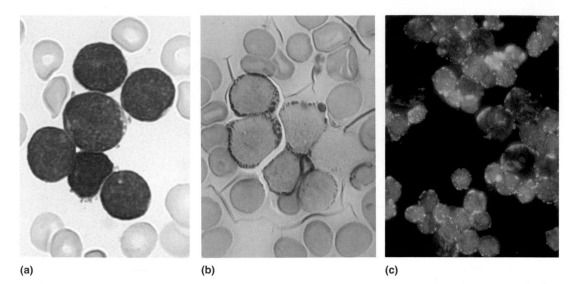

(a)   (b)   (c)

Immunological classification

The AML FAB subtypes are associated with different morphology and cytochemical staining (Fig. 11.6c, d) and in many cases characteristic surface antigens and chromosomal changes (see also Chapter 10). The blasts are usually CD13+, CD33+ and TdT− (see Table 11.4, Fig. 11.8). Special antibodies are helpful in the diagnosis of AML M_6 or M_7 (see Table 11.4). Their treatment and prognosis are basically similar but there are some clinical differences mentioned above as well as differences in treatment.

FAB subclassifies ALL into three subtypes (see Table 11.2):
1 the L_1 type show uniform, small blast cells with scanty cytoplasm;
2 the L_2 type comprise larger blast cells with more prominent nucleoli and cytoplasm and with more heterogeneity; and
3 the L_3 blasts show perinuclear and cytoplasmic vacuoles.

ALL is also subdivided according to immunological markers into:
1 *precursor B-ALL* which is CD19+, cytoplasmic CD22+ and TdT+, includes three subtypes, common-ALL which is CD10+ (Fig. 11.7c), null type which is CD10− and pre-B-ALL which shows intracytoplasmic μ chains (and may be CD10+ or CD10−);
2 *T-ALL* which shows T-cell antigens (e.g. CD7 and cytoplasmic CD3); and
3 *B-ALL* which shows surface immunoglobulin (Ig) and is TdT−.

B-ALL usually corresponds to the morphological L_3 type whereas the CD10+, null, pre-B or T types may all be L_1 or L_2 and are morphologically indistinguishable.

Fig. 11.7 Acute lymphoblastic leukaemia: precursor B type. (a) Blasts show scanty cytoplasm without granules. (b) Periodic-acid-Schiff (PAS) staining reveals coarse granules. (c) Indirect immunofluorescence reveals nuclear TdT (green) and membrane CD10 (orange). (Courtesy of Professor G. Janossy.)

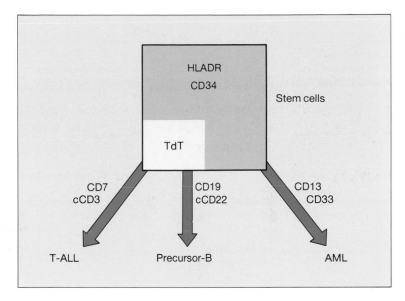

Fig. 11.8 Development of three cell lineages from pluripotential stem cells giving rise to the three main immunologic subclasses of acute leukaemia. The immunological characterization using pairs of markers is shown, as well as the three markers characterizing the early 'stem' cells. ALL, acute lymphoblastic leukaemia; AML, acute myeloid leukaemia; c, cytoplasmic.

Other investigations

Tests for DIC are positive in patients with the promyelocytic (M_3) variant of AML. Lumbar puncture shows that the spinal fluid has an increased pressure and contains leukaemic cells in patients with meningeal leukaemia.

X-rays may reveal lytic bone lesions, especially in childhood ALL; a mediastinal mass due to enlargement of the thymus and/ or mediastinal lymph nodes is characteristic of T-ALL (see Fig. 11.5), and infiltration of the lung fields due to infection or less frequently due to the leukaemia itself may be seen.

Biochemical tests may reveal a raised serum uric acid, serum lactate dehydrogenase and less commonly hypercalcaemia. Liver and renal function tests are performed as a baseline before treatment begins.

Special investigations

Differentiation of ALL from AML

In most cases, the clinical features and morphology on routine staining separate ALL from AML. In ALL the blasts show no differentiation (with the exception of B-ALL) whereas in AML some evidence of differentiation to granulocytes or monocytes is usually seen in the blasts or their progeny. Special tests are needed when the cells are undifferentiated to confirm the diagnosis of AML or ALL and to subdivide cases of AML or ALL into their different subtypes.

Cytochemistry (Table 11.3). This may help to show granule

	ALL	AML
Cytochemistry		
• Myeloperoxidase	–	+ (including Auer rods)
• Sudan Black	–	+ (including Auer rods)
• Non-specific esterase	–	+ in M_4, M_5
• Periodic-acid-Schiff (PAS)	+ (coarse in c-ALL)	+ (fine blocks in M_6)
• Acid phosphatase	+ in T-ALL (Golgi staining)	+ M_6 (diffuse)
Electron microscopy	–	+ (early granule formation)
Immunoglobulin (Ig) and TCR genes	Precursor B-ALL: clonal rearrangement of Ig genes T-ALL: clonal rearrangement of TCR genes	Germ-line configuration of Ig and TCR genes
Chromosomes (see Chapter 10)		
Immunological markers (see Table 11.4)		

Table 11.3 Special tests for acute lymphoblastic leukaemia (ALL) and acute myeloid leukaemia (AML).

development or monocytic differentiation in AML and help distinguish ALL into its subtypes.

Immunological markers (Table 11.4). These are used to distinguish AML from ALL and are particularly useful in subclassifying ALL (see earlier).

Immunoglobulin and T-cell receptors (TCR) gene rearrangements (see p. 169). Detection of clonal rearrangements of immunoglobulin or TCR genes is a sensitive method for detecting a monoclonal population of cells of B lineage (as in c-ALL or pre-B-ALL) or T lineage (as in T-ALL) (Table 10.2). Cross-lineage rearrangements occur, however, and occasional cases of AML also show aberrant immunoglobulin or TCR clonal gene rearrangements. Because of the complicated technique, gene rearrangement studies are not used routinely.

Chromosome analysis (see Table 10.2). Certain chromosome changes are typical of different subtypes of AML or ALL. They are therefore useful in diagnosis and in monitoring for residual disease during therapy. Chromosome changes may carry prognostic significance (e.g. Ph+ ALL has a poor prognosis whereas hyperdiploidy in ALL is a good prognostic feature) and therefore can be important in planning therapy.

Table 11.4 Immunological markers for classification of acute leukaemia.

Marker	AML	ALL Precursor B*	T
Myeloid			
CD13	+	−	−
CD33	+	−	−
glycophorin	+ (M$_6$)	−	−
platelet antigens	+ (M$_7$)	−	−
B lineage			
CD19	−	+	−
cCD22	−	+	−
CD10	−	+ (common) or − (null)	−
cIg	−	+ (pre-B)	
T lineage			−
CD7	−	−	+
cCD3	−	−	+
TdT	−	+	+

* B-ALL resembles precursor B-ALL immunologically but has surface Ig and is TdT−.
ALL, acute lymphoblastic leukaemia; AML, acute myeloid leukaemia; c, cytoplasmic.

Hybrid acute leukaemia

In a minority of cases of acute leukaemia, the blast cells on special testing show features of both AML and ALL. These features may be on the same cell (biphenotypic) or on separate populations (bilineal). They include inappropriate expression of immunological markers, e.g. TdT+ AML or CD13+ ALL or inappropriate gene rearrangements. Treatment is usually given on the basis of the dominant pattern.

Management

General supportive therapy for bone marrow failure includes the following.

Insertion of a central venous catheter. It is usual to insert a central venous catheter (e.g. Hickman) via a skin tunnel (to reduce the risk of infection) from the chest into the superior vena cava to give ease of access for giving chemotherapy, blood, blood products, antibiotics, intravenous feeding, etc. and for blood sampling for laboratory tests.

Prevention of vomiting. Cytotoxic drugs, radiotherapy, anaesthetics and infections are all potent causes of nausea and vomiting. Drugs used to prevent or treat this include metoclopramide, phenothiazines (e.g. chlorpromazine or prochlorperazine), steroids (e.g. dexamethasone), benzodiazepines (e.g. lorazepam), cannabinoids (e.g. nabilone) or most recently, selective 5-HT3 receptor antagonists (e.g. Ondansetrone, Kytril or Navoban).

Treatment of anaemia. Packed red cell transfusions are given.

Treatment and prophylaxis of haemorrhage. As haemorrhage is an important cause of death soon after presentation, regular platelet concentrates are given in the management of patients with repeated minor haemorrhage and in all cases with severe thrombocytopenia (platelets less than $20 \times 10^9/l$) and during initial induction therapy when severe thrombocytopenia is likely. Replacement of clotting factors with fresh frozen plasma, and multiple platelet transfusions are needed particularly in patients with DIC due to the M_3 variant of AML before and during initial chemotherapy. Heparin therapy may also be of value in the initial stages in the M_3 disorder with DIC. Tranexamic acid is often used to reduce haemorrhage by reducing fibrinolysis.

Prophylaxis and treatment of infection

Neutropenia due to bone marrow replacement by leukaemic blasts and because of intensive cytotoxic therapy renders the patient exquisitely susceptible to infection, particularly when the absolute neutrophil count falls below $0.2 \times 10^9/l$. In many patients, neutrophils are totally absent from the blood for 2 weeks or more. The infections are predominantly bacterial and usually arise from the patient's own commensal bacterial flora — most commonly Gram-positive skin organisms (e.g. *Staphylococcus* and *Streptococcus*), *Acinetobacter* or Gram-negative gut bacteria (e.g. *Pseudomonas aeruginosa, E. coli, Proteus, Klebsiella* and anaerobes). Organisms not normally considered pathogeneic, e.g. *Staphylococcus epidermidis*, may cause life-threatening infection. Moreover, in the absence of neutrophils, local superficial lesions rapidly cause severe septicaemia. Viral (e.g. herpes simplex and zoster), fungal (e.g. *Candida, Aspergillus*) and protozoal (e.g. *Toxoplasma gondii*) infections also occur with increased frequency, particularly when neutropenia is prolonged, lymphopenia is present and multiple courses of antibiotics have been used to treat possible bacterial infection.

The following measures are taken to reduce the risk of death from infection.

Prophylaxis of infection

Isolation facilities. Patients should be nursed in separate rooms preferably with reverse-barrier isolation techniques and air filtration used to prevent infection by airborne spores, e.g. *Aspergillus* species.

Reduction of gut and other commensal flora. Oral antimicrobial agents (e.g. co-trimoxazole, neomycin and colistin) and antifungal agents (e.g. amphotericin and fluconazole) may be given prophy-lactically. Oral quinolones, e.g. ciprofloxacin, have been found to reduce Gram-negative infections and are now used routinely in some units. Regular cultures should be taken from urine, faeces, sputum, throat, gums, nose, catheter sites, and axillary and perineal skin areas to document the patient's bacterial flora and its sensitivity. Topical antiseptics are used for bathing and mouthwashes and for treating any site where pathogens are detected. If these are not eliminated, systemic antibiotic therapy is considered, particularly if dangerous pathogens, e.g. *Pseudomonas* species, are isolated.

Treatment of infection
Fever is the main indication that infection is present. Blood cultures and cultures from any likely focus should be taken immediately fever occurs. Vigorous attempts should be made to identify the responsible organism by direct examination of possibly infected material as well as by culture methods. The mouth and throat, intravenous catheter site, and perineal and perianal areas are particularly likely foci. Because of the absence of neutrophils, pus is not formed and infections are not localized. The absence of a neutrophil reaction makes the severity of infections of, for example, the lungs, urine or skin more difficult to assess. Chest X-ray and urine culture are essential.

Antibiotic therapy must be started immediately after blood and other cultures have been taken. In at least 50% of febrile episodes no organisms are isolated. The combination of an aminoglycoside (e.g. gentamicin, amikacin or netilmicin) with a penicillin active against *Pseudomonas* (e.g. azlocillin, ticarcillin or piperacillin) or with a cephalosporin in high dosage (e.g. ceftazidime) have been proved excellent initial combinations. Vancomycin or teicoplanin (effective against Gram-positive organisms) combined with Gram-negative cover (e.g. ceftazidime) is particularly effective. Current trials compare chemotherapy with a single broad-spectrum agent (e.g. imipenem) against one or other of these different combinations. All these regimens cover Gram-negative organisms including *Pseudomonas* as well as some Gram-positive cocci and are effective bactericidal drugs in the face of severe neutropenia. As soon as the infective agent and its antibiotic sensitivities are known, appropriate changes in the regimen may be made. If no response occurs, the possibility of fungal or viral infection should be

considered and appropriate therapy given, e.g. with amphotericin
or acyclovir. Fungal infections are most likely to occur after
initial infective episodes have been treated and when bone
marrow recovery has not occurred. Adult respiratory distress
syndrome (ARDS) is a dangerous complication of infection,
especially with *Streptococcus mitis*.

Cytotoxic drug therapy

Most of the cytotoxic drugs used in leukaemia therapy damage
the capacity of cells for reproduction (Table 11.5). Combinations
of at least three drugs are now usually used initially to increase
the cytotoxic effect, improve remission rates and reduce the
frequency of emergence of drug resistance. These multiple drug
combinations have also been found to give longer remissions in
acute leukaemias than single agents.

Initial therapy may be accompanied by hyperkalaemia and
hyperuricaemia with urate nephropathy (the 'tumour lysis
syndrome'). Thus the patient should be given allopurinol before
starting therapy, be well hydrated and if the white cell count
is high and there is substantial organ infiltration, alkalization
of the urine should be carried out with intravenous sodium
bicarbonate.

The aim of cytotoxic therapy is first to induce a remission
(absence of any clinical or conventional laboratory evidence
of the disease) and then to eliminate the hidden leukaemic cell
population by courses of consolidation therapy (Fig. 11.9).
Cyclical combinations of two, three or four drugs are given with
treatment-free intervals to allow the bone marrow to recover.
This recovery depends upon the differential regrowth pattern of
normal haemopoietic and leukaemic cells. For ALL, long-term
(2 years) maintenance therapy has been found to reduce the
risk of relapse but this is not established in AML.

Table 11.5 Drugs used in the treatment of leukaemia.

	Mechanism of action	Particular side effects*
Antimetabolites		
• Methotrexate	Inhibit pyrimidine or purine synthesis or incorporation into DNA	Mouth ulcers, gut toxicity
• 6-Mercaptopurine†		Jaundice
• 6-Thioguanine†		Gut toxicity
• Cytosine arabinoside		CNS especially cerebellar toxicity in high doses
• Hydroxyurea		Gut toxicity, skin atrophy (rare)

Table 11.5 *Continued*

	Mechanism of action	Particular side effects*
Alkylating agents		
● Cyclophosphamide	Cross-link DNA, impede RNA formation	Haemorrhagic cystitis, cardiomyopathy, loss of hair
● Chlorambucil		Marrow aplasia, hepatic toxicity, dermatitis
● Busulphan (Myleran)		Marrow aplasia, pulmonary fibrosis, hyperpigmentation
● Nitrosoureas BCNU, CCNU		Renal and pulmonary toxicity
DNA binding		
● Daunorubicin		
● Hydroxodaunorubicin (Adriamycin)	Bind to DNA and interfere with mitosis	Cardiac toxicity, hair loss
● Mitoxantrone		
● Idarubicin		
● Bleomycin	DNA breaks	Pulmonary fibrosis, skin pigmentation
Mitotic inhibitors		
● Vincristine (Oncovin)	Spindle damage, absent metaphase	Neuropathy (peripheral or bladder or gut), hair loss
● Vinblastine		
● Vindesine		
Miscellaneous		
● Corticosteroids	Inhibition or enhancement of gene expression	Peptic ulcer, obesity, diabetes, osteoporosis, psychosis
● L-Asparaginase	Deprive cells of asparagine	Hypersensitivity, low albumin and coagulation factors, pancreatitis
● Epipodophyllotoxin (etoposide, VP-16)	Mitotic inhibitor	Hair loss, oral ulceration
● α-Interferon	Activation of RNAase and natural killer activity	Flu-like symptoms, thrombocytopenia, leucopenia, weight loss
● Deoxycoformycin	Inhibits adenosine deaminase	Renal failure, neurotoxicity
● Trans-retinoic acid	Induces differentiation	Liver dysfunction, skin hyperkeratosis, leucocytosis and hyperviscosity

* Most of the drugs cause nausea, vomiting, mucositis and bone marrow toxicity, and in large doses infertility. Tissue necrosis is a problem if the drugs are extravasated during infusion.
† Allopurinol potentiates the action and side effects of 6-mercaptopurine and 6-thioguanine.

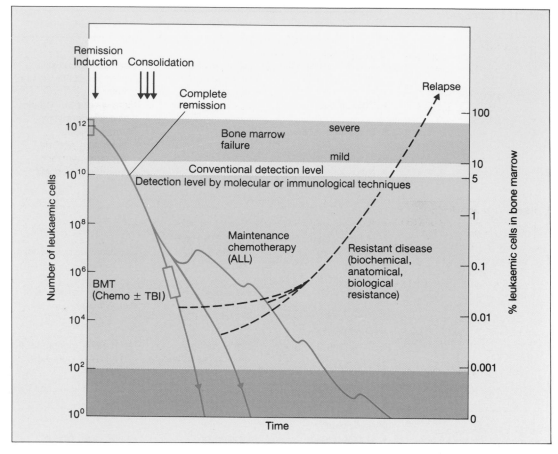

Fig. 11.9 Acute leukaemia: principles of therapy. ALL, acute lymphoblastic leukaemia; Chemo ± TBI, chemotherapy ± total body irradiation.

Cytotoxic therapy of ALL

Prednisolone, vincristine, daunorubicin and asparaginase are the drugs usually used and these achieve remission in over 90% of children and in 80–90% of adults (Fig. 11.10). Intensive consolidation therapy is then needed and a variety of drugs are used in different protocols. A typical protocol involves the use of vincristine, cytosine arabinoside, daunorubicin, etoposide and thioguanine given as 5-day blocks after induction therapy and again 2–3 months after cranial radiotherapy (early and late consolidation). Some units add cyclophosphamide and courses of high-dose methotrexate and cytosine arabinoside to the consolidation regimens.

Certain groups of patients carry a less favourable prognosis (Table 11.6). For some, e.g. B-ALL, different therapy is needed (e.g. with cyclophosphamide, high-dose methotrexate and cytosine arabinoside) and if the prognosis is considered poor (Table 11.6), allogeneic bone marrow transplantation in first remission is considered if there is a compatible sibling (Table 11.7). Overall

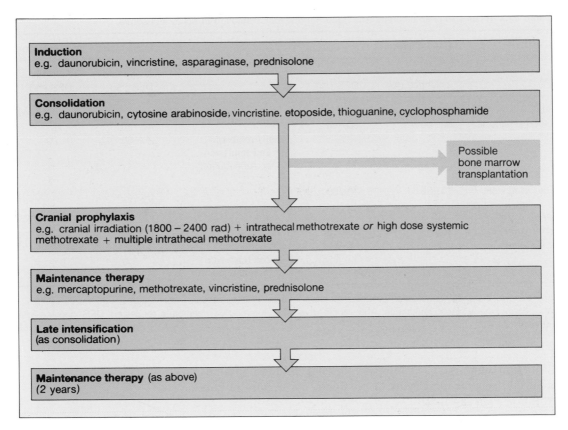

Fig. 11.10 Acute lympho-blastic leukaemia: flow chart illustrating typical treatment regimen.

60−70% of children with c-ALL are now alive and off all treatment 5 years from presentation. It seems likely that many of them are cured. In other patients, death occurs because of resistant disease or from infections or other complications during initial treatment, subsequent maintainance therapy or during re-

Table 11.6 Prognosis in acute lymphoblastic leukaemia (ALL).

	Good	Bad
WBC	Low	High (e.g. $>20 \times 10^9/l$)
Sex	Girls	Boys
Immunophenotype	c-ALL (CD10+)	B-ALL
Age	Child	Adult (or <2 years)
Cytogenetics	Normal or hyperdiploidy	Ph+, other translocations
Time to remission	<4 weeks	>4 weeks
CNS disease at presentation	Absent	Present

Ph+, Philadelphia chromosome positive; WBC, white blood cell count.

Table 11.7 Results of chemotherapy and bone marrow transplantation in acute leukaemia.

	Chemotherapy			Bone marrow transplantation	
	Remission incidence (%)	Long-term DFS (%)		Allogeneic DFS (%)	Autologous DFS (%)
ALL			*ALL*		
Good prognosis	80–90	60–80	1st CR	40–50*	? 20*
			Early relapse, 2nd remission or subsequently	20–30	0–20
Bad prognosis	70–80	20–30			
AML			*AML*		
<60 years	80	20–30	1st CR	50–60	50
>60 years	50	5–15	Early relapse, 2nd remission or subsequently	30	0–25

* % survival depends on selection of cases for bone marrow transplantation.
ALL, acute lymphoblastic leukaemia; AML, acute myeloid leukaemia; CR, complete remission; DFS, disease-free survival.

induction after relapse. Relapsed disease is more difficult to treat and second remissions, if obtained, are usually of shorter duration than the first.

CNS prophylaxis

Leukaemic cells in the meninges are beyond the reach of most of the cytotoxic drugs used in therapy unless very high doses, e.g. of cytosine arabinoside or methotrexate, are given systemically. Meningeal leukaemia used to occur in three of every four children during the first 4 years after diagnosis of ALL. Repopulation of the bone marrow from the meninges is a cause for haematological relapse.

Cranial irradiation (1800–2400 rad) and courses of intrathecal methotrexate during initial treatment and during the period of cranial irradiation after the remission has been obtained, are now used in most cases of ALL patients under 60 years old to prevent CNS relapse. In children less than 2 years old irradiation to the brain is delayed and prophylactic intrathecal methotrexate alone is used initially. Some units use methotrexate alone intrathecally with or without systemic high-dose therapy, and omit radiotherapy in good prognosis children because of its long-term effect on intellectual development. CNS relapses still occur and present with headache, vomiting, papilloedema and blasts cells in the cerebrospinal fluid. Treatment is with intrathecal methotrexate and/or cytosine arabinoside.

Testicular disease

Relapse may occur in this 'sanctuary site'. If so testicular irradiation is given with re-induction chemotherapy. Prophylactic testicular irradiation is not used.

Maintenance chemotherapy

This is given in ALL for 2 years normally with daily oral mercaptopurine and once weekly oral methotrexate and monthly intravenous injections of vincristine with a short course (5 days) of oral corticosteroids.

There is a high risk of varicella or measles during maintenance therapy in children who lack immunity to these viruses. If exposure to these infections occurs, prophylactic immunoglobulin should be given. Oral co-trimoxazole is given to reduce the risk of *Pneumocystis carinii*.

Treatment of relapse

If this occurs during maintainance therapy, the outlook is poor and marrow transplantation after re-induction chemotherapy is the only hope of cure. Relapse off maintainance therapy is less grave but nevertheless the patient is unlikely to be cured by chemotherapy alone and some form of marrow transplantation is considered.

Drug resistance

In some cases of ALL, AML or other haematological malignancies relapse is associated with the emergence of resistant clones of cells. Several mechanisms exist by which malignant cells are or become resistant to cytotoxic drugs. These include reduced uptake of the drug, increased levels of the target enzyme, selection of alternative pathways of metabolism and alteration in cell cycle. An important mechanism in human leukaemias, myeloma and lymphoma is the presence of increased levels of expression of the multi-drug resistance (MDR) gene coding for a glycoprotein, p170. This acts as a pump transporting the drug from the cell to the surrounding medium and is relevant for resistance for the anthracyclines (e.g. doxorubicin (adriamycin), daunorubicin, mitoxantrone), the vinca alkaloids (e.g. vincristine, vinblastine, vindesine), amasacrine and the epipodophyllotoxins (e.g. VP-16). Inhibitors of the action of p170 include verapamil, tamoxifen and cyclosporin A, drugs which are also pumped out by the protein. Increased levels of the enzyme glutathione transferase is another mechanism by which cells become resistant to certain drugs.

Cytotoxic therapy of AML

The most commonly used induction regimen for AML is a combination of the drugs cytosine arabinoside, daunorubicin and either 6-thioguanine or etoposide (Fig. 11.11). Cases of all the AML subtypes (FAB M_0-M_7) are treated similarly except for the promyelocytic (M_3) variant. For this, trans-retinoic acid may be used to obtain a remission (see below) and large numbers of platelet concentrates and fresh frozen plasma to provide clotting factors are used until remission is obtained. A typical good response in AML to cytotoxics is shown in Fig. 11.12. Because myelotoxic drugs are needed with less selectivity between leukaemic and normal marrow cells, marrow failure is severe and prolonged and intensive supportive care is required. Early deaths from infection, haemorrhage or other causes are common, particularly in patients over 60 years. In about 10–20% of cases remissions are not obtained even after two courses of therapy. The remission rate in patients less than 60 years is about 80%. Two or three consolidation courses of intensive chemotherapy are usually given post-remission with the same or alternative drugs, e.g. m-amasacrine, mitoxantrone and high doses of cytosine arabinoside. Maintenance therapy is not given by most units and CNS prophylaxis is not usually given in AML. A meningeal relapse occasionally occurs especially in children and young adults with M_4 or M_5 disease; prophylactic cranial therapy may be given to them.

Fig. 11.11 Acute myeloid leukaemia: flow chart illustrating typical treatment regimen.

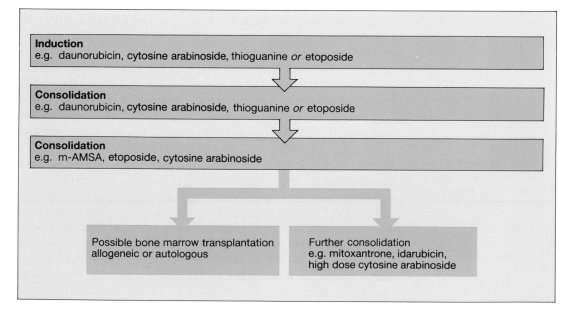

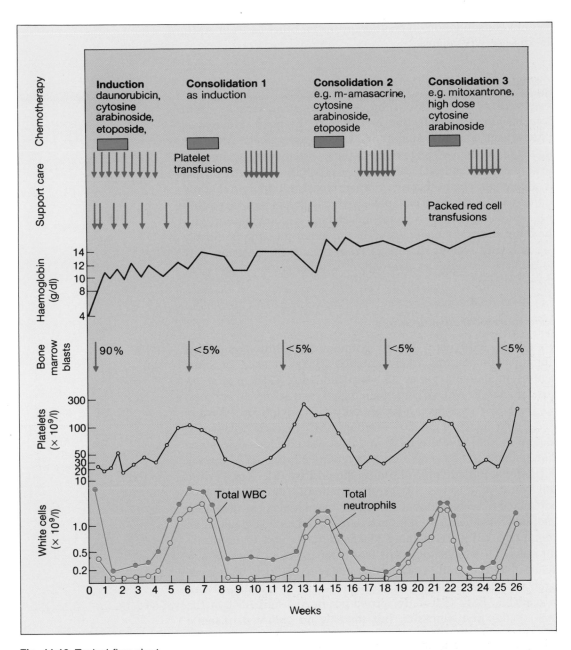

Fig. 11.12 Typical flow chart for the management with chemotherapy of acute myeloid leukaemia.

Treatment of AML M₃: all trans-retinoic acid

In patients with this disease associated with the 15;17 chromosome translocation, the drug trans-retinoic acid has been used to induce remission by causing differentiation of the malignant clone. The 15;17 translocation (which involves the retinoic acid receptor, see p. 199) may become undetectable. Nevertheless, without consolidation chemotherapy, as for other cases of AML, the disease will relapse.

Patients over 60 years of age

Results of AML therapy in the elderly are poor because death from haemorrhage, infection or failure of the heart, kidneys or other organs is more frequent than in younger patients. Attempts are made to balance the toxicity of the chemotherapy against the need to obtain remission as quickly as possible. In those regarded as suitable for chemotherapy, similar intensive induction therapy to that used in younger patients is given. Different anthracyclines (e.g. mitozantrone, epirubicin, idarubicin) in combination with the other drugs are being tested in induction therapy. In elderly patients with serious disease of other organs, the decision may be made to use support care with or without gentle, single drug chemotherapy.

Bone marrow transplantation

Allogeneic (HLA and mixed lymphocyte culture-compatible sibling) bone marrow transplantation (BMT) is used in some centres in patients under 45 years old with AML in first re-mission, and in ALL patients who relapse and achieve a success-ful second remission after re-induction cytotoxic therapy (see Table 11.7). It is also used in AML in early relapse or second or subsequent remissions. It is also considered in some ALL patients in first remission with a particularly poor prognosis (e.g. adults, Philadelphia chromosome positive (Ph+) or a white cell count of $>100 \times 10^9$ at presentation). Transplantation is performed to reconstitute the patient's haemopoietic system after total body irradiation and intensive chemotherapy is given in an attempt to kill all remaining leukaemic cells and to immuno-suppress the patient to accept the donor marrow. There is evi-dence that the graft itself further reduces the risk of relapse (graft vs leukaemia effect). If a syngeneic donor (identical twin) is available, BMT is usually carried out in ALL and AML at the time of the first remission but there is no graft-vs-leukaemia effect.

In patients without a matching sibling donor, trials of autologous BMT are being carried out. Marrow is harvested in first remission and in some centres 'purged' of residual leukaemic cells by drugs or antibodies. The autologous transplant may be performed in first remission or after relapse and re-induction therapy (second remission). Finally, BMT using unrelated but HLA-matching donors is being tried. The relative merits of these approaches are the subject of many randomized trials worldwide.

Prognosis

The prognosis of ALL in children has been improved greatly by the use of chemotherapy, radiotherapy, better supportive therapy and the development of special leukaemia units. Progress in AML has been less spectacular. The approximate survival figures are shown in Table 11.7.

Bibliography

Bain B.J. (1990) *Leukaemic Diagnosis: A Guide to the FAB Classification.* Gower Medical, London.

Bain B.J. & Catovsky D. (1990) Current concerns in haematology, 2. Classification of acute leukaemia. *Journal of Clinical Pathology*, **43**, 882–887.

Cartwright R.A. & Staines A. (1992) Acute leukaemias. *Clinical Haematology*, **5**, 1–26.

Catovsky D. (ed.) (1991) *The Leukaemic Cell*, 2nd Edition. Methods in Haematology, Vol. 2. Churchill Livingstone, Edinburgh.

Henderson E.S. & Lister T.A. (eds) (1990) *Leukaemia*, 5th Edition. W.B. Saunders, Philadelphia.

Pochedly C. & Civin C.I. (ed.) (1990) Childhood acute lymphoblastic leukaemia, Parts I & II. *Hematology Clinics of North America*, **4**, 715–1017.

Proctor S.J. (1991) Minimal residual disease in leukaemia. *Clinical Haematology*, **4**, 577–791.

Quaglino D. & Hayhoe F.G. (1992) *Haematological Oncology. Clinical Practice.* Churchill Livingstone, Edinburgh.

Whittaker J.A. (ed.) (1992) *Leukaemia*, 2nd Edition. Blackwell Scientific Publications, Oxford.

Wiernik P.H., Canellos G.P., Kyle R.A. & Schiffer C.A. (1991) *Neoplastic Diseases in the Blood.* Churchill Livingstone, Edinburgh.

Zittoun R.A. (ed.) (1991) Chemotherapy of malignant blood diseases. *Clinical Haematology*, **4**, 1–246.

Chapter 12
Chronic Leukaemias and Myelodysplastic Syndromes

Chronic myeloid leukaemia

Chronic myeloid (myelogenous) leukaemia (CML) comprises <20% of all the leukaemias and is seen most frequently in middle age. In over 95% of patients there is a replacement of normal bone marrow by cells with an abnormal chromosome — the Philadelphia or Ph chromosome (Fig. 12.1). This is an abnormal chromosome 22 due to the translocation of part of a long (q) arm of chromosome 22 to another chromosome, usually 9, with translocation of part of chromosome 9 including the *ABL* oncogene to chromosome 22. It is an acquired abnormality of haemopoietic stem cells that is present in all dividing granulocytic, erythyroid and megakaryocytic cells in the marrow and also in some B and probably a minority of T lymphocytes. The term chronic granulocytic leukaemia (CGL) is used to describe Ph+ or *BCR*-rearranged CML (see p. 200). In a minority of patients the same molecular rearrangements have occured without the Ph abnormality being seen on light microscopy (see p. 235). A great increase in total body granulocyte mass is responsible for most of the clinical features. In at least 70% of patients there is a terminal metamorphosis to acute leukaemia (myeloblastic or lymphoblastic) with an increase of blast cells in the marrow to 50% or more. The typical Ph+ case is referred to as CGL but this and a number of rarer disorders including Ph− cases are grouped under the broad heading of chronic myeloid leukaemia (Table 12.1).

Clinical features

This disease occurs in either sex (male:female, 1.4:1), most frequently between the ages of 40 and 60 years. However, it may occur in children and neonates and in the very old. In most cases there are no predisposing factors but the incidence was increased in survivors of the atom bomb exposures in Japan. Its clinical features include the following.
1 Symptoms related to hypermetabolism, e.g. weight loss, lassitude, anorexia or night sweats.
2 Splenomegaly is nearly always present and is frequently massive. In some patients splenic enlargement is associated with considerable discomfort, pain or indigestion.

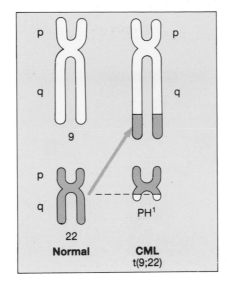

Fig. 12.1 The Philadelphia chromosome. There is translocation of part of the long (q) arms of chromosome 22 to the long arms of chromosome 9 and reciprocal translocation of part of the long arm of chromosome 9 to chromosome 22 (the Philadelphia chromosome). The molecular consequences are described on p. 235.

3 Features of anaemia may include pallor, dyspnoea and tachycardia.
4 Bruising, epistaxis, menorrhagia or haemorrhage from other sites due to abnormal platelet function.
5 Gout or renal impairment due to hyperuricaemia from excessive purine breakdown may be a problem.
6 Rare symptoms include visual disturbances and priapism.

Laboratory findings

1 Leucocytosis is usually $>50 \times 10^9/l$ and sometimes $>500 \times 10^9/l$. A complete spectrum of myeloid cells is seen in the peripheral blood. The levels of neutrophils and myelocytes exceed those of blast cells and promyelocytes (Fig. 12.2).
2 Ph chromosome on cytogenetic analysis of blood or bone marrow (Fig. 12.1).
3 Bone marrow is hypercellular with granulopoietic predominance.

Table 12.1 Classification of chronic myeloid leukaemias.

1 Chronic myeloid leukaemia, Ph positive (CML, Ph+) (chronic granulocytic leukaemia, CGL)

2 Chronic myeloid leukaemia, Ph negative (CML, Ph−)

3 Juvenile chronic myeloid leukaemia

4 Chronic neutrophilic leukaemia

5 Eosinophilic leukaemia

6 Chronic myelomonocytic leukaemia (CMML) (see myelodysplasia, p. 245)

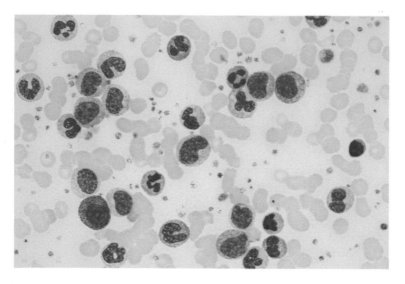

Fig. 12.2 Chronic myeloid leukaemia: peripheral blood film showing various stages of granulopoiesis including promyelocytes, myelocytes, metamyelocytes and band and segmented neutrophils.

4 Neutrophil alkaline phosphatase score is invariably low (Table 12.2).
5 Increased circulating basophils.
6 Normochromic, normocytic anaemia is usual.
7 Platelet count may be increased (most frequently), normal or decreased.
8 Serum vitamin B_{12} and vitamin B_{12}-binding capacity are increased.
9 Serum uric acid is usually raised.

Treatment of chronic phase

There is a predictable response to therapy in the chronic phase (Fig. 12.3). By reducing the total granulocyte mass, cytotoxic drugs are able to keep patients symptom-free for long periods but they do not delay the onset of acute transformation.

Busulphan (myleran). This alkylating agent is convenient and was widely used. Regular blood counts allow the dose to be titrated in individual patients. The drug may be given intermittently by daily small doses (e.g. 2—8 mg) or in higher doses

Raised in	Low in
Infections	Chronic myeloid leukaemia
Pregnancy	
Polycythaemia vera	
Myelofibrosis	
Leukaemoid reactions	

Table 12.2 Neutrophil alkaline phosphatase score (see p. 155); normal score is 20—100.

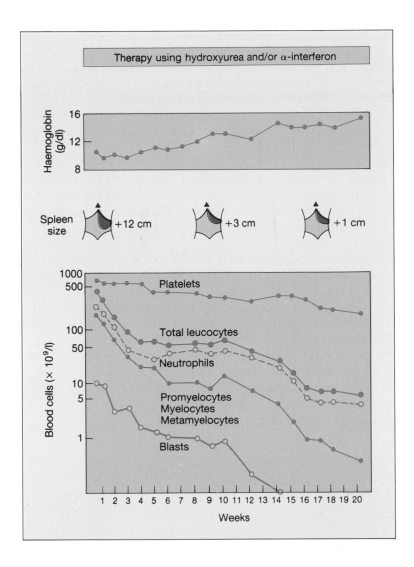

Fig. 12.3 Chronic myeloid leukaemia: typical haematological course of a patient treated with hydroxyurea and/or α-interferon.

(1–1.5 mg/kg) on a single day every 4–6 weeks. Long-term busulphan therapy may cause pulmonary fibrosis ('busulphan lung'), skin pigmentation and an Addisonian syndrome and because of these, the use of busulphan is becoming less popular.

Hydroxyurea. This is the preferred alternative to busulphan with fewer side effects. It is given daily (0.5–3.0 g) but its shorter action entails more frequent monitoring and continuous therapy is usually needed to control the white cell count.

Alpha-interferon. This controls the white cell count in most cases and in a minority causes a substantial reduction or total disappearance of Ph+ cells. It is necessary to keep the leucocyte count low (e.g. $<5 \times 10^9/l$) to achieve this effect. In some studies, it has been associated with a reduction in myeloblastic compared to lymphoblastic transformation. Whether it prolongs overall survival is the subject of current trials but those who respond well do seem to have a prolonged chronic phase. Side effects (p. 223) are a problem in some patients.

Allopurinol. This prevents high urate production which might cause gout or renal damage.

Splenic irradiation or splenectomy are usually reserved for patients whose splenic enlargement is not responsive to chemotherapy and causes clinical problems. Elective splenectomy is of no proven value.

Bone marrow transplantation (BMT). Allogeneic BMT in the chronic phase offers a 50–70% chance of cure for patients of 55 years or younger, who have an HLA-matching sibling (Fig. 12.4). This is the only treatment regularly leading to elimination of the Ph+ clone of cells. In some cases the disease recurs following BMT, however, and others die of complications of the procedure. Allogeneic BMT in the accelerated or acute phase leads to 20% or fewer long-term survivors. BMT from HLA-matched unrelated donors are now being carried out in some centres. The results are worse than with matching sibling donors.

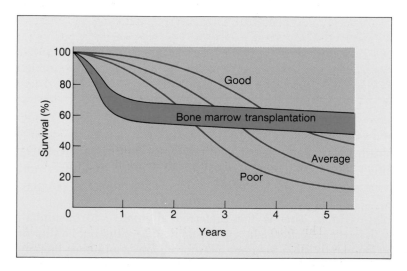

Fig. 12.4 Probability of survival for patients under the age of 35 allografted in the chronic phase with bone marrow from an HLA-identical sibling. There is an early mortality in the first 12–18 months followed by a plateau of survival. The curve has been superimposed on survival courses for patients in three prognostic groups defined according to clinical and haematological criteria and receiving busulphan or hydroxyurea therapy. (From Goldman, 1988.)

Course and prognosis

CML usually shows an excellent response to chemotherapy in the chronic phase (see Fig. 12.3). The median survival is 3–4 years. Death usually occurs from terminal acute transformation or from intercurrent haemorrhage or infection. Twenty per cent of patients survive 10 years or more. The patients may be divided into prognostic groups according to age, spleen size, platelet count, blast cell percentage on presentation and ease of response to therapy; these are only rough guides to outcome. The position of the breakpoint in M-bcr (see p. 201) on chromosome 22 was related to survival in some but not other studies.

Accelerated phase and metamorphosis (blast cell or acute transformation)

Acute transformation may occur rapidly over days or weeks. More commonly the patient becomes refractory to therapy usually with anaemia, thrombocytopenia and an increase in basophils, eosinophils or blast cells in the blood and marrow. The spleen may be enlarged despite control of the blood count and the marrow may become fibrotic. The patient may be in this accelerated phase for several months during which the disease is less easy to control than in the chronic phase. In either the accelerated or acute phase, new chromosome abnormalities (e.g. double Ph chromosome) are often present. In about one-third of cases the transformation is lymphoblastic and then there may be a temporary response to therapy with vincristine and corticosteroids. In this case, these drugs, together usually with daunorubicin and asparaginase may restore the chronic phase for months or even a year or two. In the majority, transformation is into acute myeloid leukaemia (AML) or mixed types. These are more difficult to treat. Marrow or peripheral blood stem cells stored during the chronic phase may be used to restore haemopoiesis after intensive chemotherapy with or without total body radiotherapy (autologous BMT). Survival following AML transformation is brief, however, and rarely more than 12 months.

Variants of CML

Ph– CML. This disorder divides into two groups. One with the molecular changes of CML (*ABL* oncogene moved from chromosome 9 to the *BCR* region of chromosome 22) resembles typical CGL. A second type without this translocation shows haematological differences, often with features of myelodysplasia.

Juvenile CML. A Ph– variant which occurs in young children, often with enlargement of the liver and spleen, extensive lymphadenopathy and eczema. The neutrophil alkaline phosphatase score is normal and the level of foetal haemoglobin increased. It responds poorly to treatment.

Chronic neutrophilic leukaemia. This is very rare and can only be diagnosed after all other causes of neutrophil leucocytosis have been excluded. Chromosomes are normal.

Eosinophilic leukaemia. This is often difficult to distinguish from the hypereosinophilia syndrome. Hepatosplenomegaly, rashes and cardiac and pulmonary abnormalities occur in both. In the leukaemia, more blasts are present and a variety of cytogenetic abnormalities (other than Ph) may also be seen.

Chronic myelomonocytic leukaemia. See p. 245.

Philadelphia-positive acute lymphoblastic leukaemia

About 3% of children and 20−25% of adults with acute lymphoblastic leukaemia (ALL) show the Ph chromosome (t9;22). They present without features of CML and are usually of the CD10+ (common ALL) phenotype. A proportion show an identical molecular defect to chronic phase CML with a breakpoint in the major (M) *BCR* region (of 5.8 kb) between the second and third or third and fourth exons and produce the typical tyrosine kinase protein molecular weight 210 000 (p210) (p. 200). Some have a breakpoint in the first intron of the *BCR* region minor (m)-*BCR* and these produce a different chimeric tyrosine kinase protein with a molecular weight of 190 000 (p190). Most Ph+ cases of ALL have a course typical of acute ALL of poor prognosis but a few in remission show haematological features typical of chronic phase CML. It has been suggested that p210 ALL is a form of CML presenting in acute transformation, whereas p190 ALL is a true *de novo* form of ALL, but this is controversial (see Fig. 10.7).

Chronic lymphocytic leukaemia

Chronic lymphocytic (lymphatic) leukaemia (CLL) accounts for 25% or more of the leukaemias seen in clinical practice and occurs chiefly in the elderly. Although classified as a lymphoproliferative disorder, in most patients there is little evidence of an aggressive proliferation of the abnormal lymphocytes. The accumulation of large numbers of lymphocytes to 50−100 times the normal lymphoid mass in the blood, bone marrow, spleen, lymph nodes and liver may be related to immunological nonreactivity and excessive lifespan. The cells are a monoclonal population of B lymphocytes. B- and T-cell chronic leukaemias other than (B-)CLL are all relatively uncommon. With advanced CLL there is often bone marrow failure, a tumorous syndrome with generalized discrete lymphadenopathy and sometimes soft tissue lymphoid masses; immunological failure results from reduced humoral and cellular immune processes with a tendency to infection. The disease is thought to arise by clonal expansion of a rare CD5+ B cell normally seen in the mantle zone of peripheral lymph nodes.

The classification of the chronic lymphoid leukaemias is given in Table 12.3.

Clinical features

1 The disease occurs in older subjects and is rare before 40 years. The male to female ratio is 2:1.

2 Symmetrical enlargement of superficial lymph nodes is found in many patients (Fig. 12.5). The nodes are usually discrete and non-tender.

3 Features of anaemia may be present, e.g. pallor, dyspnoea.

4 Splenomegaly and hepatomegaly are usual in later stages.

5 Bacterial or fungal infections are common in later stages because of immune deficiency and neutropenia (due to marrow infiltration, chemotherapy or hypersplenism). There is also an association with herpes zoster (Fig. 12.6). In some patients this is the presenting feature.

6 Patients with thrombocytopenia may show bruising or purpura.

7 Excessive reactions to vaccination and insect bites may occur.

8 Skin infiltration is present in a small number of patients.

9 Tonsillar enlargement may be a feature. Involvement of the salivary and lacrimal glands (Mikulicz's syndrome) is a rare presentation.

10 Many cases (usually stage 0) are diagnosed when a routine

Table 12.3 Classification of the chronic lymphoid leukaemias.

B cell	T cell
B-chronic lymphocytic leukaemia (B-CLL, CLL)	T-chronic lymphocytic leukaemia (T-CLL) (large granular lymphocyte leukaemia)
B-prolymphocytic leukaemia (B-PLL)	T-prolymphocyte leukaemia (T-PLL)
Hairy cell leukaemia (HCL)	Adult T-cell leukaemia/lymphoma
Plasma cell leukaemia	

In many cases of non-Hodgkin's lymphoma, lymphoma cells are found in the blood and in some cases the distinction between chronic leukaemia and lymphoma is arbitrary, depending on the relative proportion of the disease in soft tissue masses compared to blood and bone marrow.

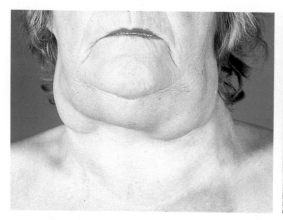 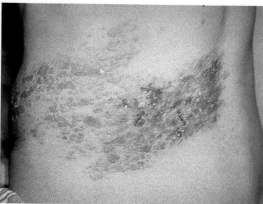

Fig. 12.5 Chronic lymphocytic leukaemia: bilateral cervical lymphadenopathy in a 67-year-old woman. Haemoglobin 12.5 g/dl; white blood count 150 × 19^9/l (lymphocytes 146 × 10^9/l); platelets 120 × 19^9/l.

Fig. 12.6 Chronic lymphocytic leukaemia: herpes zoster infection in a 68-year-old female.

blood test is performed. With increasing routine medical check-ups, this proportion is rising.

Laboratory findings

1 Lymphocytosis. The absolute lymphocyte count is >5 × 10^9/l and may be up to 300 × 10^9/l or more. Between 70% and 99% of white cells in the blood film appear as small lymphocytes (Fig. 12.7). Smudge or smear cells are also present. Immunophenotyping of the lymphocytes shows them to be B-cell (surface CD19, CD20 positive), weakly expressing surface immunoglobulin (IgM or IgD). This is shown to be monoclonal because of expression of one form of light chain (κ or λ only, see p. 189). Characteristically the cells are also surface CD5 (normally a T-cell marker) positive.

2 Normocytic, normochromic anaemia is present in later stages due to marrow infiltration or hypersplenism. Autoimmune haemolysis may also occur (see below).

3 Thrombocytopenia occurs in many patients.

4 Bone marrow aspiration shows lymphocytic replacement of normal marrow elements. Lymphocytes comprise 25–95% of all the cells. Trephine biopsy reveals either nodular, diffuse or interstitial involvement by lymphocytes.

5 Reduced concentrations of serum immunoglobulins are found and this becomes more marked with advanced disease. Rarely a paraprotein is present.

6 Trisomy 12 or 14q+ or translocation 11:14 are the most frequent chromosome findings but cytogenetic analysis is not usually performed. A submicroscopic translocation of the

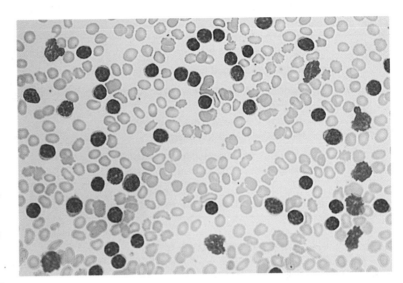

Fig. 12.7 Chronic lymphocytic leukaemia: peripheral blood film shows lymphocytes with thin rims of cytoplasm, coarse condensed nuclear chromatin and rare nucleoli. Typical smudge cells are present.

oncogene BCL-2 onto chromosome 22 or 2 in association with the immunoglobulin light chain genes has also been described.

Course and prognosis

The disease has been divided into five stages (Rai *et al.*, 1975) and into three stages by an International Working Party (Table 12.4). These stages correlate with different prognoses. Most patients with CLL live for 3–5 years. Younger patients, females and patients with earlier stage disease do better. Patients with slowly progressive disease or the 'benign' form often survive for more than 10 years (Rai stage 0, mean survival 12 years or more) while Rai stage I patients have a mean survival of 8 years). Unlike CML, CLL does not transform into acute leukaemia, although immunoblastic transformation may occur as a terminal lymphoma (Richter's syndrome). Death is usually caused by infection due to bone marrow failure and immune deficiency.

Treatment

There is no need to treat state 0 disease but patients in other stages may need treatment, particularly if there is: (a) evidence of bone marrow failure; (b) symptomatic involvement of lymph nodes or skin; (c) splenomegaly causing 'hypersplenism' or symptoms; or (d) autoimmune haemolytic anaemia or thrombocytopenia.

Corticosteroids. Patients in bone marrow failure should be

(a) Rai classification.

Table 12.4 Staging of CLL.

Stage 0	Absolute lymphocytosis $>15 \times 10^9$/l*
I	As stage 0 + enlarged lymph nodes (adenopathy)
II	As stage 0 + enlarged liver and/or spleen $\pm$ adenopathy
III	As stage 0 + anaemia (Hb <10.0 g/dl)* $\pm$ adenopathy $\pm$ organomegaly
IV	As state 0 + thrombocytopenia (platelets $<100 \times 10^9$/l)* $\pm$ adenopathy $\pm$ organomegaly

(b) International Working Party classification (Binet *et al.*, 1981).

	Organ enlargement†	Haemoglobin* (g/dl)	Platelets* ($\times 10^9$/l)
Stage A	0, 1 or 2 areas		
B	3, 4 or 5 areas	$\geqslant 10$	$\geqslant 100$
C	Not considered	<10 and/or	<100

* Secondary causes of anaemia (e.g. iron deficiency) or autoimmune haemolytic anaemia or thrombocytopenia must be treated before staging.
† One area = lymph nodes >1 cm in neck, axillae, groins or spleen, or liver enlargement.

treated initially with prednisolone alone until there is significant recovery of the platelet, neutrophil and haemoglobin levels. The peripheral lymphocyte count initially rises as infiltrated organs shrink, but later the count falls. Corticosteroids are also indicated in autoimmune haemolytic anaemia or thrombocytopenia.

Alkylating agents. Continuous or intermittent therapy with either chlorambucil or cyclophosphamide successfully reduces the total lymphocyte mass and may prevent bone marrow failure for periods of several years until the lymphocytes become refractory to this therapy.

Newer single agents. Fludarabine and chlorodeoxyadenosine are two anti-purine drugs which have been found effective even in some patients refractory to chlorambucil.

Radiotherapy may be useful for treating lymph nodes or local deposits causing pressure symptoms and also for reducing the spleen size in patients with hypersplenism. Splenic irradiation is also useful as systemic therapy in later stages.

Combination chemotherapy. For patients resistant to alkylating agents, therapy with an anthracycline drug in combination with other cytotoxic drugs is often effective. CHOP (cyclophosphamide, hydroxodaunorubicin (Adriamycin), vincristine (Oncovin) and prednisolone) is one such regime. Trials are also in progress of the use of an anthracycline with chlorambucil as initial therapy.

Splenectomy is indicated for autoimmune haemolytic anaemia which does not respond to steroids and alkylating agents and for occasional patients with massive splenomegaly which is refractory to therapy and causing symptoms or 'hypersplenism'.

Ancillary therapy includes active treatment and prophylaxis of infection with antibacterial and antifungal aspects. Regular infusions of γ-globulin may help patients with severe hypogammaglobulinaemia who are having recurrent infections. Allopurinol reduces urate production in patients with high lymphocyte counts. Supportive transfusions with red cells or platelets may be required for patients in bone marrow failure.

Variants of CLL

1 CLL may be asymptomatic and without abnormal physical signs or cytopenias. The course of this benign (stage 0) form may remain stable for many years and these patients may never need treatment.

2 A more aggressive form may be seen in younger patients aged 30−50 years, when it is characterized by fatigue, weight loss, anorexia, sweating, progressive lymphadenopathy, hepatosplenomegaly, bone marrow and immunological failure.

3 Some 10−15% of CLL patients develop a secondary autoimmune haemolytic anaemia associated with jaundice, marked reticulocytosis, spherocytosis and a positive direct antiglobulin test with IgG on the surface of the red cells. A secondary autoimmune thrombocytopenia occurs in about 5% of patients.

4 Prolymphocytic leukaemia is a variant of CLL characterized by massive splenomegaly and lymphocyte counts up to and sometimes exceeding $400 \times 10^9/l$ but with absent lymph node enlargement. The cells are large with a prominent nucleolus and immature nucleus. They are usually B cells with strong expression of surface immunoglobulin but T-cell types also occur which are more likely to show lymphadenopathy, serous effusions and skin lesions. The response to treatment is poor.

5 Chronic T-cell leukaemia (large granular lymphocyte leukaemia) is rare and occurs in younger subjects than the usual B-CLL. There is also less lymphadenopathy, more cutaneous involvement, and a poor response to therapy. The course is, however, often benign. About a third of cases are associated with clinical or serological evidence of rheumatoid arthritis. The cells have more cytoplasm than in B-CLL and show multiple granules. Anaemia, neutropenia or thrombocytopenia alone or in combination, and refractory to therapy are frequent and thought to be due to cell-mediated supression of normal haemopoiesis by the leukaemic cells. Adult T-cell leukaemia/lymphoma and cutaneous T-cell lymphomas are considered in Chapter 13.

Hairy cell leukaemia

Hairy cell leukaemia (HCL) is an unusual disease of peak age 40−60 years with a male to female ratio of 4 : 1. It is characterized clinically by features due to pancytopenia. The spleen may be moderately enlarged. There is a monoclonal proliferation of cells with an irregular cytoplasmic outline ('hairy' cells, a type of B lymphocyte) in the peripheral blood, bone marrow, liver and other organs (Fig. 12.8) The number of hairy cells in the peripheral blood is variable; they may be rare. The bone marrow trephine shows a characteristic appearance of mild fibrosis and a diffuse cellular infiltrate. A serum paraprotein may be present and the patients may have arthritis, serositis or vasculitis.

Treatment

Splenectomy may improve the haematological picture if the spleen is large. Excellent haematological responses and remission of the disease occurs in up to 80% of patients given prolonged therapy (e.g. for 1 year) with α-interferon. The mechanism is thought to be breakdown of an autocrine growth loop of the malignant B cells for tumour necrosis factor (TNF) and possibly for IL-6. An even higher remission rate occurs with the adenosine deaminase inhibitor deoxycoformycin or with chlorodeoxyadenosine. The course of HCL is often chronic, requiring only supportive therapy. With these new treatments the prognosis of patients has improved considerably and most survive for many years.

Lymphoma/leukaemia syndromes

Circulating malignant lymphoid cells occur in a variety of syndromes in association with otherwise typical cases of non-Hodgkin's lymphoma. This syndrome is most frequently seen in B-cell tumours of the follicle centre cell type (with circulating indented or cleaved nuclei) and the course is that of the non-Hodgkin's lymphoma (p. 259). Other types of lymphoma may also show tumour cells in the peripheral blood and bone marrow (Table 12.3) and in some cases it is difficult to define the disease as either lymphoma (with mainly soft tissue masses) or leukaemia. Adult T-cell leukaemia/lymphoma is discussed on p. 270.

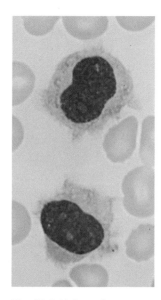

Fig. 12.8 Hairy cell leukaemia: peripheral blood film showing typical 'hairy' cells with oval nuclei and finely mottled pale grey/blue cytoplasm with an irregular edge.

Myelodysplastic syndromes (myelodysplasia)

This is a large group of acquired neoplastic disorders of the bone marrow, most common in the elderly and characterized by increasing bone marrow failure with quantitative and qualitative abnormalities of all three myeloid cell lines (red cell, granulocyte/monocyte and platelets) due to a defect of the stem cells. A hallmark of the disease is ineffective haemopoiesis so that cytopenias often accompany a marrow of normal or increased cellularlity. There is a tendency to progress to acute myeloid leukaemia, although death often occurs before this develops. In most cases, the disease arises *de novo*, but in a significant proportion chemotherapy and/or radiotherapy has previously been given for another haematological disease, lymphoma or other solid tumour.

Classification

The myelodysplastic syndromes (MDS) are classified into five subgroups (Table 12.5). The groups are arbitrarily separated according to: (a) the proportion of blasts in the blood and marrow; (b) whether or not ring sideroblasts are frequent in the marrow; and (c) the proportion of monocytes in the peripheral blood. The prognosis is substantially better in patients with a normal proportion of marrow blasts (<5%) than in those with increased marrow blasts (5% or more) (Table 12.5).

Table 12.5 Classification of the myelodysplastic syndromes.

	Peripheral blood	Bone marrow	Approximate median survival (months)
1 Refractory anaemia (RA)*	Blasts <1%	Blasts <5%	50
2 RA with ring sideroblasts (RARS)	Blasts <1%	Blasts <5% Ring sideroblasts >15% of total erythroblasts	50
3 RA with excess blasts (RAEB)	Blasts <5%	Blasts 5–20%	11
4 RAEB in transformation (RAEB-t)	Blasts >5%	Blasts 20–30% or Auer rods present	5
5 Chronic myelomonocytic leukaemia (CMML)	As any of the above with >1.0 × 10⁹/l monocytes	As any of the above with promomonocytes	11

* In some cases neutropenia or thrombocytopenia is present without anaemia. These cases are termed refractory cytopenia.

Clinical features

About half the patients are over 70 and less than 25% are less than 50 years old. Males are more commonly affected. The evolution is often slow and the disease may be found by chance when a patient has a blood count for some unrelated reason. The symptoms, if present, are those of anaemia, infections or of easy bruising or bleeding (Fig. 12.9). In some patients, transfusion-dependent anaemia dominates the course, while in others recurring infections or spontaneous bruising and bleeding is the major clinical problem. Because the neutrophils, monocytes and platelets are often functionally impaired, spontaneous infections on the one hand, or bruising or bleeding on the other, may occur out of proportion to the severity of the cytopenia. The spleen is not usually enlarged except in chronic myelomonocytic leukaemia (CMML) in which gum hypertrophy and lymphadenopathy may also occur.

Laboratory findings

Peripheral blood. Pancytopenia is a frequent finding. The red cells are usually macrocytic or dimorphic but occasionally hypochromic; normoblasts may be present. The reticulocyte count is

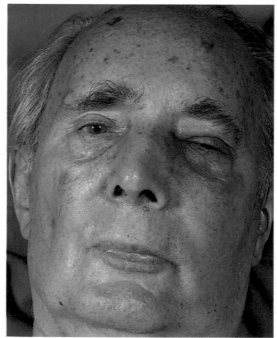

(a)

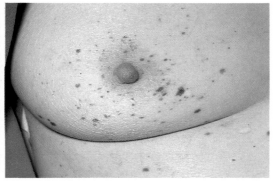

(b)

Fig. 12.9 (a) Myelodysplasia: a male 78-year-old patient with refractory anaemia had recurring infections of the face and maxillary sinuses associated with neutropenia (haemoglobin 9.8 g/dl; white cells 1.3 × 10⁹/l; neutrophils 0.3 × 10⁹/l; platelets 38 × 10⁹/l). (b) Myelodysplasia. Purpura in a female (aged 58) with refractory anaemia (haemoglobin 10.5 g/dl; white cells 2.3 × 10⁹/l; platelets 8 × 10⁹/l).

low. Granulocytes are often reduced and may show lack of granulation (Fig. 12.10). Their chemotactic, phagocytic and adhesive functions are impaired. The Pelger abnormality (single or bilobed nucleus) is often present and in CMML monocytes are $>1.0 \times 10^9/l$ in the blood and the total WBC (white blood count) may be $>100 \times 10^9/l$. The platelets may be unduly large or small and are usually decreased in number but in 10% of cases are elevated. In poor prognosis cases variable numbers of myeloblasts are present in the blood.

Bone marrow. The cellularity is usually increased. Ring sideroblasts may occur in all five FAB types but by definition constitute $>15\%$ of the normoblasts in refractory anaemia with ring sideroblasts. Multinucleate normoblasts and other dyserythropoietic features are seen (Fig. 12.10). The granulocyte precursors show defective primary and secondary granulation, and cells which are difficult to identify as either agranular myelocytes, monocytes or promonocytes are frequent. Megakaryocytes are abnormal with micro-, small binuclear or polynuclear forms. Bone marrow biopsy shows fibrosis in 10% of cases.

Chromosomal and oncogene abnormalities

Cytogenetic abnormalities are more frequent in secondary than primary MDS and most commonly constitute partial or total loss of chromosomes 5, 7 or Y or trisomy 8. The loss of chromosome 5 bands q13 to q33 in elderly females with macrocytic anaemia, normal or raised platelet counts and micro-megakaryocytes has been termed the 5q-syndrome with a relatively good prognosis. *RAS* oncogene (usually N-*RAS*) mutations occur in about 20% of cases and mutations of *FMS* in about 15%.

Management

This is often extremely difficult because no therapy has been found to regularly revert haemopoiesis to normal and intensive or even low-dose chemotherapy may, in some cases, make the situation worse rather than better.

Low-grade MDS

This is defined as those patients with less than 5% blasts in the marrow. This is usually managed conservatively with red cell transfusions, platelet transfusions or antibiotics as required. Attempts are being made to improve marrow function with haemopoietic growth factors, e.g. GM-CSF (colony-stimulating factor) or IL-3 (interleukin-3), but this therapy needs careful trials in case the onset of acute leukaemia is accelerated. Trials

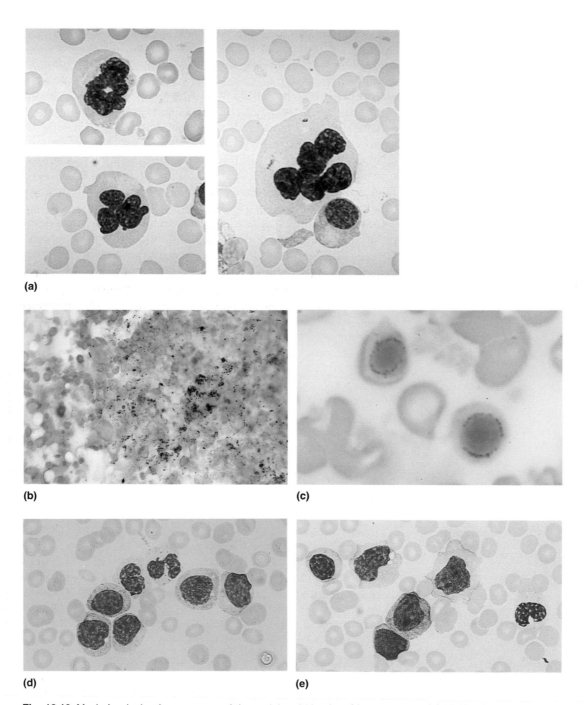

Fig. 12.10 Myelodysplasia. Appearances of the peripheral blood and bone marrow. (a) Multinucleate polychromatic erythroblasts. (b) Perls' stain. Iron overload in macrophages of a bone marrow fragment. (c) Multiple ring sideroblasts. (d) White cells showing pseudo-Pelger cells, agranular myelocytes and neutrophils. (e) Monocytoid cells and an agranular neutrophil.

with erythropoietin therapy have been disappointing but in a few patients, the anaemia has partially improved. In the long term, iron overload may be a problem after multiple transfusions; iron chelation therapy (see p. 106) should be started after 30−50 units have been transfused and if the anaemia and the need for transfusion continues to be the dominant problem.

High-risk MDS

In these patients with 5% or more blasts in the marrow, a variety of treatments have been attempted to improve the overall prognosis with varying degrees of success. These treatments extend from general support only to intensive chemotherapy.

General support care only. This is most suitable in elderly patients with other major medical problems. Transfusions of red cells and platelets, and therapy with antibiotics and antifungals are given as needed.

Low-dose cytotoxic therapy with, for example, cytosine arabinoside (ara-C). Low-dose ara-C (e.g. $10\,mg/m^2$ twice daily) subcutaneously has been used widely with the aim of reducing the proportion of blast cells and increasing differentiation of myeloid cells. Complete responses are rare and pancytopenia (with infections or bleeding) may become more marked at least temporarily. Some workers have combined low dose ara-C with 'differentiating agents', e.g. retinoic acid, or with haemopoietic growth factors, e.g. GM-CSF or IL-3, but these are not of established additional benefit.

Single agent oral chemotherapy. Hydroxyurea, etoposide or mercaptopurine may be given with some benefit to patients with CMML or with RAEB (refractory anaemia with excess blasts) or RAEB-t (RAEB in transformation) with high circulating white cell counts.

Intensive chemotherapy. Chemotherapy as given in AML (p. 228) may be tried in younger bad-risk patients, e.g. under the age of 60. Full remission is less frequent than in *de novo* AML and the risks of intensive chemotherapy are greater since prolonged pancytopenia may occur in some cases without normal haemopoietic regeneration, presumably because normal stem cells are not present.

Bone marrow transplantation (BMT). In younger patients (less than 50−55 years) with an HLA-matching brother or sister or an unrelated but HLA-matching donor, BMT offers a prospect of complete cure. BMT is usually carried out in MDS without a complete remission being first obtained with chemotherapy, although in high-risk cases initial chemotherapy may be tried to reduce the blast proportion and the risk of recurrence of the MDS after the BMT. Because of the usual old age of the MDS patient, BMT is only feasible in a small minority of the patients.

Bibliography

Bennett J.M., Catovsky D., Daniel M.T. *et al.* (1982) Proposals for the classification of the acute leukaemias. *British Journal of Haematology*, **51**, 189–199.

Bennett J.M., Catovsky D., Daniel M.T. *et al.* (1989) Proposals in the classification of chronic (mature) B and T lymphoid leukaemias. *Journal of Clinical Pathology*, **42**, 567–584.

Binet J.L., Auquier A., Dighiero G. *et al.* (1981) A new prognostic classification of chronic lymphocytic leukemia derived from a multivariate survival analysis. *Cancer*, **48**, 198–206.

Canellos G.P. (ed.) (1990) Chronic leukemias. *Hematology/Oncology Clinics of North America*, **4**, 319–502.

Catovsky D. & Foa R. (1990) *The Lymphoid Leukaemias*. Butterworth, London.

Cheson B.D. (ed.) (1992a) *Chronic Lymphocytic Leukemia*. Marcel Dekker, New York (in press).

Cheson B.D. (1992b) Therapy of chronic B-cell leukaemias. In *Recent Advances in Haematology*, 6 (eds A.V. Hoffbrand & M.K. Brenner). Churchill Livingstone, Edinburgh, pp. 107–130.

Culligan D., Jacobs A. & Padua R.A. (1993) The genetic basis of myelodysplasia. In *Recent Advances in Haematology*, 7 (eds M.K. Brenner & A.V. Hoffbrand). Churchill Livingstone, Edinburgh (in press).

Finch S.C. & Linet M.S. (1992) Chronic leukaemias. *Clinical Haematology*, **5**, 27–56.

Galvani D.W. & Cawley J.C. (1990) The current status of interferon α in haemic malignancy. *Blood Reviews*, **4**, 175–180.

Goldman J.M. (ed.) (1987) Chronic myeloid leukaemia. *Clinical Haematology*, **1**, 869–1080.

Goldman J.M. (1988) Chronic myeloid leukaemia: pathogenesis and management. In *Recent Advances in Haematology*, 5 (ed A.V. Hoffbrand). Churchill Livingstone, Edinburgh, pp. 131–152.

Heslop H.E., Hoffbrand A.V. & Brenner M.K. (1992) Interferons in haematological malignancies. In *Recent Advances in Haematology*, 6 (eds A.V. Hoffbrand & M.K. Brenner). Churchill Livingstone, Edinburgh, pp. 131– 148.

Hughes T.P. & Goldman J.M. (1991) Chronic myloid leukemia. In *Hematology: Basic Principles and Practice* (eds R. Hoffman, E.J. Benz, S.J. Shattil, B. Furie & H.J. Cohen). Churchill Livingstone, New York, pp. 854–869.

Koeffler H.P. (ed.) (1992) Myelodysplastic syndromes. *Hematology/Oncology Clinics of North America*, **6**, 485–728.

Mufti G.I. & Galton D.A.G. (Eds) (1992) *The Myelodysplastic Syndromes*. Churchill Livingstone, Edinburgh.

Polliack A. & Catovsky D. (eds) (1988) *Chronic Lymphocytic Leukaemia*. Harwood Academic Publishers, London.

Rai K.R., Sawitsky A., Cronkite E.P., Chanana A.D., Levy R.N. & Pasternack B.S. (1975) Clinical staging of chronic lymphocytic leukemia. *Blood*, **46**, 219–234.

Chapter 13
Malignant Lymphomas

This group of diseases is divided into Hodgkin's disease and non-Hodgkin's lymphomas. In both, there is replacement of normal lymphoid structure by collections of abnormal cells, Hodgkin's disease being characterized by the presence of Reed — Sternberg (RS) cells and the non-Hodgkin's lymphomas by diffuse or nodular collections of abnormal lymphocytes or, rarely, histiocytes.

Hodgkin's disease

Pathogenesis

Hodgkin's disease is a malignant tumour closely related to the other malignant lymphomas. In many patients, the disease is localized initially to a single peripheral lymph node region and its subsequent progression is by contiguity within the lymphatic system. It is likely that the characteristic RS cells and the associated abnormal and smaller mononuclear cells are neoplastic and that the associated inflammatory cells represent a hypersensitivity response by the host, the effectiveness of which determines the pattern of evolution. After a variable period of containment within the lymph nodes, the natural progression of the disease is to disseminate to involve non-lymphatic tissue.

The origin of the malignant cell in Hodgkin's disease is not firmly established. Although RS cells express features of cellular activation, markers of definite T- or B-cell lineage have not been demonstrated except in the lymphocyte-predominant sub-type in which the RS cells are clearly of B cell type. The RS cells regularly express MHC (major histocompatibility complex) class II antigens and IgG Fc receptors but are not phagocytic. They express CD15, CD25 (IL-2 receptor) and transferrin receptor. Monoclonal antibodies detecting activation antigens of the CD30 group, e.g. Ki-1, which react with Hodgkin's cells also react with some high-grade T-cell lymphomas, activated T lymphocytes and EBV (Epstein—Barr virus)-transformed B-cell lines. Clonal immunoglobulin gene rearrangements have been demonstrated in a minority of cases but these have not been the typical heavy and light chain rearrangements of B-cell tumours. It seems most likely that the malignant cell is an early lymphoid cell genotypically although phenotypically it has developed some later markers.

The EBV genome has been detected in about 20−50% of cases in Hodgkin tissue and it is possible that this or other viral infections, acquired later in life than usual, underlie the condition. This is supported by the increased frequency of Hodgkin's disease in individuals with higher social status, less density of housing and smaller number of siblings.

Clinical features

The disease can present at any age but is rare in children. It has a bimodal age incidence, one peak in young adults (age 20−30 years) and a second after the age of 50. In developed countries the ratio of young adult to child cases and of nodular sclerosing disease to other types is increased. There is an almost 2 : 1 male predominance. The following symptoms are common.

1 Most patients present with painless, non-tender, asymmetrical, firm, discrete and rubbery enlargement of the superficial lymph nodes. The cervical nodes are involved in 60−70% of patients, axillary nodes in about 10−15% and inguinal nodes in 6−12%. In some cases the size of the nodes decreases and increases spontaneously. They may become matted. Retroperitoneal nodes are also often involved but usually only diagnosed by computerized tomography (CT) scan.

2 Clinical splenomegaly occurs during the course of the disease in 50% of patients. The splenic enlargement is seldom massive. The liver may also be enlarged due to liver involvement.

3 Mediastinal involvement is found in 6−11% of patients at presentation. This is a feature of the nodular sclerosing type, particularly in young women. There may be associated pleural effusions or superior vena cava obstruction.

4 Cutaneous Hodgkin's disease occurs as a late complication in about 10% of patients. Other organs (e.g. gastrointestinal tract, bone, lung, spinal cord or brain) may also be involved even at presentation but this is unusual.

5 Constitutional symptoms are prominent in patients with widespread disease. The following may be seen.

   (a) Fever occurs in about 30% of patients and is continuous or cyclic. In the latter type, a few days of high swinging pyrexia may alternate with a few days when the patient is afebrile (Pel−Ebstein fever).

   (b) Pruritus, which is often severe, occurs in *c.* 25% of cases.

   (c) Alcohol-induced pain in the areas where disease is present occurs in some patients.

   (d) Other constitutional symptoms include weight loss, profuse sweating (especially at night), weakness, fatigue, anorexia and cachexia. Haematological and infectious complications are discussed below.

Haematological findings

1 Normochromic, normocytic anaemia is most common. With marrow infiltration, bone marrow failure may occur with a leuco-erythroblastic anaemia.
2 One-third of patients have a leucocytosis due to a neutrophil increase.
3 Eosinophilia is frequent.
4 Advanced disease is associated with lymphopenia.
5 The platelet count is normal or increased during early disease, and reduced in later stages.
6 The ESR (erythrocyte sedimentation rate) is usually raised and is useful in monitoring disease progress.
7 Bone marrow involvement is unusual in early disease. It may be demonstrated by trephine biopsy, usually in patients with disease at many sites. Bilateral trephine biopsy is performed in some units.

Immunological findings

There is a progressive loss of immunologically competent T lymphocytes with reduced cell-mediated immune reactions. Antibody production is maintained until the later stages of the disease. Infections are common, particularly herpes zoster, cyto-megalovirus and fungal, e.g. *Cryptococcus* and *Candida*. Tuber-culosis may occur.

Biochemical findings

Patients with bone disease may show hypercalcaemia, hypo-phosphataemia and increased levels of serum alkaline phospha-tase. Serum LDH (lactate dehydrogenase) is raised initially in 30–40% of cases and indicates a poor prognosis. Elevated levels of serum transaminases may indicate liver involvement, while serum bilirubin may be raised due to biliary obstruction caused by large lymph nodes at the porta hepatis. Hyperuricaemia may occur.

Diagnosis and histological classification

The diagnosis is usually made by histological examination of an excised lymph node. The distinctive multinucleate, polyploid RS cell is central to the diagnosis (Figs 13.1 and 13.2). Inflam-matory components consist of lymphocytes, histiocytes, polymorphs, eosinophils, plasma cells and variable fibrosis. Histological classification is into four types (Table 13.1), each of which implies a different prognosis. Patients with lymphocyte-predominant histology have the most favourable prognosis. It is possible that they have a more effective cellular immune re-sponse than those with a lymphocyte-depleted histology who have a relatively poor prognosis. Nodular sclerosis may be

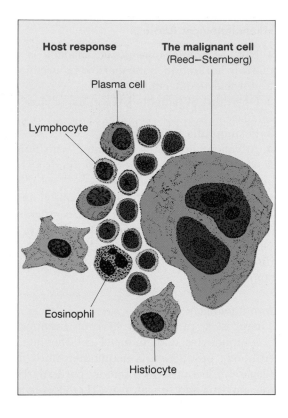

Fig. 13.1 Diagrammatic representation of the different cells seen histologically in Hodgkin's disease.

associated with each of the other three histological types and then carries the corresponding prognosis.

The nodular sclerosis type predominates in young adults; the other types have a bimodal age distribution with a second peak in old age. Lymphocyte predominance occurs mostly in children; lymphocyte depletion in the elderly.

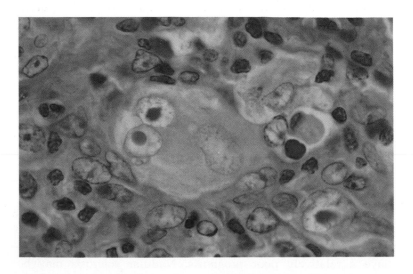

Fig. 13.2 Hodgkin's disease: high power view of lymph node biopsy showing two typical multinucleate Reed–Sternberg cells, one with a characteristic owl eye appearance, surrounded by lymphocytes, histiocytes and an eosinophil.

Table 13.1 Histological classification of Hodgkin's disease.

---

1 *Lymphocyte predominant*
Lymphocyte proliferation dominates. Few Reed—Sternberg cells are seen. Nodular and diffuse patterns are recognized

2 *Nodular sclerosis*
Collagen bands extend from the node capsule to encircle nodules of abnormal tissue. A characteristic 'lacunar cell' variant of the Reed—Sternberg cell is often found. The cellular infiltrate may be of the lymphocyte-predominant, mixed cellularity or lymphocyte-depleted type; eosinophilia is frequent

3 *Mixed cellularity*
The Reed—Sternberg cells are numerous and lymphocyte numbers are intermediate

4 *Lymphocyte depleted*
There is either a 'reticular' pattern with dominance of Reed—Sternberg cells and sparse numbers of lymphocytes or a 'diffuse fibrosis' pattern where the lymph node is replaced by disordered connective tissue containing few lymphocytes. Reed—Sternberg cells may also be infrequent in this latter subtype

---

Clinical staging

The selection of appropriate treatment depends on accurate staging of the extent of disease. Figure 13.3 shows the scheme now recommended. Thorough clinical examination and the following procedures are employed.

1 *Chest X-ray* to detect mediastinal, hilar node or lung involvement (Fig. 13.4).

2 *Bone marrow trephine*. This and/or liver biopsy may be needed to establish the diagnosis.

3 *Liver biopsy* (percutaneous needle or wedge at laparotomy).

4 *CT scan:* CT scanning is used to detect intrathoracic, intra-abdominal or pelvic disease (Fig. 13.5). It is also used to monitor response to therapy. Magnetic resonance imaging (MRI) scanning may be needed in difficult cases.

5 *Lymphangiography* may detect clinically silent pelvic and retroperitoneal para-aortic node involvement (Fig. 13.6).

6 Staging laparotomy and splenectomy were previously recommended in cases thought to be stage I or stage II. The excellence of contrast-assisted CT or MRI scanning in detecting occult abdominal disease and the use of combination chemotherapy in patients with less extensive disease have reduced the need for these procedures. Moreover, the immunological defect produced by splenectomy has been associated with a significant mortality due to widespread sepsis.

7 The patients are also classified as 'A' or 'B' according to whether or not constitutional features (fever or weight loss) are present (see Fig. 13.3).

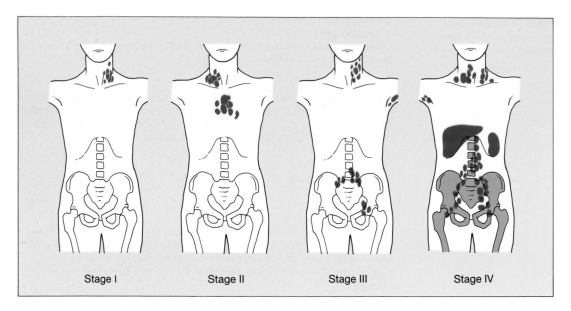

Stage I   Stage II   Stage III   Stage IV

Fig. 13.3 Staging of Hodgkin's disease. *Stage I* indicates node involvement in one lymph node area. *Stage II* indicates disease involving two or more lymph nodal areas confined to one side of the diaphragm. *Stage III* indicates disease involving lymph nodes above and below the diaphragm. Splenic disease is included in stage III but this has special significance (see below). *Stage IV* indicates involvement outside the lymph node areas and refers to disease in the bone marrow, liver and other extranodal sites.

NB The stage number in all cases is followed by the letter A or B—indicating the absence (A) or presence (B) of one or more of the following: unexplained fever above 38°C; night sweats; and loss of more than 10% of body weight within 6 months. Localized extranodal extension from a mass of nodes does not advance the stage but is indicated by the subscript$_E$. Thus mediastinal disease with contiguous spread to the lung or spinal theca would be classified as I$_E$. As involvement of the spleen is often a prelude to widespread haematogenous spread of the disease, patients with lymph node and splenic involvement are staged as III$_S$. Bulky disease (widening of the mediastinum by more than one-third, or the presence of a nodal mass >10 cm in diameter) is relevant to therapy at any stage.

Treatment

Radiotherapy

This may be the treatment used in some patients with stage I and II disease, and is also used in some stage III and IV patients in combination with chemotherapy. Patients with stage I and IIA Hodgkin's disease may be cured by radiotherapy alone. A total dose of not less than 4000 rad (40 Gy) is able to destroy lymph node Hodgkin's tissue in most of these patients. Improved high voltage radiotherapy techniques allow the treatment of all lymph node areas above or below the diaphragm by single 'upper mantle' or 'inverted Y' blocks. Radiotherapy also has a role in the treatment of particularly bulky tumour masses, e.g. media-

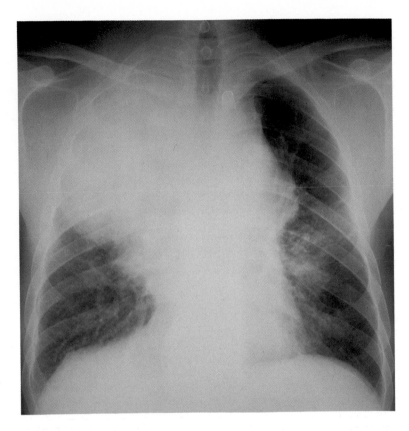

Fig. 13.4 Chest X-ray in Hodgkin's disease showing widespread enlargement of hilar and mediastinal lymph nodes with associated collapse of the right upper lobe and infiltration or possibly pneumonic changes in the mid zone of the left lung.

stinal disease in nodular sclerosing disease, or painful skeletal, nodal or soft tissue deposits and ulcerating skin lesions in stage II, III or IV patients following or between courses of chemotherapy.

Chemotherapy
Cyclical chemotherapy is used for stage III and IV disease and also in stage I and II patients who have bulky disease or B symptoms. Quadruple therapy with mustine, vincristine (Oncovin), procarbazine and prednisolone (MOPP) was the mainstay of treatment. Combinations of other drugs, e.g. Adriamycin, bleomycin, vinblastine and dacarbazine (ABVD), which are less likely than MOPP to cause sterility or secondary leukaemia, have proved to be successful and many workers now alternate these regimens or use MOPP-ABVD hybrid regimens, or use ABVD alone or other combinations (e.g. with chlorambucil instead of mustine) as initial therapy. It is usual to give six cycles (or four after full remission).

Relapsed cases
The patient is treated with an alternative combination chemotherapy to the initial regimen and, if necessary, with radiotherapy

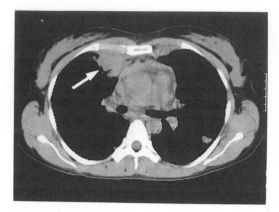

Fig. 13.5 Hodgkin's disease (nodular sclerosing type): CT scan of chest showing anterior mediastinal mass of enlarged lymph nodes (arrowed).

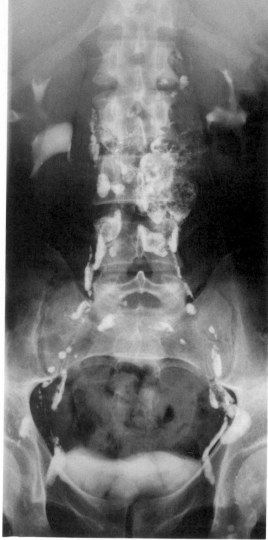

Fig. 13.6 Abdominal X-ray following lymphangiography in Hodgkin's disease. There is marked enlargement of the para-aortic lymph nodes with disruption of the normal nodal pattern. The pelvic lymph nodes appear normal. An intravenous pyelogram, performed on the second day of the lymphangiography study, demonstrates the relation of the kidneys and ureters to the associated enlarged lymph nodes.

to sites of bulky disease. Autologous bone marrow transplantation (BMT) provides a technique for administering high doses of chemotherapy with or without total body radiotherapy and leads to long-term survival in about 25% of relapsed cases.

Prognosis

Approximate 5-year survival rates are: stages I and II, 85%; stage IIIA, 70%; stages IIIB and IV, 50%. As mentioned above, the histological grading also affects prognosis within each of the clinical stages.

There is an increased incidence (but <2%) of myelodysplasia or AML (acute myeloid leukaemia) with a peak at 4 years after treatment for Hodgkin's disease with alkylating agents, especially if radiotherapy has also been given. Non-Hodgkin's lymphomas and other cancers also occur with greater frequency than in controls. Non-malignant complications include sterility (semen storage should be carried out before therapy is commenced), intestinal complications, myocardial infarction and other cardiac or pulmonary complications of the mediastinal radiation and chemotherapy.

Non-Hodgkin's lymphomas

The clinical presentation and natural history of these malignant lymphomas are more variable than in Hodgkin's disease, the pattern of spread is not as regular, and a greater proportion of patients present with extranodal disease or leukaemic manifestations.

Classification and histopathology

No area of diagnostic histopathology has been associated with greater confusion than the classification of non-Hodgkin's lymphomas. The recognition that the majority of non-Hodgkin's lymphomas arise from germinal follicle centre cells (FCC) and that these tumours may have either follicular (nodular) or diffuse architecture, was a major conceptual advance in their understanding and classification. Immunological marker and molecular biological studies including gene rearrangement analysis of tumour cells have contributed to our knowledge.

A scheme of normal lymphocyte development appears in Figure 13.7. In malignant lymphoma it is assumed that the tumour represents a clone of cells, whose maturation is fixed at a particular stage of development, with an inability to proceed further.

The two most frequently used classifications, the Kiel and the National Cancer Institute's Working Formulation are shown in Table 13.2.

The non-Hodgkin's lymphomas are a diverse group of diseases varying from highly proliferative and rapidly fatal diseases, to some of the most indolent and well-tolerated malignancies found in man. Patients with centrocytic lymphomas with a follicular

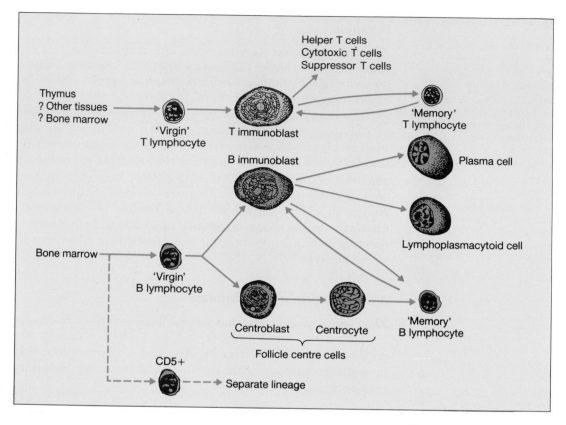

Fig. 13.7 Lymphocyte development after antigenic stimulation (see also Fig. 9.10). The CD5+ cell is thought to give rise to chronic lymphocytic leukaemia. (From Lennert, 1981.)

pattern and patients with relatively small lymphoid cells (lymphocytes and lympho-plasmacytoid cells) have a more favourable natural history and survival. The intermediate and high-grade malignancy group of tumours characterized by larger cells and 'blast' forms carry with them a poorer prognosis although in a minority a 'cure' is possible.

Practically all follicular and most diffuse lymphomas are derived from B lymphocytes. Less than 10% carry membrane features of T cells; some have neither B- nor T-cell markers and are designated as 'null' cell tumours, but may show B- or T-lineage commitment on gene rearrangement analysis.

Small lymphocytic lymphomas are closely related to chronic lymphocytic leukaemia (CLL) and many regard this lymphoma as a tissue phase of the latter disease. The characteristic small, mature-appearing lymphocyte is typically surface CD5+ and is related to B cells which give rise to autoantibodies in auto-immune disease. Many patients with this condition are elderly with slowly progressive disease, which may not require treatment for extended periods. Some lymphoplasmacytoid lymphomas may be associated with the production of mono-clonal paraproteins. If there are significant amounts of IgM,

Table 13.2 Classification of lymphomas.

(a) Kiel classification (updated).

B cell	T cell
Low-grade malignancy	*Low-grade malignancy*
Lymphocytic	Lymphocytic
Lymphoplasmacytic	Small cerebriform cell
Plasmacytic	mycosis fungoides
Centroblastic/centrocytic	Sézary's syndrome
follicular	Lymphoepithelioid
diffuse	(Lennert's lymphoma)
Centrocytic	Angioimmunoblastic
	T zone
High-grade malignancy	Pleomorphic small cell*
Centroblastic	
Immunoblastic	*High-grade malignancy*
Large cell anaplastic	Pleomorphic medium
(Ki-1+)	and large cell*
Burkitt's lymphoma	Immunoblastic*
Lymphoblastic	Large cell anaplastic
	(Ki-1+)†
Rare types	Lymphoblastic
	Rare types

* These tumours may be HTLV-1 positive.
† Anti Ki-1 is an antibody which detects activated CD30 and reacts with these primitive cell tumours and also with Reed–Sternberg cells.

(b) National Cancer Institute's Working Formulation.

Low-grade malignancy
A Small lymphocytic with or without
   plasmacytoid differentiation
B Follicular, small cleaved
C Follicular, mixed small cleaved and large cell

Intermediate-grade malignancy
D Follicular, large cell
E Diffuse, small cleaved
F Diffuse, mixed small and large cell
G Diffuse, large cell

High-grade malignancy
H Large cell immunoblastic
I Lymphoblastic (convoluted or non-
   convoluted)
J Small non-cleaved cell (Burkitt and non-
   Burkitt types)

Miscellaneous
Composite
Histiocytic
Mycosis fungoides
Hairy cell
Unclassifiable
Others

the condition is known as Waldenström's macroglobulinaemia (see p. 278).

Follicular centre cell lymphomas are composed of cells resembling normal follicle centre B cells, with a background of dendritic and T-helper cells. Patients with follicular tumours are likely to be middle-aged and their disease is often characterized by a benign course for many years. However, sudden transformation may occur to aggressive blast cell and diffuse tumours which are sometimes associated with a leukaemic phase.

The intermediate and high-grade malignancy group of lymphomas are associated with a fast rate of cellular proliferation. Histologically, in immunoblastic and centroblastic types, there is widespread destruction of nodal architecture often with extension through the capsule to surrounding perinodal tissues. Progressive infiltration may affect the gastrointestinal tract, the spinal cord, the kidneys or other organs. The lymphoblastic lymphomas occur mainly in children and young adults and these conditions merge clinically and morphologically with acute lymphoblastic leukaemia (ALL). Young patients presenting with mediastinal masses may be labelled as T-cell lymphoblastic lymphoma or T-cell lymphoblastic leukaemia (T-ALL) depending on the degree of bone marrow and peripheral blood involvement at presentation.

It is now clear from marker studies that tumours of true histiocytes or monocyte-derived cells are rare. These tumours are discussed later in this chapter.

Predisposing diseases

In AIDS there is an increased incidence of lymphomas, often at unusual sites, e.g. in the central nervous system. The lymphomas are usually of B-cell origin, of high-grade or intermediate histology. Other immune deficiencies, inherited or acquired, e.g. due to therapeutic immunosuppression following renal, marrow or cardiac transplantation or following treatment of Hodgkin's disease with radiotherapy and chemotherapy, also predispose to B-cell lymphomas. EBV is usually present in the post-transplant lymphomas which may begin with a polyclonal B-cell proliferation, which resolves if immunosuppression is discontinued. Coeliac disease, dermatitis herpetiformis and angioimmunoblastic lymphadenopathy predispose to T-cell lymphomas, while infections may play a role in development of some intestinal lymphomas since antibiotics may cause resolution of the pre-malignant α-chain disease. In some MALT (mucosa associated lymphoid tumours) of the stomach *Helicobactor* infection has been implicated as a predisposing factor. Autoimmune diseases may all be complicated by non-Hodgkin's lymphoma.

Clinical features

1 *Superficial lymphadenopathy*. The majority of patients present with asymmetric painless enlargement of lymph nodes in one or more peripheral lymph node regions.
2 *Constitutional symptoms*. Fever, night sweats and weight loss occur less frequently than in Hodgkin's disease and their presence is usually associated with disseminated disease. Anaemia and infections of the type seen in Hodgkin's disease may occur.
3 *Oropharyngeal involvement*. In 5−10% of patients there is disease of the oropharyngeal lymphoid structures (Waldeyer's ring) which may cause complaints of a 'sore throat' or noisy or obstructed breathing.
4 *Anaemia*, neutropenia with infections or thrombocytopenia with purpura may be presenting features in patients with diffuse bone marrow disease. Cytopenias may be autoimmune in origin.
5 *Abdominal disease*. The liver and spleen are often enlarged and involvement of retroperitoneal or mesenteric nodes is fre-

quent (see Fig. 13.11). The gastrointestinal tract is the most commonly involved extranodal site after the bone marrow, and patients may present with acute abdominal symptoms.

6 *Other organs.* Skin, brain, testis, gastrointestinal tract or thyroid involvement is not infrequent. The skin is also primarily involved in two unusual, closely related T-cell lymphomas, mycosis fungoides and Sézary's syndrome.

The median age at presentation is 50 years.

Haematological findings

1 A normochromic, normocytic anaemia is usual but auto-immune haemolytic anaemia may also occur.

2 In advanced disease with marrow involvement there may be neutropenia, thrombocytopenia (especially if the spleen is enlarged) or leuco-erythroblastic features.

3 Lymphoma cells ('cleaved follicular lymphoma' or 'blast' cells) with variable nuclear abnormalities may be found in the peripheral blood in some patients.

4 Trephine biopsy of marrow shows focal involvement, usually paratrabecular, in 20% of cases (see Fig. 13.12). Diffuse infiltration often accompanied by fibrosis may also occur. Paradoxically, bone marrow involvement is found more frequently in low-grade malignant lymphomas. Immunological marker studies using fluorescence or peroxidase techniques may detect minimal involvement (e.g. with a clonal population of B cells shown by restricted Ig light chain (κ or λ) usage) not easily recognized by conventional microscopy.

Immunological markers
Monoclonal antibodies to antigens expressed on cells at sequential stages of lymphoid development and in different lineages or states of activation are used in the classification of malignant lymphoma (Table 13.3).

Chromosome findings
Follicular B-cell lymphoma (and rarely other B-cell lymphomas) are associated with the translocation 14;18 in which the onco-gene BCL-2 is moved from chromosome 18 into the heavy chain immunoglobulin locus on chromosome 14 and expressed excessively. In small or large cell diffuse lymphomas the t(11;14) translocation is frequent. The oncogene BCL-1 is translocated from chromosome 11 to chromosome 14. Translocations involving chromosome 14 and the T-cell receptor α and δ genes are frequent in T-cell lymphoma. Various other cytogenetic abnormalities have been described in both B- and T-cell lymphomas.

264

CHAPTER 13

T cell	B cell	Activation markers	Leucocyte common antigen
CD2	CD19	CD23	CD45
CD3	CD20	CD25	
CD5	CD22	CD30	
CD7	CD24		
T-cell	*Rare*		
subsets	*B cell*		
CD4	CD5		
CD8			

Other antigens which may be useful in lymphoma diagnosis include CD10, TdT and adherence molecules

TdT, terminal deoxynucleotidyl transferase.

Table 13.3 Cluster differentiation (CD) antigens useful in lymphoma diagnosis.

Gene rearrangements

In B-cell lymphomas the immunoglobulin genes are clonally rearranged, usually involving both heavy and light chain genes; whereas in T-cell lymphomas, the immunoglobin genes are in germ-line configuration but there is clonal rearrangement of the T-cell receptor genes.

Blood chemistry

Elevation of serum uric acid may occur. Abnormal liver function tests suggest disseminated disease. The serum LDH level is raised in more rapidly proliferating and extensive disease and may be used as a prognostic marker.

(a)

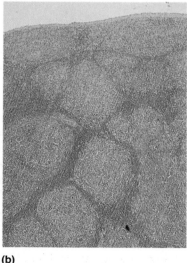

(b)

Fig. 13.8 Non-Hodgkin's lymphoma: histological sections of lymph nodes showing: (a) a diffuse pattern of involvement in lymphocytic lymphoma with the normal architecture totally replaced by neoplastic lymphocytic cells; (b) a follicular or nodular pattern in centrocytic/centroblastic lymphoma—the 'follicles' or 'nodules' of neoplastic cells compress surrounding tissue and lack a mantle of small lymphocytes.

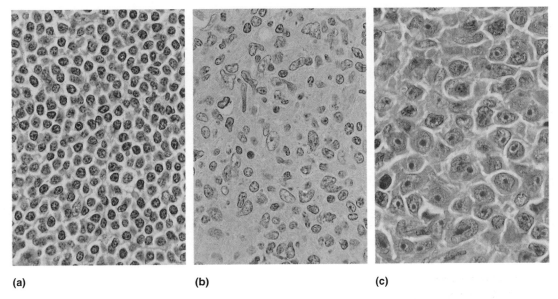

(a)   (b)   (c)

Fig. 13.9 Non-Hodgkin's lymphoma: high power view of lymph node biopsies showing: (a) lymphocytic lymphoma showing predominantly small lymphocytes with round nuclei containing densely clumped heterochromatin; (b) centrocytic lymphoma showing medium-sized cells with nuclear pleomorphism but characteristically having a cleaved nucleus and pale indistinct cytoplasm. The nuclei have a light chromatin pattern and may contain nucleoli;
(c) immunoblastic lymphoma showing large neoplastic cells with a single prominent nucleolus and abundant darkly staining cytoplasm.

Diagnostic investigations and clinical staging

The diagnosis is made by histological examination of excised lymph nodes (Figs 13.8–13.10) or extranodal tumour. The staging system is the same as that described for Hodgkin's disease but is less clearly related than histological type to prognosis.

Staging procedures include chest X-ray to detect thoracic involvement, liver biopsy, CT scanning (Fig. 13.11) or MRI to detect abdominal disease, and bone marrow aspiration and trephine (Fig. 13.12).

Because of the early haematogenous spread in the majority of patients with non-Hodgkin's lymphoma there is usually no need for exploratory laparotomy, except when required to make the initial diagnosis.

In 10–15% of patients there is initial extranodal disease, e.g. involvement of the gastrointestinal tract, lung and other organs such as the skin, brain or testis. If a careful search fails to show evidence of disseminated disease these patients are graded as having stage I_E rather than stage IV.

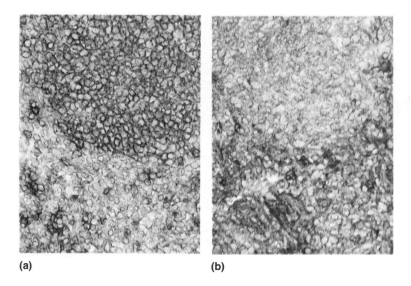

(a)   (b)

Fig. 13.10 Non-Hodgkin's lymphoma: lymph node stained by immunoperoxidase shows (a) brown ring staining for κ in the malignant lymphoid nodule, and (b) no labelling for λ confirming the monoclonal origin of the lymphoma.

Prognostic features

Apart from histology and stage, a variety of clinical and laboratory findings are relevant to the outcome of therapy. Poor prognostic factors include: the patient being older than 60–65 years, poor performance status, multiple sites of extranodal disease, elevated serum LDH, bulky disease (major mass >5 cm in diameter), and prior history of low-grade disease or of AIDS.

Treatment

Low-grade malignancy group
Some patients with low-grade malignant tumours, particularly the lymphocytic group, require no initial treatment if they are asymptomatic and the size and location of the lymphadenopathy poses no major threat. Local radiotherapy may be used for stages I, I_E or stage II. Continuous or intermittent chlorambucil or cyclophosphamide or repeated courses of fludarabine produce good results in patients with advancing disease or systemic symptoms but cure is not achieved. Trials of more aggressive combinations or even autologous BMT in an attempt to cure some patients with low-grade disease are in progress. Alpha-interferon is also used experimentally in some centres in remission induction or maintenance in non-Hodgkin's lymphomas of all grades of malignancy.

Intermediate-grade malignancy group
Patients with localized disease may be treated with initial combination therapy, e.g. cyclophosphamide, hydroxodaunorubicin (Adriamycin), vincristine (Oncovin) and prednisolone (CHOP),

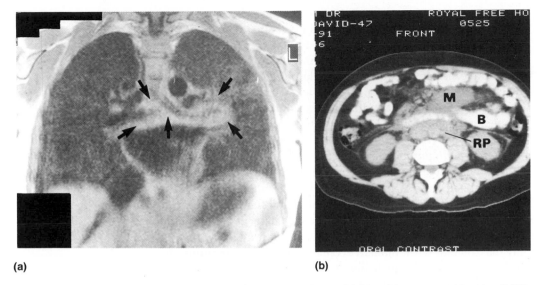

(a)   (b)

Fig. 13.11 Non-Hodgkin's lymphoma. (a) Magnetic resonance imaging (MRI) scan of the chest showing large mediastinal lymph nodes (white and arrowed) adjacent to the great vessels (black). (b) CT scan of the abdomen showing enlarged mesenteric (M) and retroperitoneal (RP; para-aortic) lymph nodes. B, bowel. (Courtesy of Dr L. Berger.)

followed by irradiation to the involved areas. In older subjects, trials of single agent therapy may be used. In patients with stage I or II bulky disease or with advanced disease (stage III or IV), intensive cyclical chemotherapy with CHOP or with one or other 'second generation' combination, e.g. M-BACOD (high- or intermediate-dose methotrexate, bleomycin, Adriamycin, cyclophosphamide, vincristine (Oncovin) and dexamethasone), has produced remission rates of 75% and long-term disease-free survival of 30–50% of patients. Paradoxically, cure seems more possible in intermediate- and high-grade lymphomas than in

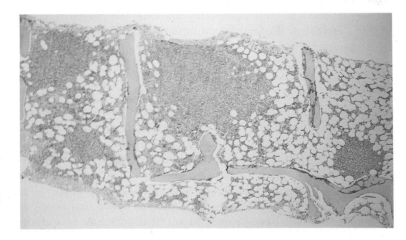

Fig. 13.12 Iliac crest trephine biopsy in lymphocytic lymphoma. Four prominent nodules of lymphoid tissue are seen in the intertrabecular space.

low-grade disease. Local irradiation for major bulky sites of the disease is considered if the disease results in anatomical obstruction. Third generation regimens, e.g. PROMACE (prednisolone, methotrexate, Adriamycin, cyclophosphamide, etoposide)-MOPP have been introduced in the hope of improving results, but controlled trials do not suggest an overall increased long-term disease-free survival with these second or third generation regimens compared with CHOP.

High-grade malignancy group
Patients with large cell lymphomas, e.g. immunoblastic, that are truly localized stage I may be cured by radiotherapy. However, the disease is usually widespread and chemotherapy is advised in all, as for the patients in the intermediate group. Patients with lymphoblastic lymphoma, including Burkitt's lymphoma, may be treated with intensive chemotherapy programmes including, for example, high doses of methotrexate and cytosine arabinoside together with cycles of cyclophosphamide, Adriamycin and vincristine (MACHO); similar regimens are used for B-ALL. There is usually a dramatic response but the relapse rate is high. Central nervous system prophylaxis employing intrathecal (or high-dose systemic) methotrexate or cytosine arabinoside, with or without cranial irradiation, is required to prevent meningeal relapse in young subjects including those with T-cell disease. Allogeneic or autologous BMT in first complete remission is considered.

Relapsed cases
As in Hodgkin's disease, re-induction chemotherapy followed by intensive chemotherapy/radiotherapy with autologous bone marrow infusion as rescue, may be used in an attempt to cure patients who have relapsed after initial therapy. Some units 'purge' the harvested marrow of possible residual tumour cells using monoclonal antibodies or other techniques. Drugs which are often used in intensive combinations for relapsed cases include cisplatin, ifosfamide, cyclophosphamide, mitoxantrone, cytosine arabinoside and etoposide.

Prognosis

The majority of patients with low-grade malignant disease and follicular patterns of architecture survive for longer than 5 years and many are alive more than 10 years after diagnosis. Some patients with localized high-grade malignancy disease are cured by radiotherapy. With intensive chemotherapy, patients with widespread high-grade malignant lymphomas have a 40–50% disease-free survival at 2 years and it seems likely that some of these patients will have prolonged survival and may be cured.

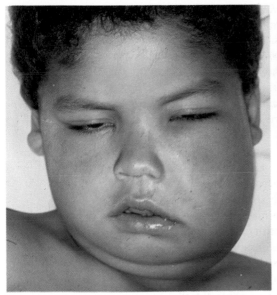

Fig. 13.13 Burkitt's lymphoma: characteristic facial swelling due to extensive tumour involvement of the mandible and surrounding soft tissues.

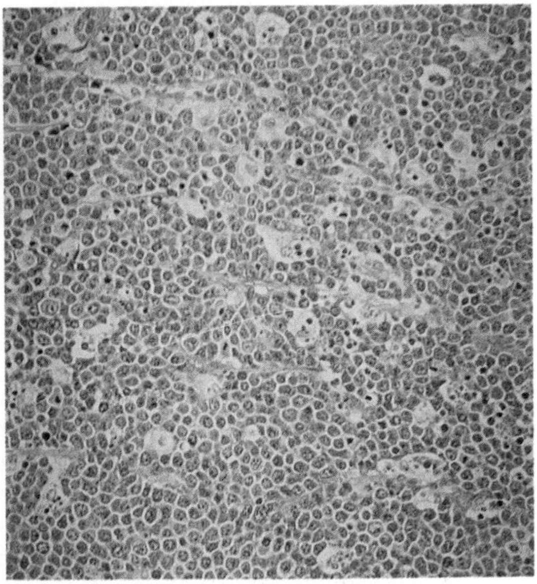

Fig. 13.14 Burkitt lymphoma: histological section of lymph node showing sheets of lymphoblasts and 'starry sky' tingible body macrophages.

Rare syndromes

Burkitt's ('African') lymphoma

This unusual B-lymphoblastic lymphoma which is found particularly in young African children has a peculiar predilection for massive jaw lesions (Fig. 13.13), extranodal abdominal involvement and, in girls, ovarian tumours.

Isolated histiocytes in the masses of abnormal lymphoblasts produce a characteristic 'starry sky' appearance in tissue sections (Fig. 13.14). The EBV has been identified in Burkitt cell culture and the chromosome translocation t(8;14) is usual. Other translocations involving the immunoglobulin genes and c-*MYC* (t8;22, t2;8) occur in a minority of patients (see Chapter 10). Sporadic cases of Burkitt's lymphoma occur in other races.

Chemotherapy produces dramatic initial clinical remissions but relapses are frequent, with only 30% of patients being cured. Autologous BMT may be used as salvage therapy.

Mycosis fungoides and Sézary's syndrome

Mycosis fungoides is a chronic cutaneous T-cell lymphoma which presents with severe pruritus and psoriasis-like lesions. Ultimately deeper organs are affected, particularly lymph nodes, spleen, liver and bone marrow. In Sézary's syndrome, there is

characteristically exfoliative dermatitis, erythrodermia, generalized lymphadenopathy and circulating T-lymphoma cells. The
cells are usually CD4+ and have a folded or cerebriform nuclear
chromatin. Initial treatment of these conditions is by local
irradiation, topical chemotherapy or photochemotherapy with
psoralen and ultraviolet light (PUVA). Subsequently chemotherapy may be needed. Deoxycoformycin produces partial or
complete remissions in 50% of cases of Sézary's syndrome.

Adult T-cell leukaemia/lymphoma

This is a widespread disease of adults of either sex, usually presenting with lymphadenopathy, hepatic and splenic enlargement, cutaneous infiltrations and hypercalcaemia. The disease
is frequent in Japan, the Caribbean and South America but
occurs in countries of Africa, the USA and sporadically elsewhere. It has a rapid clinical course. The blood, bone marrow
and other tissues are infiltrated with lymphoma cells with
lobulated nuclei, which have been shown to be CD3+ T cells
infected with the human T-cell leukaemia/lymphoma virus,
HTLV-1.

The virus is an exogenous human chronic leukaemia retrovirus. The site of integration into the host cell DNA varies
between patients, but in any one patient, is clonal. The mechanism by which the virus causes malignant transformation in a
proportion of infected subjects is uncertain since the virus lacks
a transforming oncogene (v-onc) (see Chapter 10). Serological
studies show that many apparently healthy persons have also
been infected with the virus and are carriers. They are found
most frequently among close contacts of the patients with overt
disease. The disease responds poorly to chemotherapy.

Close contact appears to be necessary for HTLV-1 transmission.
The related virus HIV is the cause of AIDS (see p. 179). This
latter virus also infects T cells, specifically the CD4 subset, but
also kills them, leading to immune suppression rather than to
malignant transformation.

Angioimmunoblastic lymphadenopathy

This disease usually occurs in elderly patients with generalized
lymphadenopathy, hepatosplenomegaly, skin rashes and a polyclonal increase in serum IgG. In the majority, the malignant cell
has been identified as an abnormal T cell. Occasionally, the
condition appears to be precipitated by exposure to drugs. Histologically, the lymph node shows replacement by a mixed cellular
infiltrate, comprising immunoblasts, plasma cells, macrophages
and granulocytes, around proliferating small blood vessels. The
condition may transform into an immunoblastic lymphoma.

Malignant histiocytic tumours

True histiocytic tumours of the lymphoid system are rare. Histiocytic lymphoma is a high-grade lymphoma which may terminate with a leukaemic phase. Disseminated malignant histiocytosis is a rapidly fatal disease. Patients present with fever, weight loss, anorexia, hepatosplenomegaly and bone marrow failure. In the variant known as histiocytic medullary reticulosis, the malignant histiocytes phagocytose red cells causing a haemolytic anaemia with prominent jaundice. In these syndromes survival beyond 6 months is rare.

Sinus histiocytosis with massive lymphadenopathy

This occurs particularly in young Africans and is characterized by massive cervical lymphadenopathy, fever, leucocytosis and a polyclonal increase in IgG. The nodes show sinusoidal dilation with plasma cell and macrophage infiltration. The condition appears to be due to virus infection and recovers spontaneously usually over several months or years.

Bibliography

Aisenberg A.C. (1991) *Malignant Lymphoma: Biology, Natural History and Treatment*. Lea & Febiger, Philadelphia.

American Journal of Clinical Pathology. (1993) Special Issue: A tribute to Henry Rappaport. **99**, 359–525.

Armitage J.O. (ed.) (1991) Non-Hodgkin's lymphoma. *Hematology/Oncology Clinics of North America*, **5**, 845–1093.

Bonadonna G. & Santoro A. (1990) Current issues in the management of advanced Hodgkin's disease. *Blood Reviews*, **4**, 69–73.

Collins R.H. (1990) The pathogenesis of Hodgkin's disease. *Blood Reviews*, **4**, 61–72.

Goldstone A.H. & Linch D.C. (1992) Bone marrow transplantation in the malignant lymphomas. In *Recent Advances in Haematology*, 6 (eds A.V. Hoffbrand & M.K. Brenner). Churchill Livingstone, Edinburgh, pp. 149–172.

Jarrett R.F. (1992) Hodgkin's disease. *Clinical Haematology*, **5**, 57–80.

Kaplan H.S. (1980) *Hodgkin's Disease*, 2nd Edition. Harvard University Press, Cambridge, Mass.

Lennert K. (1981) *Histopathology of Non-Hodgkin's Lymphomas*. Springer-Verlag, New York.

Lukes R.J. & Collins R.D. (1992) *Tumors of the Hematopoietic System*. Armed Forces Institute of Pathology, Washington.

Magrath I.T. (1990) *The Non-Hodgkin's Lymphomas*. Edward Arnold, London.

Ramot B. & Rechavi G. (1992) Non-Hodgkin's lymphomas and paraproteinaemias. *Clinical Haematology*, **5**, 81–100.

Swerdlow S.H. (1992) *Biopsy Interpretation of Lymph Nodes*. Raven, New York.

Urba W.J. & Longo D.L. (1992) Medical progress: Hodgkin's disease. *New England Journal of Medicine*, **326**, 618–687.

Williams S.F., Farah R. & Golomb H.M. (1989) Hodgkin's disease. *Hematology/Oncology Clinics of North America*, **3**, 187–367.

Chapter 14
Multiple Myeloma and Related Disorders

Multiple myeloma

Multiple myeloma (myelomatosis) is a neoplastic monoclonal proliferation of bone marrow plasma cells, characterized by lytic bone lesions, plasma cell accumulation in the bone marrow, and the presence of monoclonal protein in the serum and urine. Ninety-eight per cent of cases occur over the age of 40 with a peak incidence in the seventh decade. In Britain there is a mean annual death rate of nine per million of the population.

The cell of origin is unknown although small TdT− (terminal deoxynucleotidyl transferase negative), CD10+ lymphoid cells of the bone marrow or post-germinal centre cells have been suggested. The myeloma cells have clonally rearranged immuno-globulin genes and show on their surface the same paraprotein that is present in serum. Whether these cells arise in the bone marrow or peripherally in lymphoid germinal centres and then home to the marrow is controversial. A variety of clonal chromosomal changes have been found as well as mutations of the RAS oncogenes. Interleukin (IL)-6 is a potent growth factor for myeloma, possibly by an autocrine mechanism. The osteolytic lesions in this disease are probably the result of osteoclast-activating factor (OAF) now thought to be tumour necrosis factor (TNF) and/or IL-1 secreted by the myeloma cells.

Clinical features

1 Bone pain (especially backache) and pathological fractures.
2 Features of anaemia: lethargy, weakness, dyspnoea, pallor, tachycardia, etc.
3 Repeated infections; these are related to deficient antibody production and, in advanced disease, to neutropenia.
4 Features of renal failure and/or hypercalcaemia: polydipsia, polyuria, anorexia, vomiting, constipation and mental disturbance.
5 Abnormal bleeding tendency: myeloma protein may interfere with platelet function and coagulation factors; thrombocytopenia occurs in advanced disease.
6 Occasionally there is macroglossia, carpal tunnel syndrome and diarrhoea due to amyloid disease.
7 In about 2% of cases there is a hyperviscosity syndrome with

purpura, haemorrhages, visual failure, CNS symptoms and neuropathies, and heart failure. This results from polymerization of the abnormal immunoglobulin (Ig) and is particularly likely when this is IgA, IgM or IgD.

Diagnosis

This depends on three principal findings.

1 In 98% of patients monoclonal protein occurs in the serum or urine or both (Fig. 14.1). The serum paraprotein is IgG in two-thirds, IgA in one-third, with rare IgM or IgD or mixed cases. Other causes of a serum paraprotein are listed in Table 14.1. In doubtful cases, follow-up studies will show a progressive rise in paraprotein concentration in untreated myeloma. Normal serum immunoglobulins (IgG, IgA and IgM) are depressed. The urine contains Bence-Jones protein in two-thirds of cases. This consists of free light chains, either κ or λ, of the same type as the serum paraprotein. In 15% of cases, however, Bence-Jones proteinuria is present without a serum paraprotein.

2 The bone marrow shows increased plasma cells (>4% and usually >30%), often with abnormal forms — 'myeloma cells' (Fig. 14.2). Immunological testing shows these cells to be monoclonal B cells and to express the same immunoglobulin heavy and light chains as the serum monoclonal protein.

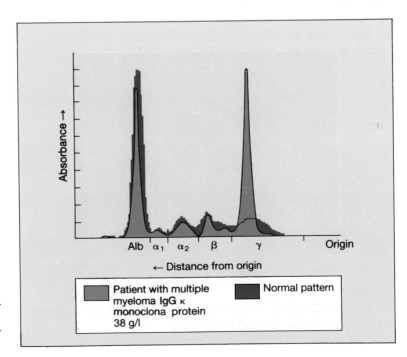

Fig. 14.1 Serum protein electrophoresis in multiple myeloma showing an abnormal paraprotein in the γ-globulin region with reduced levels of background β- and γ-globulins.

Malignant or uncontrolled production
Multiple myeloma
Waldenström's macroglobulinaemia
Malignant lymphoma
Chronic lymphocytic leukaemia
Primary amyloidosis
Plasma cell leukaemia
Heavy chain disease
Benign or stable production
Benign monoclonal gammopathy
Chronic cold haemagglutinin disease
Transient M proteins
Acquired immune deficiency syndrome (AIDS)
Rarely with carcinoma and other conditions

Table 14.1 Diseases associated with M proteins.

3 Skeletal survey shows osteolytic areas without evidence of surrounding osteoblastic reaction or sclerosis in 60% of patients (Fig. 14.3) or generalized bone rarefaction (20%) (Fig. 14.4). Pathological fractures are common. No bone lesions are found in 20% of patients.

Usually at least two of the three diagnostic features mentioned above are present.

Other laboratory findings
1 There is usually a normochromic, normocytic or macrocytic anaemia. Rouleaux formation is marked in most cases (Fig. 14.5). Neutropenia and thrombocytopenia occur in advanced disease. Abnormal plasma cells appear in the blood film in 15% of patients. Leuco-erythroblastic changes are occasionally seen.
2 High erythrocyte sedimentation rate (ESR).

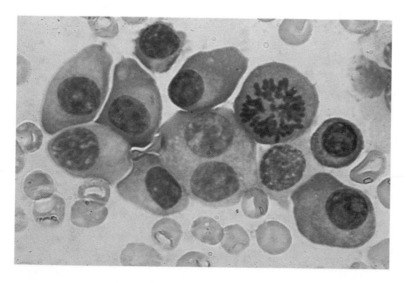

Fig. 14.2 The bone marrow in multiple myeloma showing large numbers of plasma cells, with many abnormal forms.

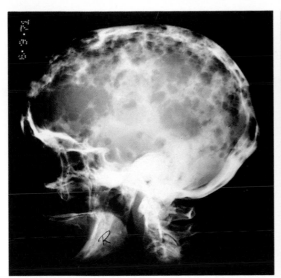

Fig. 14.3 Skull X-ray in multiple myeloma showing many 'punched-out' lesions.

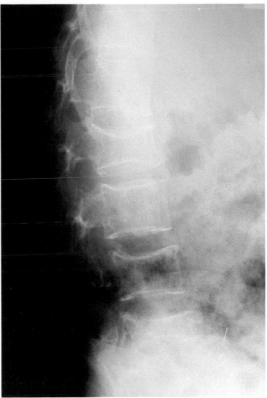

Fig. 14.4 Multiple myeloma: X-ray of lumbar spine showing severe demineralization with partial collapse of L3.

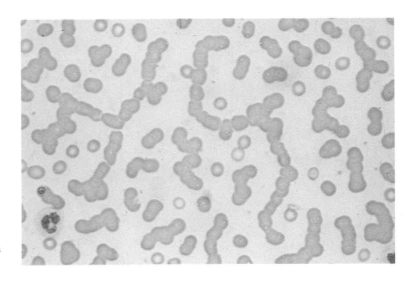

Fig. 14.5 The peripheral blood film in multiple myeloma showing rouleaux formation.

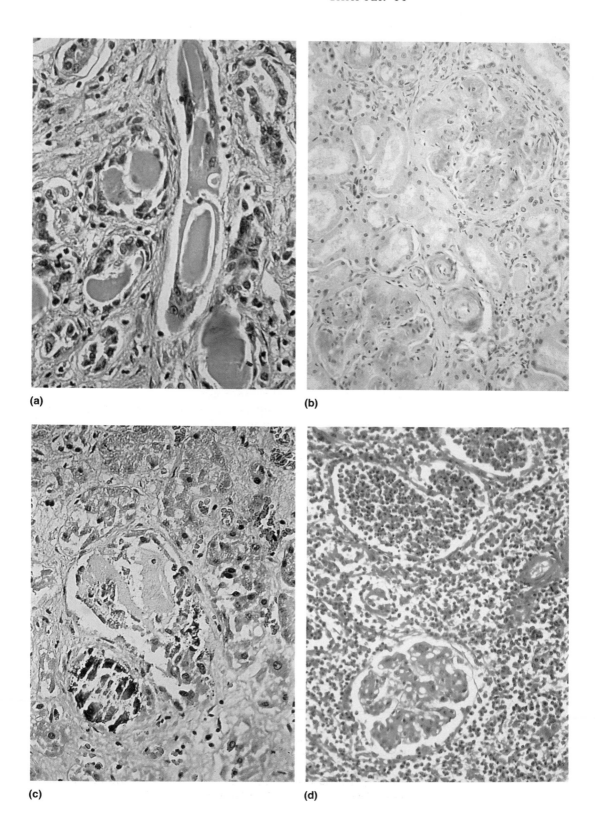

(a)

(b)

(c)

(d)

3 Serum calcium elevation occurs in 45% of patients. There is a normal serum alkaline phosphatase (except following pathological fractures).

4 The blood urea is raised above 14 mmol/l and serum creatinine raised in 20% of cases. Proteinaceous deposits from heavy Bence-Jones proteinuria, hypercalcaemia, uric acid, amyloid and pyelonephritis may all contribute to renal failure (Fig. 14.6).

5 A low serum albumin occurs with advanced disease.

6 Serum β_2-microglobulin (the light chain of the HLA class 1 antigens) is a useful indicator of prognosis. It partly reflects renal function. Levels less than 4 mg/l imply a relatively good prognosis.

Treatment

Emergency situations

1 Uraemia: rehydrate and treat underlying cause (e.g. hypercalcaemia, hyperuricaemia). Haemodialysis is considered in some patients.

2 Acute hypercalcaemia: rehydrate with isotonic saline and give prednisolone intravenously or orally. Mithramycin or calcitonin may also be beneficial. Diphosphonates may be used to try to prevent or reverse bone absorption.

3 Compression paraplegia: decompression laminectomy, irradiation or chemotherapy.

4 Single painful skeletal lesion: chemotherapy or irradiation.

5 Severe anaemia: transfusion of packed red cells.

6 Bleeding due to paraprotein interference with coagulation and hyperviscosity syndrome may be treated by repeated plasmapheresis.

7 Severe recurrent infections: prophylactic infusions of immunoglobulin concentrates together with oral broad-spectrum antibiotics and antifungal agents may be needed.

Chemotherapy

Alkylating agents relieve pain, reduce plasma cell proliferation in the marrow and so reduce the serum paraprotein levels. As plasma cells are killed, normal bone marrow function improves. In older patients (over the age of 65) melphalan or cyclophos-

---

Fig. 14.6 (*Opposite*) The kidney in multiple myeloma. (a) *Myeloma kidney* — the renal tubules are distended with hyaline protein (precipitated light chains or Bence-Jones protein). Giant cells are prominent in the surrounding cellular reaction. (b) *Amyloid deposition* — both glomeruli and several of the small blood vessels contain an amorphous pink-staining deposit characteristic of amyloid (Congo red stain). (c) *Nephrocalcinosis* — calcium deposition (dark 'fractured' material) in the renal parenchyma. (d) *Pyelonephritis* — destruction of renal parenchyma and infiltration by acute inflammatory cells.

phamide, with or without prednisolone, are the drugs of choice. Melphalan is given daily for 4–7 days every 6–8 weeks. Allopurinol is also given to prevent urate nephropathy. Because of the likelihood of resistance developing to alkylating agent therapy, treatment of symptomless patients with early disease is not justified. Regular clinical and laboratory assessment should be made of disease progression. Treatment may be delayed until the development of signs or symptoms of bone marrow failure, until there is a rise in blood urea or Bence-Jones protein appears in the urine, or until bone lesions are extensive or cause symptoms.

In younger subjects (under 60 years) many units now prefer to use repeated courses of combination chemotherapy initially, e.g. the combination ABCM (Adriamycin and BCNU on day 1 and cyclophosphamide and melphelan on day 22). Some units use an even more intensive regimen, e.g. VAD (vincristine and Adriamycin given by slow continuous infusion and dexamethasone) over a 4-day period. Multiple courses (usually four to six) are given to reduce the disease to a minimum, assessed clinically and by paraprotein measurement. Autologous bone marrow transplantation (BMT) following a high single dose of melphelan may then be given. In some cases this leads to complete remission of the disease lasting several years.

Trials are currently underway to assess the value of α-interferon therapy in combination with other drugs in the induction phase; there is evidence that it may also prolong the plateau phase.

Prognosis

The median survival is 2 years with a 20% 4-year survival. The most serious prognostic feature is the blood urea concentration: if the blood urea is more than 14 mmol/l at presentation the median survival is only a few months. If the blood urea is less than 7 mmol/l at presentation the median survival is 33 months. Severe anaemia, a low serum albumin at presentation, heavy Bence-Jones proteinuria and increased β_2-microglobulin levels are also bad prognostic features.

Waldenström's macroglobulinaemia

This is an uncommon condition, seen most frequently in men over 50 years of age, which behaves clinically as a slowly progressive lymphoma. There is proliferation of cells which produce a monoclonal IgM paraprotein and bear some resemblance both to lymphocytes and plasma cells.

The term Waldenström's macroglobulinaemia is often restricted to cases where the dominant clinical features are the result of macroglobulinaemia and diffuse cellular infiltrates.

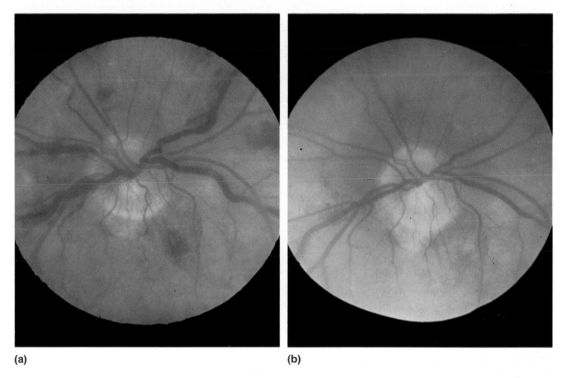

(a)   (b)

Fig. 14.7 Waldenström's macroglobulinaemia: hyperviscosity syndrome. The retina before plasmapheresis (a) shows distension of retinal vessels, particularly the veins which show bulging and constriction (the 'linked sausage' effect) and areas of haemorrhage; (b) following plasmapheresis the vessels have returned to normal and the areas of haemorrhage have cleared.

Those cases with dominant tumour masses are often referred to as malignant lymphoma with macroglobulinaemia. In both cases, the malignant cells are a monoclonal B-cell population.

Clinical features

1 There is usually an insidious onset, with fatigue and weight loss.
2 Hyperviscosity syndrome (see p. 284): IgM paraprotein increases blood viscosity more than equivalent concentrations of IgG or IgA, and small increases above 30 g/l in concentration lead to large increases in viscosity. The retina may show a variety of changes: engorged veins, haemorrhages, exudates and a blurred disc (Fig. 14.7). If the macroglobulin is a cryoglobulin, features of cryoprecipitation, e.g. Raynaud's phenomenon, may be present.
3 A bleeding tendency may result from macroglobulin interference with coagulation factors and platelet function.
4 Anaemia due to haemodilution, decreased red cell survival, blood loss and bone marrow failure in advanced disease.
5 Moderate lymphadenopathy and enlargement of the liver and spleen are frequently seen.

Diagnosis

1 Serum monoclonal IgM is usually greater than 15 g/l.

2 Bone marrow shows pleomorphic infiltration by small lymphocytes, plasma cells, plasmacytoid forms, immature lymphoid cells, mast cells and histiocytes. Trephine biopsy may show nodular disease which implies a better prognosis than the diffuse infiltration.

3 High ESR.

4 Often a peripheral blood lymphocytosis with some plasmacytoid lymphocytes.

5 Lymph node histology shows preserved sinus architecture, loss of follicular pattern with cellular infiltration similar to that found in the bone marrow.

Treatment

1 Acute hyperviscosity syndrome: give repeated plasmapheresis. As IgM is mainly intravascular, plasmapheresis is more effective than with IgG or IgA paraproteins when much of the protein is extravascular and so rapidly replenishes the plasma compartment.

2 Supportive therapy: transfusions for anaemia, antibiotics for infections, etc.

3 Alkylating agents, chlorambucil or cyclophosphamide, with prednisolone are the most widely used drugs; chlorodeoxyadenosine is a new effective agent. These reduce bone marrow infiltration and lower the serum concentration of IgM. No therapy is needed for patients without symptoms, significant hepatosplenomegaly or adenopathy or anaemia.

Other plasma cell tumours

Solitary plasmacytoma of bone

In this rare disease there is no plasma cell proliferation in parts of the skeleton beyond the primary lesion, and marrow aspirates distant from the primary tumour are usually normal. An associated M protein disappears following radiotherapy to the primary lesion.

Soft-tissue plasmacytoma

These tumours are found most frequently in the mucosa of the upper respiratory and gastrointestinal tracts, in the cervical lymph nodes, central nervous system and in the skin. They tend to remain localized and the majority are well controlled by excision or by local irradiation.

Plasma cell leukaemia

This occurs either as a late complication of myeloma or, often in younger patients, as a primary disease characterized by the presence of 20% or more plasma cells in the blood, with an absolute count of $>2.0 \times 10^9/l$. There is more liver and spleen involvement and less bone involvement than in myeloma. The paraprotein concentration in serum is often low. The results of therapy are poor.

Heavy chain disease

In these rare disorders the neoplastic cells secrete only immuno-globulin heavy chains (γ, α or μ) and these chains are usually incomplete.

Gamma-heavy chain disease presents in a similar way to malignant lymphoma. The disease is most often found in elderly males and lymphadenopathy, fever and anaemia are usually present with a monoclonal protein in the serum.

Alpha-heavy chain disease, the most common form, occurs mainly in the Mediterranean area and North Africa; particularly in Arabs and in areas where there is a heavy infestation with intestinal parasites. Malabsorption is associated with an initial benign lymphoproliferation in the gastrointestinal tract which is often followed by a poorly differentiated lymphoma arising in the small intestine. The serum monoclonal protein is found in 50% of cases in either the α or β position on electrophoresis and may also be found in the urine. A rare form of α-heavy chain disease may involve the respiratory tract.

Mu-heavy chain disease, the rarest form, is found in parasite-infected areas of Africa and may resemble chronic lymphocytic leukaemia with plasmacytoid lymphoid cells in the marrow and enlargement of the liver and spleen.

Benign monoclonal gammopathy

A paraprotein may be found in the serum, particularly of older subjects, with no definite evidence of myeloma, macro-globulinaemia or lymphoma. There are no bone lesions, usually no Bence-Jones proteinuria, and the proportion of plasma cells in the marrow is normal (<4%) or only slightly raised (<10%). The concentration of monoclonal immunoglobulin in serum is usually less than 20 g/l and remains stationary when followed over a period of 2 or 3 years. Other serum immunoglobulins are not depressed. After many years of follow-up, however, a substantial proportion of these patients develop overt myeloma.

The distinguishing features of benign and malignant paraproteinaemia are listed in Table 14.2.

	Benign	Malignant
Bence-Jones proteinuria	Absent	May be present
Serum paraprotein concentration	Usually <20 g/l and stationary	Usually >20 g/l and rising
Immuneparesis	Absent	Present
Underlying lymphoproliferative disease or myeloma	Absent	Present
Bone lesions	Absent	Present
Plasma cells in marrow	<10%	>10%

Table 14.2 Features of benign and malignant paraproteinaemia.

Amyloidosis

This is a homogenous deposit in tissues, staining pink with haematoxylin and eosin (H&E) and red with Congo red, and exhibiting green birefringence. Amyloid has a fibrillary structure.

The pathogenesis of amyloidosis is shown in Fig. 14.8. Amyloid deposition is usually due to overproduction, reduced degradation or reduced excretion of protein. Rarely variant proteins produced as a result of genetic abnormality may be the cause. Proteolysis of larger molecules produces low-molecular-weight fragments that polymerize and assume a β-conformation to form extra-

Fig. 14.8 Pathogenesis of amyloidosis (from Stone, 1990). SAA, serum amyloid-A protein (see p. 283).

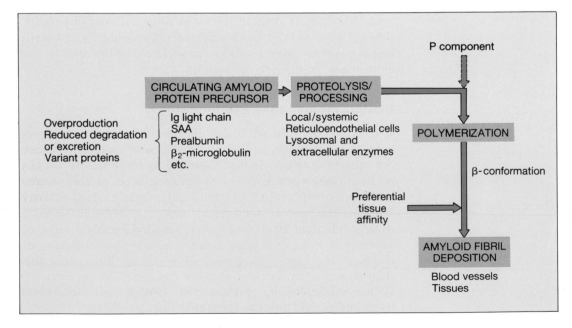

Table 14.3 Classification of amyloidosis: types, structure and organ involvement.

Type	Chemical nature	Organs involved
Immunocyte-related		
Myeloma	Ig light chains and/or	Tongue
Waldenström's	parts of their	Skin
macroglobulinaemia	variable regions	Heart
Heavy-chain disease	(AL)	Nerves
Primary amyloidosis		Connective tissue
		Kidneys
		Liver
		Spleen
Reactive systemic		
Rheumatoid arthritis	Protein A (acute	Liver
Tuberculosis	reactive, AA)	Spleen
Bronchiectasis		Kidneys
Chronic osteomyelitis		Bone marrow
Hodgkin's disease		
Carcinomas		
Familial Mediterranean fever		
Localized		
Involvement of a single	Hormones	Endocrine
organ	Protein A with other	tumours
	constituents	Skin
		Heart
		CNS
		(Alzheimer's
		disease)

cellular amyloid tissue deposits. Except for intracerebral amyloid plaques, all amyloid deposits contain a non-fibrillary glycoprotein amyloid P (AP) which is derived from a normal serum precursor structurally related to C-reactive protein. Amyloidosis is classified as follows (Table 14.3).

Amyloid associated with monoclonal immunocyte proliferation

This type consists of light chains and/or the N terminal V_L domains of the light chains. This is termed the AL type and occurs in association with myeloma, Waldenström's macroglobulinaemia, heavy-chain disease and in a 'primary' form. The clinical features are due to involvement of the heart, tongue (Fig. 14.9), peripheral nerves and kidneys, and the patient may present with heart failure, macroglosia, peripheral neuropathy or the carpal tunnel syndrome, or with renal failure.

Reactive systemic amyloidosis

This type consists of a protein A which is derived from serum amyloid-A (SAA) protein (protein A), an apolipoprotein. It is

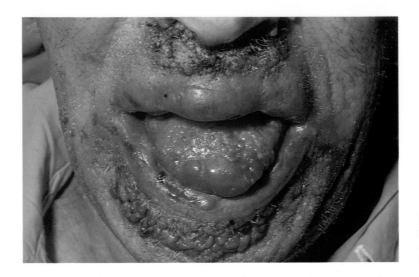

Fig. 14.9 Multiple myeloma: the tongue and lips are enlarged due to nodular and waxy deposits of amyloid.

termed the AA type. It occurs in association with chronic infections (e.g. tuberculosis), rheumatoid arthritis and neoplastic diseases, including Hodgkin's disease. It is also common in association with familial Mediterranean fever. The clinical features are due to reticuloendothelial involvement with enlargement of the liver and spleen; kidney involvement may occur with renal vein thrombosis and the nephrotic syndrome.

Amyloid due to deposition of other proteins

A variety of proteins may be degraded and deposited as localized amyloid in the central nervous system (e.g. in Alzheimer's disease), in certain endocrine tumours, the heart, and in the skin in the elderly. In some chronic dialysis patients, β_2-microglobulin deposition may occur as generalized amyloid.

Hyperviscosity syndrome

The commonest cause is polycythaemia (see p. 286). Hyperviscosity may also occur in patients with myeloma or Waldenström's macroglobulinaemia or in patients with chronic or acute leukaemias associated with very high white cell counts. Rarely, haemophiliac patients with circulating inhibitors, being treated with massive doses of cryoprecipitate, have developed hyperviscosity because of the large volumes of fibrinogen infused.

The clinical features of the hyperviscosity syndrome include visual disturbances, lethargy, confusion, muscle weakness, nervous system symptoms and signs, and congestive heart failure. The retina may show a variety of changes: engorged veins, haemorrhages, exudates and a blurred disc (see Fig. 14.7).

Emergency treatment varies with the cause: venesection or isovolaemic exchange of a plasma substitute for red cells in a polycythaemic patient; plasmapheresis in myeloma, Waldenström's disease or hyperfibrinogenaemia; and leucapheresis or chemotherapy in leukaemias associated with high white counts. The long-term treatment depends on control of the primary disease with specific therapy.

Bibliography

Barlogie B. (ed.) (1992) Multiple myeloma. *Hematology/Oncology Clinics of North America*, **6**, 211–484.

Barlogie B., Epstein J., Selvanayagam P. & Alexanian R. (1989) Plasma cell myeloma—new biological insights and advances in therapy. *Blood*, **73**, 865–879.

Cohen A.S. & Skinner M. (1990) New frontiers in the study of amyloidosis. *New England Journal of Medicine*, **323**, 542–543.

Delamore I.W. (ed.) (1986) *Multiple Myeloma and Other Paraproteinanaemias*. Churchill Livingstone, Edinburgh.

Durie B.G.M. (1988) Plasma cell disorders: recent advances in the biology and treatment. In *Recent Advances in Haematology*, 5 (ed. A.V. Hoffbrand). Churchill Livingstone, Edinburgh, pp. 305–327.

Greipp P.R. (1989) Monoclonal gammopathies: new approaches to clinical problems in diagnosis and prognosis. *Blood Reviews*, **3**, 222–236.

Hawkins P.N. (1988) Amyloidosis. *Blood Reviews*, **3**, 270–280.

Kyle R.A. (1991) Plasma cell proliferative diseases. In *Hematology: Basic Principles and Practice* (eds R. Hoffman, E.J. Benz, S.J. Shattil, B. Furie & H.J. Cohen). Churchill Livingstone, New York, pp. 1021–1038.

Mandelli F., Avvisati G., Amadori S. *et al.* (1992) Maintenance treatment with recombinant interferon alpha-2b in patients with multiple myeloma responding to conventional induction chemotherapy. *New England Journal of Medicine*, **322**, 1430–1434.

Stone M.J. (1990) Amyloidosis: a final common pathology for protein deposition in tissues. *Blood*, **75**, 531–545.

Warburton P., Joshua D.E., Gibson J. & Brown R.D. (1989) CD10-(CALLA)-positive lymphocytes in myeloma: evidence that they are a malignant precursor population and are of germinated centre origin. *Leukaemia and Lymphoma*, **1**, 11–20.

Chapter 15
Myeloproliferative Disorders

The term myeloproliferative disorders describes a group of conditions characterized by clonal proliferation of one or more haemopoietic components in the bone marrow and, in many cases, the liver and spleen. These disorders are closely related to each other; transitional forms occur and, in many patients, an evolution from one entity into another occurs during the course of the disease (Fig. 15.1). Polycythaemia vera (PV), essential thrombocythaemia and myelofibrosis are collectively known as the non-leukaemic myeloproliferative disorders and are discussed here; chronic myeloid leukaemia is discussed in Chapter 12.

Polycythaemia

Polycythaemia (erythrocytosis) refers to a pattern of blood cell changes that includes an increase in haemoglobin above 17.5 g/dl in adult males and 15.5 g/dl in females usually with an accompanying rise in red cell count (above $6.0 \times 10^{12}/l$ in males and $5.5 \times 10^{12}/l$ in females) and haematocrit (above 55% in males and 47% in females). The causes of polycythaemia are listed in Table 15.1. Studies with ^{51}Cr-labelled red cells to measure total red cell volume (TRCV) (mass) and ^{125}I-albumin (to measure plasma volume) are required to establish whether the polycythaemia is 'real', where there is an increase in TRCV, or 'relative', where there is no increase in TRCV but the circulating plasma volume is decreased (Table 15.1). Polycythaemia is considered 'real' if the TRCV is greater than 36 ml/kg in men and 32 ml/kg in women (Table 15.2).

Polycythaemia vera

In polycythaemia vera (polycythaemia rubra vera), the increase in red cell volume is caused by endogenous myeloproliferation. The stem cell origin of the defect is suggested in many patients by an overproduction of granulocytes and platelets as well as of red cells. A variety of techniques have been used to show the clonal nature of the disease (Chapter 10). Chromosomal changes, non-specific for the disease, may occur in the marrow.

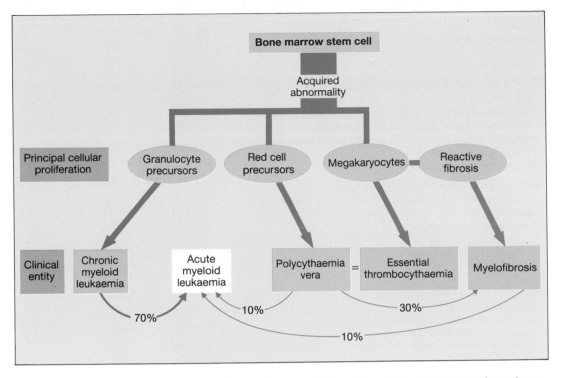

Fig. 15.1 Schematic representation of the relationship between the various myeloproliferative diseases. They may all arise by somatic mutation in the pluripotential stem and progenitor cells. Many transitional cases occur showing features of two conditions and, in other cases, the disease transforms during its course from one of these diseases to another or to acute myeloid leukaemia. Chronic myeloid leukaemia may also transform into acute lymphoblastic leukaemia.

Clinical features

This is a disease of older subjects with an equal sex incidence. Clinical features are the result of hyperviscosity, hypervolaemia or hypermetabolism.

1 Headaches, pruritus (especially after a hot bath), dyspnoea, blurred vision and night sweats.

2 Plethoric appearance — ruddy cyanosis (Fig. 15.2), conjunctival suffusion and retinal venous engorgement.

3 Splenomegaly in two-thirds of patients (Fig. 15.3a).

4 Haemorrhage (e.g. gastrointestinal, uterine, cerebral) or thrombosis either arterial (e.g. cardiac, cerebral, peripheral) or venous (e.g. deep or superficial leg veins, cerebral, portal or hepatic veins) are frequent.

5 Hypertension in one-third of patients.

6 Gout (due to raised uric acid production) (Fig. 15.4).

7 Peptic ulceration occurs in 5–10% of patients.

PRIMARY
Polycythaemia vera

SECONDARY

Due to compensatory erythropoietin increase in:
- High altitudes
- Cardiovascular disease, especially congenital with cyanosis
- Pulmonary disease and alveolar hypoventilation
- Increased affinity haemoglobin (familial polycythaemia) (see Chapter 6)
- Heavy cigarette smoking
- Methaemoglobinaemia (rarely)

Due to inappropriate erythropoietin increase in:
- Renal diseases, e.g. hydronephrosis, vascular impairment, cysts, carcinoma
- Massive uterine fibromyoma
- Hepatocellular carcinoma
- Cerebellar haemangioblastoma

RELATIVE
- Stress or pseudo- polycythaemia
- Cigarette smoking
- Dehydration: water deprivation, vomiting
- Plasma loss: burns, enteropathy

Table 15.1 Causes of polycythaemia.

Total red cell volume (^{51}Cr or ^{99m}Tc)	Men	25–35 ml/kg
	Women	22–32 ml/kg
Total plasma volume (^{125}I-albumin)		40–50 ml/kg

Table 15.2 Normal adult blood volume: radiodilution methods.

Laboratory findings

1 The haemoglobin, haematocrit and red cell count are increased. The TRCV is increased.

2 A neutrophil leucocytosis is seen in over half the patients, and some have increased circulating basophils.

3 A raised platelet count is present in about half the patients.

4 The neutrophil alkaline phosphatase score is usually increased above normal (see Table 12.2).

5 Increased serum vitamin B_{12} and vitamin B_{12}-binding capacity due to an increase in transcobalamin I.

6 The bone marrow is hypercellular with prominent mega-karyocytes, best assessed by a trephine biopsy (Fig. 15.5a). Clonal cytogenetic abnormalities may occur, but there is no single characteristic change.

7 Blood viscosity is increased.

8 Plasma urate is often increased.

9 Circulating erythroid progenitors (CFU-E, BFU-E) (see p. 2) are increased and grow *in vitro* independently of added erythropoietin.

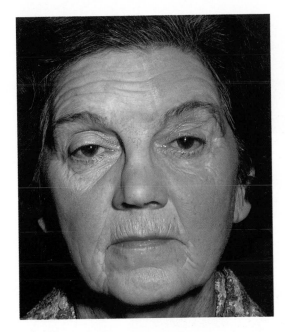

Fig. 15.2 Polycythaemia vera: facial plethora and conjunctival suffusion in a 63-year-old woman. Haemoglobin 18 g/dl; total red cell volume 45 ml/kg.

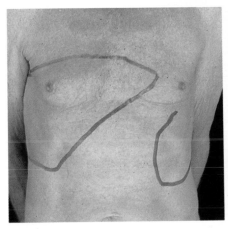

(a)

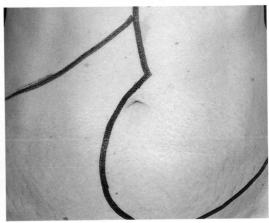

(b)

Fig. 15.3 Splenomegaly: enlarged spleens in male patients with polycythaemia vera (a) and myelofibrosis (b).

Treatment

Treatment is aimed at maintaining a normal blood count. The PCV (packed cell volume) should be maintained at about 45% and the platelet count below $400 \times 10^9/l$.

Venesection

This form of therapy is particularly useful when a rapid reduction of red cell volume is required, e.g. at the start of therapy. It is especially indicated in younger patients and those with mild disease. The resulting iron deficiency may limit erythropoiesis. Venesection does not control the platelet count.

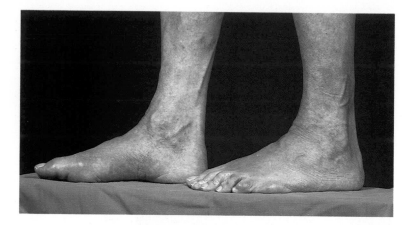

Fig. 15.4 The feet of a 72-year-old man with polycythaemia rubra vera. There is inflammation of the right metatarsophalangeal and other joints due to uric acid deposits.

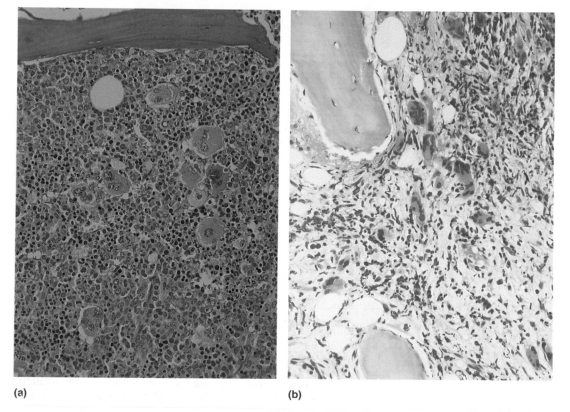

(a)   (b)

Fig. 15.5 Iliac crest trephine biopsies. (a) Polycythaemia vera: fat spaces are almost completely replaced by hyperplastic haemopoietic tissue. All haemopoietic cell lines are increased with megakaryocytes particularly prominent. (b) Myelofibrosis: normal marrow architecture is lost and haemopoietic cells are surrounded by increased fibrous tissue and intercellular substance.

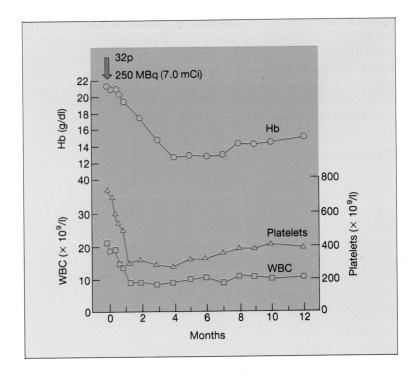

Fig. 15.6 Haematological response to therapy with radioactive phosphorus (^{32}P) in polycythaemia vera. Hb, haemoglobin; WBC, white blood cell count.

Cytotoxic myelosuppression
Continuous daily or intermittent high-dose therapy with busulphan or hydroxyurea. This therapy requires close supervision and regular blood counts to prevent overdosage. Hydroxyurea is preferred in younger patients since it is less likely to cause long-term side effects.

Phosphorus-32 (^{32}P) therapy
This is excellent therapy for older patients with severe disease. ^{32}P is a β-emitter, with a half-life of 14.3 days. It is concentrated in bone and is a most effective myelosuppressive agent. A typical response to ^{32}P is shown in Fig. 15.6. The usual remission time after a single dose is 2 years.

Course and prognosis

Thrombosis and haemorrhage are common and vascular accidents are a frequent cause of death. Increased viscosity, vascular stasis and high platelet levels may all contribute to thrombosis. Vascular distension, infarcts of small vessels, and defective platelet function may promote haemorrhage. Median survival times (10–16 years) are similar for venesection, chemotherapy or ^{32}P-treated groups of patients.

Transition from PV to myelofibrosis occurs in 30% and from PV to acute leukaemia in about 5% of patients. ^{32}P and alkylating agents (e.g. busulphan or chlorambucil) have been implicated in causing higher rates of conversion to acute leukaemia, although it is generally accepted that transition is mainly due to the natural history of PV. Nevertheless, busulphan and ^{32}P are avoided if possible in younger subjects.

Secondary polycythaemia

The causes of secondary polycythaemia are listed in Table 15.1. Hypoxia due to chronic obstructive airways disease is one of the commonest and is easily diagnosed on clinical grounds. Cyanotic heart disease usually presents no diagnostic problems. In cases of doubt the measurement of arterial oxygen saturation will provide a clue to the diagnosis. Renal and tumour causes of inappropriate erythropoietin secretion are rare. Patients with a high affinity haemoglobin often have a family history of polycythaemia and present at a young age.

Relative (stress or pseudo-) polycythaemia

Relative polycythaemia, also known as stress polycythaemia or pseudopolycythaemia, is the result of plasma volume contraction. The TRCV is normal. The cause is uncertain. This condition is far more common than PV. It occurs particularly in young or middle-aged men and may be associated with cardiovascular problems, e.g. myocardial ischaemia or cerebral transient ischaemic attacks. In association with hypertension it has been termed Gaisbock's syndrome. Diuretic therapy and heavy smoking are frequent associations. Trials of repeated venesection to maintain a PCV of 45% or less are in progress to see if survival is improved.

Cigarette smoking and polycythaemia

The association of cigarette smoking and polycythaemia is well recognized. Some heavy smokers have an elevated red cell volume but the majority have a form of relative polycythaemia with the main factor being a reduction in plasma volume. Hypoxia caused by binding of carbon monoxide to haemoglobin may increase erythropoietin production in smokers and result in an elevated red cell volume. When plasma volume contraction is present, cessation of smoking may cause a significant fall in haemoglobin level within 24 hours.

Differential diagnosis of polycythaemia

The cause of a persistently high haemoglobin level may be evident from the clinical history and from a physical examination. An enlarged spleen is a particularly valuable sign of PV. Severe PV, severe lung disease, cardiac shunt disorders and smoker's polycythaemia are relatively simple to confirm. In heavy smokers, cessation of the habit for 24 hours may result in a return of the plasma volume towards normal and a significant fall in haemoglobin level.

Tests that are usually needed include:

1 Blood count and blood chemistry: leucocytosis, thrombocytosis, elevated neutrophil alkaline phosphatase score, increased serum levels of vitamin B_{12}, vitamin B_{12}-binding capacity and of serum uric acid all support a diagnosis of PV.

2 Bone marrow aspirate and trephine examination: features of myeloproliferative disease also confirm a diagnosis of PV.

3 Measurement of TRCV and plasma volume: before proceeding with intensive investigations it is necessary to establish whether the polycythaemia is 'real' with an increased red cell volume or whether it is 'relative' and due to plasma volume contraction.

4 Oxygen-dissociation studies: in patients, particularly the young, with a family history of polycythaemia and suspected of having a high affinity haemoglobin variant, measurement of P_{50} (the oxygen tension at which the haemoglobin is half saturated) and analysis of the oxygen-dissociation curve may confirm the characteristic fall in the P_{50} and shift to the left of the curve (see Fig. 2.9, p. 20).

5 Erythropoietin assay: immunoassays may confirm high levels in patients with secondary polycythaemia. Results are normal to low in PV but are not performed routinely for this because of the difficulties in the assay and interpreting the results.

6 Blood gas analysis: arterial hypoxaemia provides supporting evidence for a secondary polycythaemia due to respiratory or cardiac disease. Carboxyhaemoglobin levels may be raised in heavy smokers.

7 Other investigations: more detailed examination may be necessary to establish a formal diagnosis, e.g. cardiac catheterization, respiratory function tests, ultrasound, CT scan or X-ray of the renal tract.

Essential thrombocythaemia

Megakaryocyte proliferation and overproduction of platelets is the dominant feature of this condition; there is a sustained increase in platelet count above normal ($400 \times 10^9/l$). The condition is closely related to PV. Some cases show patchy myelofibrosis. Recurrent haemorrhage and thrombosis are the principal

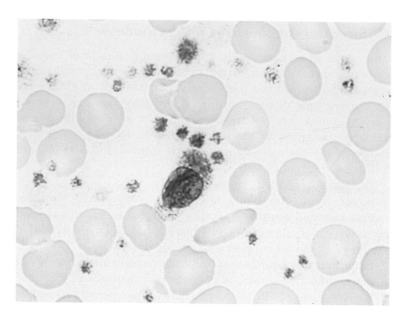

Fig. 15.7 Peripheral blood film in essential thrombocythaemia showing increased numbers of platelets and a nucleated megakaryocytic fragment.

clinical features. Splenic enlargement is frequent in the early phase but splenic atrophy due to platelets blocking the splenic microcirculation is seen in some patients.

There may be anaemia (e.g. due to iron deficiency from chronic gastrointestinal or uterine haemorrhage or due to the marrow disorder itself) or the thrombocythaemia may be accompanied by polycythaemia.

Laboratory findings

Abnormal large platelets and megakaryocyte fragments may be seen in the blood film (Fig. 15.7). The bone marrow is similar to that in PV. Cytogenetics are analysed to exclude chronic myeloid leukaemia. The condition must be distinguished from other causes of a raised platelet count (Table 15.3). Platelet

Table 15.3 Causes of a raised platelet count.

Reactive
Haemorrhage, trauma, post-operative
Chronic iron deficiency
Malignancy
Chronic infections
Connective tissue diseases, e.g. rheumatoid arthritis
Post-splenectomy

Endogenous
Essential thrombocythaemia
In some cases of polycythaemia vera, myelofibrosis and chronic myeloid leukaemia

function tests (see p. 331) are consistently abnormal, failure of aggregation with adrenaline being particularly characteristic.

Treatment

In severe cases with a platelet count above $1000 \times 10^9/l$ and spontaneous haemorrhage or thrombosis, it is important to lower the platelet count to normal with hydroxyurea or α-interferon. Busulphan and ^{32}P were used but are not now favoured because of possible long-term complications. Platelet pheresis may be helpful in the short-term management of high platelet counts in the interval before the cytotoxic therapy becomes effective.

In younger patients with platelet counts less than $1000 \times 10^9/l$ and no history of haemorrhage, low-dose aspirin is often used to reduce the risk of thrombosis. Alpha-interferon is also effective in controlling the platelet count but requires ingestion and is expensive. It is not established that hydroxyurea predisposes to leukaemic transformation.

Course

Providing death does not occur from haemorrhage or thrombosis patients may transform after a number of years to PV, myelo-fibrosis or acute leukaemia. Often the disease is stationary for 10–20 years or more.

Myelofibrosis

This condition has many names: (chronic) myelofibrosis, myelo-sclerosis, agnogenic myeloid metaplasia, or myelofibrosis with myeloid metaplasia (MMM). Haemopoietic stem cell prolifer-ation is generalized with splenic and hepatic involvement.

There is an increase in circulating stem cells associated with the establishment of extramedullary haemopoiesis. There is re-active fibrosis in the bone marrow secondary to hyperplasia of abnormal megakaryocytes. There is stimulation of fibroblasts probably by platelet-derived growth factor secreted by mega-karyocytes and platelets and inhibition of collagenase by platelet factor IV.

A third or more of the patients have a previous history of PV and some patients present with clinical and laboratory features of both disorders.

Clinical features

1 An insidious onset in older people is usual with symptoms of anaemia.

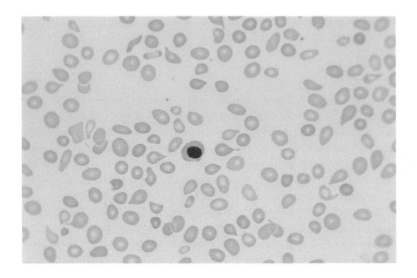

Fig. 15.8 Peripheral blood film in myelofibrosis. Leuco-erythroblastic change with 'tear-drop' cells and an erythroblast.

2 Symptoms due to massive splenomegaly (e.g. abdominal discomfort, pain or indigestion) are frequent; splenomegaly is the main physical finding (see Fig. 15.3b).
3 Loss of weight, anorexia and night sweats are common.
4 Bleeding problems, bone pain or gout occur in a minority of patients.

Myelofibrosis and chronic myeloid leukaemia are responsible for most cases of massive (>20 cm) splenic enlargement in Britain and North America.

Laboratory findings

1 Anaemia is usual but a normal or increased haemoglobin level may be found in some patients.
2 The white cell and platelet counts are frequently high at the time of presentation. Later in the disease leucopenia and thrombocytopenia are common.
3 A leuco-erythroblastic blood film is found. The red cells show characteristic 'tear-drop' poikilocytes (Fig. 15.8).
4 Bone marrow is usually unobtainable by aspiration. Trephine biopsy (see Fig. 15.5b) may show a hypercellular marrow with an increase in reticulin-fibre pattern; in other patients there is an increase in intercellular substance and variable collagen deposition. Increased megakaryocytes are frequently seen. In some cases there is increased bone formation with increased bone density on X-ray.
5 Low serum and red cell folate, raised serum vitamin B_{12} and vitamin B_{12}-binding capacity, and an increased neutrophil alkaline phosphatase score are usual.
6 High serum urate, LDH (lactate dehydrogenase) and hydroxy-

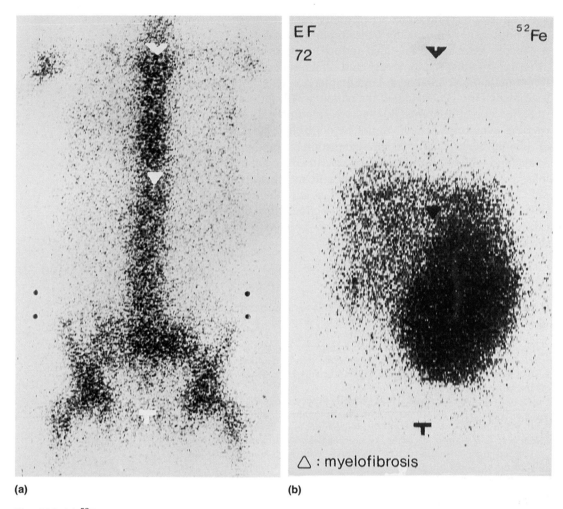

(a) (b)

Fig. 15.9 (a) ^{52}Fe scan in polycythaemia vera. The uptake of the isotope in the axial skeleton indicates the sites of bone marrow erythropoiesis. (b) ^{52}Fe scan in myelosclerosis. The heavy concentration of isotope in the splenic and liver areas indicates extramedullary erythropoiesis in these organs.

butyrate dehydrogenase levels reflect the increased but largely ineffective turnover of haemopoietic cells. The serum LDH is normal in PV.

7 Extramedullary erythropoiesis may be documented by radio-iron studies (Fig. 15.9) or by liver biopsy, but these are not routine tests.

8 Transformation to acute myeloid leukaemia occurs in 10−20% of patients.

Treatment

1 Supportive blood transfusions and regular folic acid therapy are used in severely anaemic patients.

2 Cytotoxic agents, e.g. hydroxyurea, are used in patients with evidence of gross myeloproliferation and hypermetabolism.

3 Allopurinol is indicated in virtually all patients to prevent gout and urate nephropathy from hyperuricaemia.

4 Splenic irradiation may also reduce myeloproliferation temporarily; it reduces splenic size and alleviates symptoms due to hypermetabolism and the enlarged spleen.

5 Splenectomy is considered for patients with: (a) unacceptable transfusion requirements; (b) massive splenomegaly causing distressing symptoms which cannot be controlled by radiotherapy or chemotherapy; and (c) severe thrombocytopenia which is associated with recurrent haemorrhage. In advanced disease with massive splenomegaly there is a significant operative risk; the patients are in poor general condition and there is a risk of post-operative haemorrhage and infection. Post-splenectomy thrombocytosis should be controlled to prevent a high risk of thromboembolism.

Bibliography

Hoffman R. & Boswell H.S. (1991) Polycythemia vera. In *Hematology: Basic Principles and Practice* (eds R. Hoffman, E.J. Benz, S.J. Shattil, B. Furie & H.J. Cohen). Churchill Livingstone, New York, pp. 834–854.

Hoffman R. & Silverstein M.N. (1991) Agnogenic myeloid metaplasia. In *Hematology: Basic Principles and Practice* (eds R. Hoffman, E.J. Benz, S.J. Shattil, B. Furie & H.J. Cohen). Churchill Livingstone, New York, pp. 870–881.

Hoffman R. & Silverstein M.N. (1991) Airway polycythaemia. In *Hematology: Basic Principles and Practice* (eds R. Hoffman, E.J. Benz, S.J. Shattil, B. Furie & H.J. Cohen). Churchill Livingstone, New York, pp. 881–889.

Löfzenberg E. & Wahlin A. (1988) Management of polycythaemia vera, essential thrombocythaemia and myelofibrosis with hydroxyurea. *European Journal of Haematology*, **41**, 375–381.

Reid C.D.L. & Kirk A. (1988) Endogenous erythroid classes (EEC) in polycythaemia and their relationship to diagnosis and response to treatment. *British Journal of Haematology*, **68**, 395–400.

Talpaz M., Kurzrock R., Kantarjian H., O'Brien S. & Gutterman J.U. (1989) Recombinant interferon-alpha therapy of Philadelphia chromosome negative myeloproliferative disorders with thrombocytosis. *American Journal of Medicine*, **86**, 554–558.

Tobelem G. (1989) Essential thrombocythaemia. *Clinical Haematology*, **3**, 719–728.

Chapter 16
Platelets, Blood Coagulation and Haemostasis

Platelets

Platelet production

Platelets are produced in the bone marrow by fragmentation of the cytoplasm of megakaryocytes. The precursor of the mega-karyocyte — the megakaryoblast — arises by a process of differen-tiation from the haemopoietic stem cell. The megakaryocyte matures by endomitotic synchronous nuclear replication, en-larging the cytoplasmic volume as the number of nuclear lobes increase in multiples of two. At a variable stage in development, most commonly at the eight nucleus stage, further nuclear repli-cation and cell growth ceases, the cytoplasm becomes granular and platelets are then liberated (Fig. 16.1). A mature polyploid megakaryocyte is shown in Fig. 16.2. Platelet production follows formation of microvesicles in the cytoplasm of the cell which coalesce to form platelet demarcation membranes. Each mega-karyocyte is responsible for the production of about 4000

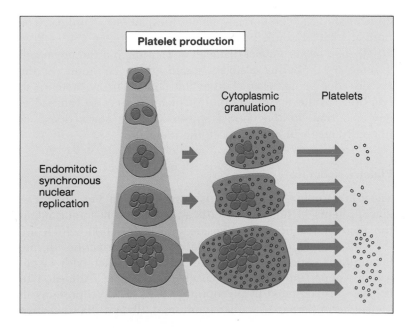

Fig. 16.1 A simplified diagram to illustrate platelet production from megakaryocytes.

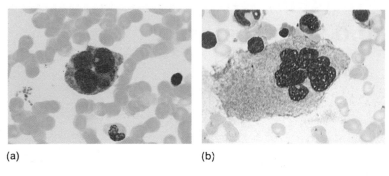

(a)   (b)

Fig. 16.2 Megakaryocytes: (a) immature form with basophilic cytoplasm; (b) mature form with many nuclear lobes and pronounced granulation of the cytoplasm.

platelets. The time interval from differentiation of the stem cell to the production of platelets average about 10 days in man.

Platelet production is under the control of humoral agents. Thrombopoietin is synthesized in the liver and to a less extent kidneys. It has structural homology with erythropoietin. It increases the number of megakaryocytes, their maturation and the release of platelets. Other growth factors act at various stages of platelet formation. IL-6 has thrombopoietin activity and IL-3 and GM-CSF also exhibit megakaryocyte colony stimulating activity. Platelet production may be increased by increasing the number of megakaryocytes and also by increasing the mean volume or nuclear units of the total megakaryocyte population.

Platelet circulation

Platelets can be labelled *in vitro* with ^{51}Cr and ^{111}In or *in vivo* with DF^{32}P (di-isopropyl-fluorophosphate) or ^{75}Se-seleno-methionine. ^{51}Cr and ^{111}In are the most satisfactory labels for clinical studies. The normal platelet lifespan is 7−10 days. The normal platelet count is about 250×10^9/l (range 150−400 × 10^9/l). The mean platelet diameter is 1−2 μm and the mean cell volume 5.8 fl. Young platelets spend up to 36 hours in the spleen after being released from the bone marrow, and up to one-third of the marrow output of platelets may be trapped at any one time in the normal spleen. Splenic stasis does not normally result in any injury to the platelet.

Platelet structure

The ultrastructure of platelets is represented in Fig. 16.3. The glycoproteins of the surface coat are particularly important in the platelet reactions of adhesion and aggregation which are the initial events leading to platelet plug formation during haemostasis. Specific glycoprotein receptors react with aggregating agents, inhibitors and coagulation factors. Adhesion to collagen is facilitated by glycoprotein (GP) Ia. Glycoproteins Ib (defective in Bernard−Soulier syndrome), IIb and IIIa (defective

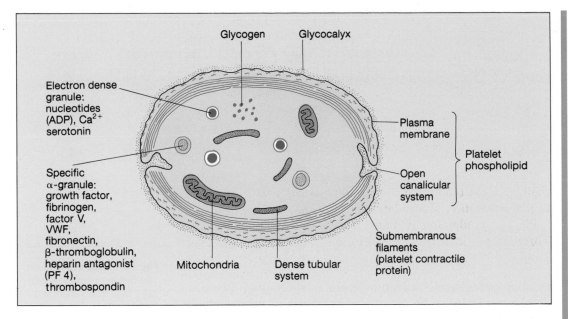

Glycogen   Glycocalyx

Electron dense granule: nucleotides (ADP), Ca²⁺ serotonin

Plasma membrane

Platelet phospholipid

Specific α-granule: growth factor, fibrinogen, factor V, VWF, fibronectin, β-thromboglobulin, heparin antagonist (PF 4), thrombospondin

Open canalicular system

Mitochondria   Dense tubular system

Submembranous filaments (platelet contractile protein)

Fig. 16.3 Diagrammatic representation of the ultrastructure of platelets. ADP, adenosine diphosphate; PF, platelet factor; VWF, von Willebrand factor.

in thrombasthenia) are important in the attachment of platelets to von Willebrand factor (VWF) and hence to vascular subendothelium (Fig. 16.4). The binding site for IIb−IIIa is also the receptor for fibrinogen which is important in platelet−platelet aggregation. The plasma membrane invaginates into the platelet interior to form an open membrane (canalicular) system which provides a large reactive surface to which the plasma coagulation proteins may be selectively absorbed. The membrane phospholipids (platelet factor 3) are of particular importance in the conversion of coagulation factor X to Xa and prothrombin to thrombin (see Fig. 16.6). The contractile protein complex system comprises microfilaments in the sub-membranous area and throughout the platelet cytoplasm. A circumferential skeleton of microtubules is responsible for the maintenance of the normal circulating discoid shape.

In the platelet interior calcium, nucleotides (particularly ADP), and serotonin are contained in electron-dense granules. Specific (α) granules contain a heparin antagonist (platelet factor 4), platelet-derived growth factor (PDGF), β-thromboglobulin, fibrinogen, VWF and other clotting factors. Other specific organelles include lysosomes which contain hydrolytic enzymes, and peroxisomes which contain catalase. During the release reaction described below, the contents of the granules are discharged into the open canalicular system. Energy for platelet reactions is derived from oxidative phosphorylation in mitochondria and also from anaerobic glycolysis utilizing platelet glycogen. The dense tubular system of platelets which represents

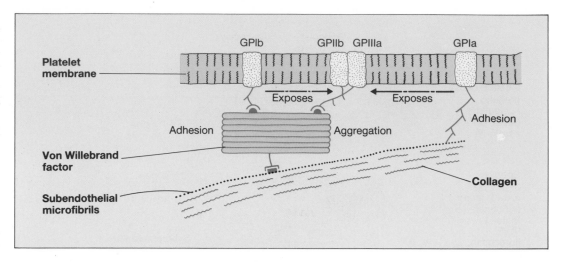

Fig. 16.4 Platelet adhesion. The binding of glycoprotein (GP) Ib to von Willebrand factor leads to adhesion to the subendothelium and also exposes the GPIIb/IIIa binding sites to fibrinogen and von Willebrand factor leading to platelet aggregation. The GPIa site permits direct adhesion to collagen.

residual endoplasmic reticulum contains substantial quantities of calcium and may be the site of synthesis of prostaglandins and thromboxane A_2.

Platelet antigens

Platelets have specific surface antigens, now called HPA1−5, each consisting of a or b alleles. They also express ABO and HLA class I antigens.

Platelet function

The main function of platelets is the formation of mechanical plugs during the normal haemostatic response to vascular injury. Central to this function are the platelet reactions of adhesion, secretion, aggregation and fusion as well as their pro-coagulant activity.

Platelet adhesion

Following blood vessel injury, platelets adhere to the exposed subendothelial connective tissues. Subendothelial microfibrils bind the larger multimers of VWF and through these react with platelet membrane GPIb (Fig. 16.4). A large number of adhesion proteins (see p. 147) are involved in platelet–vessel wall and platelet–platelet interactions. The GPIIb/GPIIIa receptor complex becomes exposed and forms a secondary binding site with VWF further promoting adhesion. Adhesion to collagen is facilitated by GPIa. Platelet adhesion induces a series of metabolic reactions which initiate the platelet release reactions, shape change and aggregation. Following adhesion, platelets become more spherical and extrude long pseudopods which enhance interaction between adjacent platelets.

Von Willebrand factor. VWF is involved in platelet adhesion to the vessel wall and to other platelets (aggregation). It also carries factor VIII (see later). It is a large complex multimeric molecule (MW $0.8-20 \times 10^6$) made up of several subunit chains ranging from dimers (MW 5×10^5) to multimers (MW 20×10^6) linked by disulphide bonds. VWF is encoded by a gene on chromosome 12 and is synthesized by endothelial cells and megakaryocytes. It is stored in Weibel–Palade bodies in endothelial cells and in specific platelet α-granules. Release of VWF from endothelial cells occurs under the influence of several hormones. Stress and exercise or infusion of either adrenaline or desmopressin (DDAVP) produces considerable increase in the level of circulating VWF.

Release reaction

Collagen exposure or thrombin action results in the secretion of platelet granule contents which include ADP, serotonin, fibrinogen, lysosomal enzymes, β-thromboglobulin and heparin neutralizing factor (platelet factor 4). Collagen and thrombin activate platelet prostaglandin synthesis. There is release of diacylglycerol (which activates protein phosphorylation via protein kinase C) and inositol triphosphate (which causes release of intracellular calcium ions). There is also arachidonate release from the cell membrane leading to the formation of a labile substance, thromboxane A_2, which lowers platelet cyclic AMP levels and initiates the release reaction (Fig. 16.5). Thromboxane A_2 not only potentiates platelet aggregation but also has powerful vasoconstrictive activity. The release reaction is inhibited by substances which increase the level of platelet cyclic AMP. One such substance is the prostaglandin prostacyclin (PGI_2) which is synthesized by vascular endothelial cells. It is a potent inhibitor of platelet aggregation and probably prevents their deposition on normal vascular endothelium.

Platelet aggregation

Released ADP and thromboxane A_2 cause additional platelets to aggregate at the site of vascular injury. ADP causes platelets to swell and encourages the platelet membranes of adjacent platelets to adhere to each other. As they do so further release reactions occur liberating more ADP and thromboxane A_2 causing secondary platelet aggregation. This positive feedback process results in the formation of a platelet mass large enough to plug the area of endothelial injury.

Platelet procoagulant activity

After platelet aggregation and release the exposed membrane phospholipid (platelet factor 3) is available for two reactions of coagulation protein complex formation. Both phospholipid-mediated reactions are calcium ion dependent. The first (tenase)

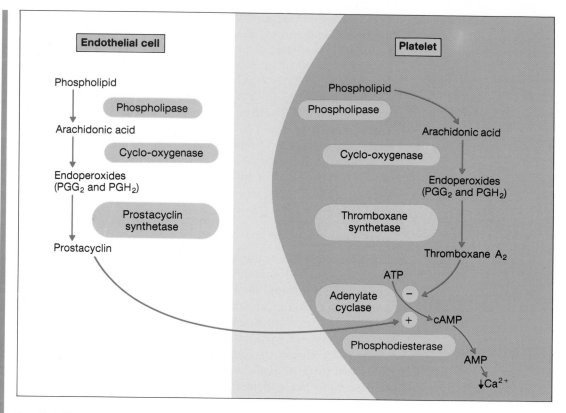

Fig. 16.5 The synthesis of prostacylin and thromboxane. The opposing effects of these agents are mediated by changes in the concentration of cyclic AMP in platelets via stimulation or inhibition of the enzyme adenylate cyclase. Cyclic AMP controls the concentration of free calcium ions in the platelet which are important in the processes which cause adhesion and aggregation. High levels of cyclic AMP lead to low free calcium ion concentrations and prevent aggregation and adhesion. AMP, adenosine monophosphate; ATP, adenosine triphosphate; Ca, calcium; PG, prostaglandin (G_2 and H_2).

involves factors IXa, VIII and X in the formation of factor Xa. The second (prothrombinase) results in the formation of thrombin from the interaction of factors Xa, V and II. The phospholipid surface forms an ideal template for the crucial concentration and orientation of these proteins.

Irreversible platelet aggregation
High concentrations of ADP, the enzymes released during the release reaction, and platelet contractile proteins contribute to irreversible fusion of platelets aggregated at the site of vascular injury. Thrombin also encourages fusion of platelets, and fibrin formation reinforces the stability of the evolving platelet plug.

Growth factor
Platelet-derived growth factor (PDGF) found in the specific

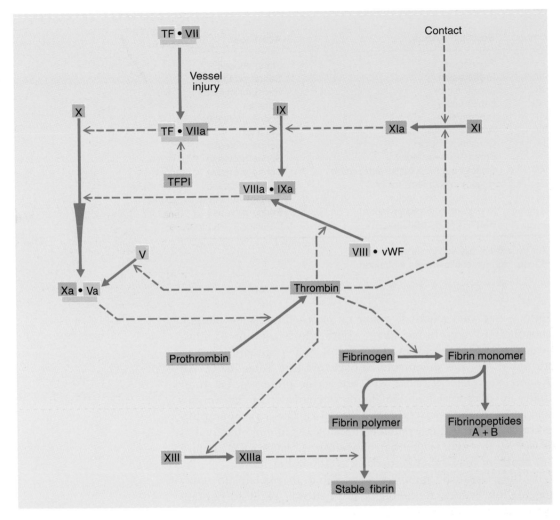

Fig. 16.6 The pathway of blood coagulation initiated by tissue factor (TF) on the cell surface. When plasma comes into contact with TF, factor (F) VII binds to TF. The complex of TF and activated VII (VIIa) activates X and IX. TF pathway inhibitor (TFPI) is an important inhibitor of TF/VIIa. VIIIa.IXa complex greatly amplifies Xa production from X. The generation of thrombin from prothrombin by the action of Xa/Va complex leads to fibrin formation. Thrombin also activates XI, V and XIII. Thrombin cleaves VIII from its carrier von Willebrand's factor (vWF). Blue, serine proteases; green, co-factors.

granules of platelets stimulates vascular smooth muscle cells to multiply and this may hasten vascular healing following injury.

Blood coagulation

Blood coagulation involves a biological amplification system in which relatively few initiation substances sequentially activate by proteolysis a cascade of circulating precursor proteins (the coagulation factor enzymes) which culminates in the generation of thrombin; this, in turn, converts soluble plasma fibrinogen into fibrin (Fig. 16.6). Fibrin enmeshes the platelet aggregates at the sites of vascular injury and converts the unstable primary platelet plugs to firm, definitive and stable haemostatic plugs. A list of the coagulation factors appears in Table 16.1.

The operation of this enzyme cascade requires local concentration of circulating coagulation factors at the site of injury.

Table 16.1 The coagulation factors.

Factor number	Descriptive name	Active form
I	Fibrinogen	Fibrin subunit
II	Prothrombin	Serine protease
III	Tissue factor	Receptor/cofactor*
V	Labile factor	Cofactor
VII	Proconvertin	Serine protease
VIII	Antihaemophilic factor	Cofactor
IX	Christmas factor	Serine protease
X	Stuart–Prower factor	Serine protease
XI	Plasma thromboplastin antecedent	Serine protease
XII	Hageman (contact) factor	Serine protease
XIII	Fibrin stabilizing factor	Transglutaminase
—	Prekallikrein (Fletcher factor)	Serine protease
—	HMWK (Fitzgerald factor)	Cofactor*

* Active without proteolytic modification.
HMWK, high-molecular-weight kininogen.

Surface-mediated reactions occur on exposed collagen, platelet phospholipid and tissue factor. With the exception of fibrinogen, which is the fibrin clot subunit, the coagulation factors are either enzyme precursors or cofactors (see Table 16.1). All the enzymes, except factor XIII, are serine proteases, i.e. their ability to hydrolyse peptide bonds depends upon the amino-acid serine at their active centre (Fig. 16.7). The scale of amplification achieved in this system is dramatic, e.g. 1 mol of activated factor XI through sequential activation of factors IX, X and prothrombin may generate up to 2×10^8 mol of fibrin.

In the 'classical' pathway formulated to explain *in vitro* coagulation testing, initiation of the pathway required contact reactions between factor XII, Kallikrein and high molecular weight kininogen (HMWK) leading to the activation of factor XI.

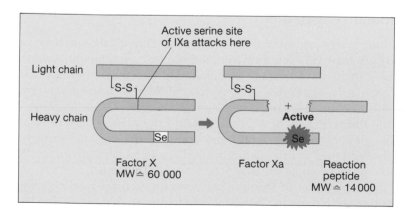

Fig. 16.7 Serine (Se) protease activity. This example shows the activation of factor X by factor IX.

However, the lack of abnormal bleeding in individuals with hereditary deficiencies of these contact factors suggested that these reactions are not required for physiological coagulation *in vivo*.

Coagulation is now thought to be initiated *in vivo* by tissue factor, found on the surface of perivascular tissue, binding to coagulation factor VII (see Fig. 16.6). This activates factor VII which then activates both factor IX and factor X. Activation of factor X leads to generation of small amounts of thrombin which amplify the coagulation process by activating co-factors V and VIII. Thrombin also activates factor XI which may increase production of activated factor IX. This amplification pathway involving factors VIII and IX assumes the dominant role of consolidating the production of activated factor X.

Coagulation factor VIII is a single chain protein with a molecular weight of 350 000 (see Fig. 16.10). It is coded by a 186-kb gene located in the long arm (q2.8 region) of the X chromosome. Factor VIII is bound in plasma to VWF. It is synthesized in the liver, probably by the hepatocytes.

Factor XI does not seem to play a role in the physiological initiation of coagulation. However, its supplementary role in the activation of factor IX may be important at major sites of trauma or at operations.

Activated factor X in association with co-factor V on the phospholipid surface and calcium converts prothrombin into

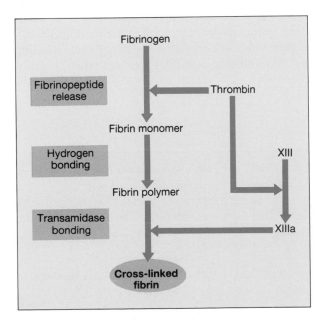

Fig. 16.8 The formation and stabilization of fibrin.

thrombin. Thrombin hydrolyses fibrinogen, releasing fibrinopeptides A and B to form fibrin monomers (Fig. 16.8). Fibrin
monomers link spontaneously by hydrogen bonds to form a loose,
insoluble fibrin polymer. Factor XIII is also activated by thrombin
together with calcium. Activated factor XIII stabilizes the fibrin
polymers with the formation of covalent bond crosslinks.

Fibrinogen has a molecular with of 340 000 and consists of two
identical subunits, each containing three dissimilar polypeptide
chains (Aα, Bβ and τ) which are linked by disulphide bonds
(Fig. 16.9). After cleavage by thrombin of fibrinopeptides A and
B, fibrin monomer consists of three paired α, β and τ chains.

One of the physiological inhibitors of coagulation, protein C is
also activated by thrombin (see p. 310). Tissue factor pathway
inhibitor (TFPI) plays a key role in limiting coagulation but in
contrast to the other inhibitors, pathological abnormalities of
TFPI leading to a thrombotic tendency have not been described.

Some of the properties of the coagulation factors are listed in
Table 16.2. The activity of factors II, VII, IX and X is dependent
upon vitamin K which is responsible for a post-ribosomal
carboxylation of a number of terminal glutamic acid residues on
each of these molecules (see Fig. 18.8). The carboxylation facilitates the binding of calcium required to form complexes with
phospholipid. In the absence of vitamin K, no carboxylation of
glutamic acid residues occurs, calcium is not bound and these
factors are not linked to platelet phospholipid. Without the
concentration and orientation of these reacting coagulation
factors the rate of prothrombin conversion to thrombin is
minimal.

The serine protease coagulation factors along with those of
the fibrinolytic system (see later) have a high degree of homology and contain characteristic structural domains (Fig. 16.10),
such as the kringles which are concerned with substrate binding
and the carboxylated glutamic acid (gla) residues which bind to

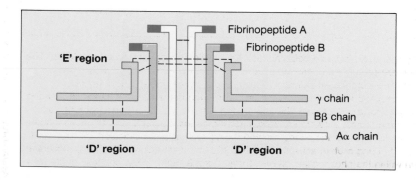

Fig. 16.9 A simplified
diagram of a fibrinogen
molecule. The dashed lines
show sites of cleavage by
thrombin. (From Hutton,
1989.)

Table 16.2 The coagulation factors.

Factor	Plasma half-life (hours)	Plasma concentration (mg/l)	Comments
II	65	100	Prothrombin group;
VII	5	0.5	vitamin K needed for
IX	25	5	synthesis; require Ca^{2+}
X	40	10	for activation; stable
I	90	3000	Thrombin interacts with them;
V	15	10	increase in inflammation,
VIII	10	0.1	pregnancy, oral contraceptives
XI	45	5	
XII	50	30	

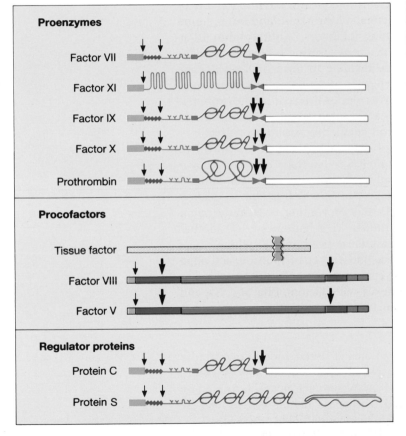

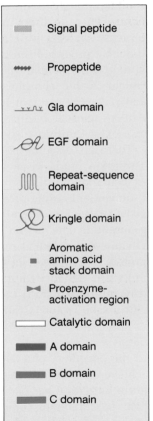

Fig. 16.10 Domains of the enzymes, receptors and cofactors involved in blood coagulation and regulation. The components of blood coagulation are proenzymes, procofactors and regulatory proteins. The proenzymes, including protein C, contain a catalytic domain, an activation region and a signal peptide. The vitamin K-dependent proteins include a propeptide and a γ-carboxyglutamic acid (Gla) domain. Other important domains include the epidermal growth factor-like (EGF) domain, the kringle domain and the repeat-sequence domain. Tissue factor is an integral membrane protein unrelated to other known proteins. Factor V and VIII have marked similarities in structure. Sites of intracellular peptide bonds cleaved during synthesis are indicated by thin arrows, and sites of peptide bonds cleaved during protein activation are indicated by thick arrows. The transmembrane domain of tissue factor is shown within the phospholipid bilayer. (From Furie & Furie, 1992, courtesy of the *New England Journal of Medicine*.)

phospholipid. There are also regions of homology with fibronectin (finger regions) and with epidermal growth factor. Although factor VIII and V cofactors are not protease enzymes they circulate in a precursor form that requires limited cleavage by thrombin for expression of full cofactor activity.

Physiological limitation of blood coagulation

Unchecked blood coagulation would lead to dangerous occlusion of blood vessels (thrombosis) if the following protective mechanisms were not in operation.

Plasma inhibitors of activated factors

It is important that the effect of thrombin is limited to the site of injury. There is direct inactivation of thrombin (and other serine protease factors) by circulating inhibitors. Antithrombin III is the most potent of these. It inactivates serine proteases by combining with them by peptide bonding to form high-molecular-weight, stable complexes. Heparin potentiates its action markedly. Another protein, heparin cofactor II, also inhibits thrombin. Alpha$_2$-macroglobulins, α_2-antiplasmin and α_2-antitrypsin also exert inhibitory effects on circulating serine proteases.

There are also inhibitors of coagulation cofactors V and VIII. Thrombin binds to an endothelial cell-surface receptor known as thrombomodulin. The resulting complex activates the vitamin K-dependent serine protease protein C, which is able to destroy activated factors V and VIII, thus preventing further thrombin generation. The action of protein C is enhanced by another vitamin K-dependent protein known as protein S, which binds protein C to the platelet surface (Fig. 16.11). In addition, activated protein C enhances fibrinolysis (see below). Tissue factor pathway inhibitor (TFPI) complexes with factors VIIa and Xa and with tissue factor to limit the main *in vivo* pathway.

Blood flow

At the periphery of a damaged area of tissue, blood flow rapidly achieves a dilution and dispersal of activated factors before fibrin formation has occurred. Activated factors are destroyed by liver parenchymal cells and particulate matter is removed by liver Kupffer cells and other reticuloendothelial (RE) cells.

Plasmin and fibrin split products

When in pathological excess, plasmin generation (see below) at the site of injury also limits the extent of the evolving thrombus by digesting fibrin, fibrinogen and factors V and VIII. The split products of fibrinolysis are competitive inhibitors of thrombin and fibrin polymerization. Normally α_2-antiplasmin inhibits any local free plasmin.

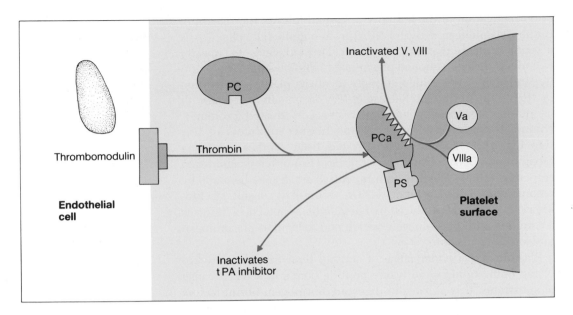

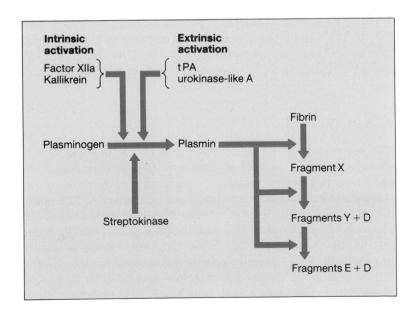

Fig. 16.11 Activation and action of protein C (PC) by thrombin which has bound to thrombomodulin on the endothelial cell surface. Protein S (PS) is a cofactor which facilitates binding of activated protein C (PCa) to the platelet surface. The inactivation of factors Va and VIIIa results in the inhibition of blood coagulation. The inactivation of tPA (tissue plasminogen activator) inhibitor (PAI-1) enhances fibrinolysis.

Fibrinolysis

Fibrinolysis (like coagulation) is a normal haemostatic response to vascular injury. Plasminogen, a β-globulin proenzyme in blood and tissue fluid, is converted to the serine protease plasmin by activators either from the vessel wall (intrinsic activation) or from the tissues (extrinsic activation) (Fig. 16.12). Intrinsic blood activation of fibrinolysis involving factor XII, factor XI and HMWK and kallikrein is probably of only minor importance.

Fig. 16.12 The fibrinolytic system.

Major activation of the fibrinolytic system follows the release of
tissue plasminogen activator (tPA) from endothelial cells. tPA is
a serine protease that binds to fibrin. This enhances its capacity
to convert thrombus-bound plasminogen into plasmin. This fibrin
dependence of tPA action strongly localizes plasmin generation
by tPA to the fibrin clot. Release of tPA occurs after such stimuli
as trauma, exercise or emotional stress. Activated protein C
stimulates fibrinolysis by destroying plasma inhibitors of tPA
(see Fig. 16.11). Therapeutic tPA has been synthesized using
recombinant DNA technology. Urokinase is a tissue plasminogen
activator initially isolated from human urine. It may be made by
recombinant DNA technology. The fibrinolytic agent streptokinase is a peptide produced by haemolytic streptococci. It forms
a complex with plasminogen, which converts other plasminogen
molecules to plasmin.

Plasmin has a wider range of activity than thrombin, hydro-
lysing both arginine and lysine peptide bonds in a wider range
of substrates. It is capable of digesting fibrinogen, fibrin, factors
V and VIII and many other proteins. Cleavage of peptide bonds
in fibrin and fibrinogen produces a variety of split (degradation)
products (see Fig. 16.12). The largest split product, fragment X,
which is released from early digestion of fibrinogen or fibrin,
retains thrombin susceptible sites and thus is a competitive
inhibitor of thrombin. A later and smaller digestion fragment, Y,
is a competitive inhibitor of fibrin polymerization. Large amounts
of the smallest fragments D and E are detected in the plasma of
patients with disseminated intravascular coagulation.

Inactivation of plasmin

Tissue plasminogen activator is inactivated by PAI-1 (see
Fig. 16.11). Circulating plasmin is inactivated by potent inhibitors α_2-antiplasmin and α_2-macroglobulin. This prevents widespread destruction of fibrinogen and other coagulation factor
proteins.

Endothelial cells

The active role of the endothelial cell in the maintenance of
vascular integrity is well established. This cell provides the
basement membrane, collagen, elastin and fibronectin of the
subendothelial connective tissue. Loss or damage to the endothelial lining results in both haemorrhage and activation of the
haemostatic mechanism. The endothelial cell also has an active
role in the haemostatic response. Synthesis of tissue factor,
prostacyclin, VWF, plasminogen activator, antithrombin III and
thrombomodulin, the surface protein responsible for activation
of protein C, provides agents which are vital to both platelet

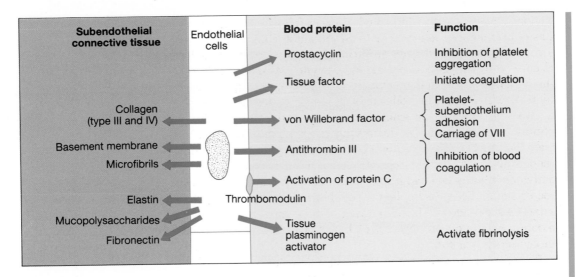

Subendothelial connective tissue	Endothelial cells	Blood protein	Function
		Prostacyclin	Inhibition of platelet aggregation
		Tissue factor	Initiate coagulation
Collagen (type III and IV)		von Willebrand factor	Platelet-subendothelium adhesion / Carriage of VIII
Basement membrane		Antithrombin III	Inhibition of blood coagulation
Microfibrils		Activation of protein C	
Elastin	Thrombomodulin		
Mucopolysaccharides		Tissue plasminogen activator	Activate fibrinolysis
Fibronectin			

Fig. 16.13 The role of the endothelial cell in protecting blood from coagulation and platelets from subendothelial aggregating substances.

reactions and blood coagulation (Fig. 16.13). There is also evidence that endothelial cells, especially in the pulmonary microcirculation, remove potential vasoactive and platelet aggregating agents such as serotonin, bradykinin and angiotensin I from the circulating blood.

Haemostatic response

The normal haemostatic response to vascular damage depends on closely linked interaction between the blood vessel wall, circulating platelets and blood coagulation factors (Fig. 16.14).

Vasoconstriction

An immediate vasoconstriction of the injured vessel and reflex constriction of adjacent small arteries and arterioles is responsible for an initial slowing of blood flow to the area of injury. When there is widespread damage this vascular reaction prevents exsanguination. The reduced blood flow allows contact activation of platelets and coagulation factors. The vasoactive amines and thromboxane A_2 from platelets, and the fibrinopeptides liberated during fibrin formation, may also have vasoconstrictive activity.

Platelet reactions and primary haemostatic plug formation

Following a break in the endothelial lining, there is an initial adherence of platelets to exposed connective tissue. This platelet adhesion is potentiated by VWF. Collagen exposure and thrombin produced at the site of injury cause the adherent platelets to release their granule contents which include ADP, serotonin,

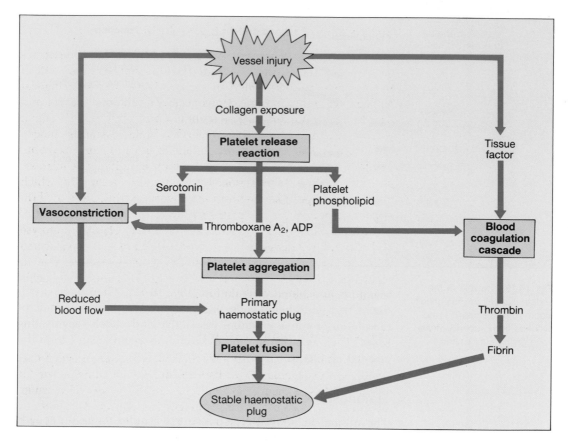

Fig. 16.14 Reactions involved in haemostasis.

fibrinogen, lysosomal enzymes and heparin-neutralizing factor (PF-4). Collagen and thrombin activate platelet prostaglandin synthesis leading to the formation of thromboxane A_2 which potentiates platelet release reactions, platelet aggregation and also has powerful vasoconstrictive ability. Released ADP causes platelets to swell and aggregate. Additional platelets from the circulating blood are drawn to the area of injury. This continuing platelet aggregation promotes the growth of the haemostatic plug which soon covers the exposed connective tissue. Released platelet granule enzymes, ADP and thrombosthenin may all contribute to the consolidation of the accumulated platelet plug. It seems likely that prostacyclin, produced by endothelial and smooth muscle cells in the vessel wall adjacent to the area of damage, is important in limiting the extent of the initial platelet plug. The unstable primary haemostatic plug produced by these platelet reactions in the first minute or so following injury is usually sufficient to provide temporary control of bleeding.

Definitive haemostasis is achieved when fibrin formed by blood coagulation is added to the platelet mass and by platelet-induced clot retraction/compaction.

Stabilization of the platelet plug by fibrin

Following vascular injury, activation of tissue factor activates factor VII of the extrinsic system and this activates factor IX of the intrinsic system, which in turn activates factor X. Platelet aggregation and release reactions accelerate the coagulation process by providing abundant membrane phospholipid. Thrombin generated at the injury site converts soluble plasma fibrinogen into fibrin and also potentiates platelet aggregation and secretion. Thrombin also activates factor XI which amplifies the intrinsic pathway activity. Furthermore, it activates factor XIII which covalently cross-links the fibrin meshwork. A meshwork of fibrin anchors and extends the platelet plug. The fibrin component of the haemostatic plug increases as the fused platelets autolyse and after a few hours the entire haemostatic plug is transformed into a solid mass of cross-linked fibrin. Nevertheless, due to incorporation of plasminogen and tPa (p. 312) this plug begins to autodigest during the same time frame.

Tests of haemostatic function

Defective haemostasis with abnormal bleeding may result from: (a) thrombocytopenia, (b) a disorder of platelet function, or (c) defective blood coagulation. Patients with a variety of vascular disorders may also suffer from a bleeding disorder. A number of simple tests are employed to assess the platelet, vessel wall and coagulation components of haemostasis.

Blood count and blood film examination

As thrombocytopenia is a common cause of abnormal bleeding, patients with suspected bleeding disorders should initially have a blood count including platelet count and blood film examination. In addition to establishing the presence of thrombocytopenia, the cause may be obvious, e.g. an acute leukaemia.

Bleeding time

When the blood count, platelet count and blood film examination are normal the bleeding time is done to detect abnormal platelet function. The test measures platelet plug formation *in vivo*. In the Ivy template method, after the application of 40 mmHg pressure to the upper arm with a blood pressure cuff, two 1-mm deep, 1-cm long incisions are made in the flexor surface forearm skin. Bleeding stops normally in 3−8 minutes and there is a progressive prolongation with platelet counts less than $75 \times 10^9/l$. Long times are also found in patients with disorders of platelet function.

Screening tests	Abnormalities indicated by prolongation	Commonest cause of disorder
Thrombin time (TT)	Deficiency or abnormality of fibrinogen or inhibition of thrombin by heparin or FDPs	Disseminated intravascular coagulation Heparin therapy
Prothrombin time (PT)	Deficiency or inhibition of one or more of the following coagulation factors: VII, X, V, II, fibrinogen	Liver disease Warfarin therapy (+ conditions above)
Activated partial thromboplastin time (APTT or PTTK)	Deficiency or inhibition of one or more of the following coagulation factors: XII, XI, IX, VIII, X, V, II, fibrinogen	Haemophilia Christmas disease (+ conditions above)

Table 16.3 Screening tests used in the diagnosis of coagulation disorders

FDPs, fibrin degradation products.

Screening tests of blood coagulation

Screening tests may provide an assessment of the extrinsic and intrinsic systems of blood coagulation and also the central conversion of fibrinogen to fibrin (Table 16.3). In general, prolongation of clotting times beyond those of normal 'control' plasmas in the test system will indicate a deficiency.

The prothrombin time (PT) measures factors VII, X, V, prothrombin and fibrinogen. Tissue thromboplastin (brain extract) and calcium are added to citrated plasma. The normal time for clotting is 10−14 seconds. It may be expressed as the international normalized ratio (INR) (see p. 359).

The activated partial thromboplastin time (APTT) measures the factors VIII, IX, XI and XII in addition to factors X, V, prothrombin and fibrinogen. Three substances — phospholipid, a surface activator (e.g. kaolin) and calcium — are added to citrated plasma. The normal time for clotting is about 30−40 seconds.

Prolonged clotting times in the PT and APTT due to factor deficiency are corrected by the addition of normal plasma to the test plasma. If there is no correction or incomplete correction with normal plasma the presence of an inhibitor of coagulation is suspected.

The thrombin clotting time (TT) is sensitive to a deficiency of fibrinogen or inhibition of thrombin. Diluted bovine thrombin is added to citrated plasma at a concentration giving a time of 14−16 seconds with normal subjects.

Specific assays of coagulation factors

Most factor assays are based on an APTT or PT in which all factors except the one to be measured are present in the substrate plasma. This usually requires a supply of plasma from patients with hereditary deficiency of the factor in question or artificially produced factor-deficient plasma. The corrective effect of the unknown plasma on the prolonged clotting time of the deficient substrate plasma is then compared with the corrective effect of normal plasma. Results are expressed as a percentage of normal activity. A number of chemical and immunological methods are available for quantitation of plasma fibrinogen, and immune assays have been developed to measure other coagulation factors, particularly VWF and factor VIII. Factor XIII activity can be assessed by testing for clot solubility in urea. Only uncross-linked clots are soluble, indicating factor XIII deficiency.

Test of fibrinolysis

Increased levels of circulating plasminogen activator may be detected by demonstrating shortened euglobulin clot lysis times. A number of immunological methods are available to detect fibrinogen or fibrin degradation products in serum. In patients with enhanced fibrinolysis, low levels of circulating plasminogen may be detected.

Bibliography

Bloom A.L. & Thomas D.P. (ed.) (1987) *Haemostasis and Thrombosis*, 2nd Edition. Churchill Livingstone, Edinburgh.

Colman R.W., Hirsh J., Marder V.J. & Salzman E.W. (eds) (1982) *Hemostasis and Thrombosis: Basic Principles and Clinical Practice*. J.B. Lippincott, Philadelphia.

Furie B. & Furie B.C. (1992) Molecular and cellular biology of blood coagulation. *New England Journal of Medicine*, **326**, 800–806.

Halkier T. (1991) *Mechanisms in Blood Coagulation, Fibrinolysis and the Complement System*. Cambridge University Press, Cambridge.

Hutton R. (1992) New developments in the detection of haemostatic disorders. In *Recent Advances in Haematology*, 6 (eds A.V. Hoffbrand & M.K. Brenner). Churchill Livingstone, Edinburgh, pp. 19–44.

Machin S.J. & Mackie I.J. (1989) Haemostasis. In *Laboratory Haematology* (ed. I. Chanarin). Churchill Livingstone, Edinburgh, pp. 263–399.

Patthy L. (1990) Evolution of blood coagulation and fibrinolysis. *Blood Coagulation and Fibrinolysis*, **2**, 153–166.

Poller L. (ed.) (1991) *Recent Advances in Blood Coagulation*, 5. Churchill Livingstone, Edinburgh.

Ratnoff O.D. & Forbes C.D. (eds) (1991) *Disorders of Hemostasis*, 2nd Edition. W.B. Saunders, Philadelphia.

Thomson JK.M. (ed.) (1991) *Blood Coagulation and Haemostasis. A Practical Guide*, 4th Edition. Churchill Livingstone, Edinburgh.

Tuddenham E.G.D. (ed.) (1989) Molecular biology of coagulation. *Clinical Haematology*, **2**, 787–1046.

Chapter 17
Bleeding Disorders due to Vascular and Platelet Abnormalities

Abnormal bleeding may result from vascular disorders, thrombocytopenia, platelet function defects or defective coagulation. The first three categories are discussed in this chapter and the disorders of blood coagulation follow in Chapter 18.

Vascular bleeding disorders

The vascular disorders are a heterogeneous group of conditions characterized by easy bruising and spontaneous bleeding from the small vessels. The underlying abnormality is either in the vessels themselves or in the perivascular connective tissues. Most cases of bleeding due to vascular defects alone are not severe. Frequently the bleeding is mainly in the skin causing petechiae, ecchymoses, or both. In some disorders there is also bleeding from mucous membranes. In some of these conditions the standard screening tests show little or no abnormality. The bleeding time is normal and the other tests of haemostasis are also normal. Vascular defects may be inherited or acquired.

Hereditary haemorrhagic telangiectasia

In this uncommon disorder, which is transmitted as an autosomal dominant trait, there are dilated microvascular swellings which appear during childhood and become more numerous in adult life. These telangiectasia develop in the skin, mucous membranes (Fig. 17.1) and internal organs. Recurrent gastrointestinal tract haemorrhage may cause chronic iron deficiency anaemia.

Acquired vascular defects

Vascular defects from many disorders may result in abnormal bleeding.
1 *Simple easy bruising* is a common benign disorder which occurs in otherwise healthy women, especially those of child-bearing age.
2 *Senile purpura* due to atrophy of the supporting tissues of cutaneous blood vessels is seen mainly on dorsal aspects of the forearm and hand.

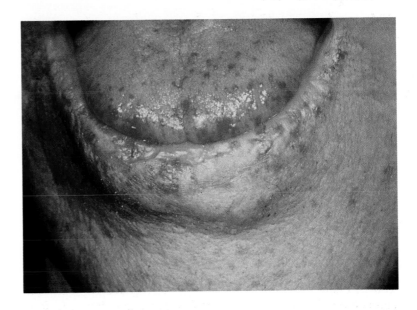

Fig. 17.1 Hereditary haemorrhagic telangiectasia: the characteristic small vascular lesions are obvious on the lips and tongue.

3 *Purpura associated with infections.* Many bacterial, viral or rickettsial infections may cause purpura from vascular damage by the organism or as a result of immune complex formation, e.g. measles, Dengue fever or meningococcal septicaemia. Purpura may also result from thrombocytopenia and disseminated intravascular coagulation (DIC) due to septicaemia.

4 *The Henoch—Schönlein syndrome* is an immune complex (type III) hypersensitivity reaction usually found in children and often follows an acute infection. The characteristic purpuric rash accompanied by localized oedema and itching is often most prominent on the buttocks and extensor surfaces of the lower legs and elbows. Painful joint swelling, haematuria and abdominal pain may also occur. It is usually a self-limiting condition but occasional patients develop renal failure.

5 *Scurvy.* In vitamin C deficiency, defective collagen may cause perifollicular petechiae, bruising and mucosal haemorrhage.

6 *Steroid purpura.* The purpura which is associated with long-term steroid therapy or Cushing's syndrome is caused by defective vascular supportive tissue.

7 *Connective tissue disorders.* In the Ehlers—Danlos syndrome there are hereditary collagen abnormalities, hyperextensibility of joints and hyperelastic friable skin. The bleeding tendency is most severe in type IV disease, in which type III collagen is defective. Pseudoxanthoma elasticum is associated with arterial haemorrhage and thrombosis. Mild cases may present with superficial bruising and purpura following minor trauma.

8 *Other causes.* Uncommon causes of purpura include auto-erythrocyte sensitization (which is probably always factitious), DNA sensitivity and fat embolism.

Thrombocytopenia

Abnormal bleeding associated with thrombocytopenia or abnormal platelet function is also characterized by spontaneous skin purpura and haemorrhage (Fig. 17.2) and prolonged bleeding after trauma. The main causes of thrombocytopenia are listed in Tables 17.1 and 17.2.

Failure of platelet production

This is the commonest cause of thrombocytopenia and is usually associated with a failure of red cell and white cell production. Selective megakaryocyte depression may result from drug toxicity, e.g. from phenylbutazone, co-trimoxazole or penicillamine (Table 17.2), or from viral infections. Decreased numbers of megakaryocytes may be part of a generalized bone marrow failure in aplastic anaemia, leukaemia, myelodysplasia, myelosclerosis, marrow infiltrations or after chemotherapy or radiotherapy. Ineffective platelet production from normal or increased numbers of megakaryocytes is a feature of megaloblastic anaemia. Diagnosis of these causes of thrombocytopenia is made from the peripheral blood count, the blood film and bone marrow examination.

Increased destruction of platelets

Chronic autoimmune thrombocytopenic purpura (ITP)

This is a relatively common disorder with the highest incidence in women aged 15–50 years. It is the commonest cause of thrombocytopenia without anaemia or neutropenia. It is usually

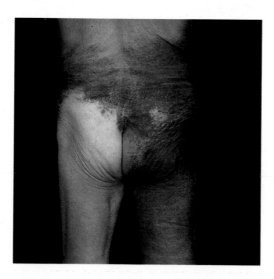

Fig. 17.2 Massive subcutaneous haemorrhage in a patient with drug-induced thrombocytopenia.

Table 17.1 Causes of thrombocytopenia.

Failure of platelet production
- Selective megakaryocyte depression
    Drugs, chemicals, viral infections
- Part of general bone marrow failure
    Cytotoxic drugs
    Radiotherapy
    Aplastic anaemia
    Leukaemia
    Myelodysplastic syndromes
    Myelosclerosis
    Marrow infiltration, e.g. carcinoma, lymphoma
    Multiple myeloma
    Megaloblastic anaemia
    HIV infection

Increased consumption of platelets
- Immune
    Autoimmune (idiopathic)
    Drug-induced
    Systemic lupus erythematosus
    Chronic lymphocytic leukaemia and lymphoma
    Infections: HIV, other viruses, malaria
    Heparin
    Post-transfusional purpura
    Neonatal (isoimmune) purpura
- Disseminated intravascular coagulation
- Thrombotic thrombocytopenic purpura

Abnormal distribution of platelets
- Splenomegaly

Dilutional loss
- Massive transfusion of stored blood to bleeding patients

Table 17.2 Thrombocytopenia due to drugs or toxins.

Bone marrow suppression
- Predictable (dose-related)
    Ionizing radiation, cytotoxic drugs, ethanol
- Occasional
    Chloramphenicol, co-trimoxazole, idoxuridine, phenylbutazone, penicillamine, organic arsenicals, benzene, etc.

Immune mechanisms (proven or probable)
- Analgesics, anti-inflammatory drugs
    Phenacetin, gold salts, rifampicin
- Antimicrobials
    Penicillins, sulphonamides, trimethoprim, *para*-aminosalicylate
- Sedatives, anticonvulsants
    Diazepam, sodium valproate
- Diuretics
    Acetazolamide, chlorathiazides, frusemide
- Antidiabetics
    Chlorpropamide, tolbutamide
- Others
    Digitoxin, heparin, methyldopa, oxyprenolol, quinine, quinidine

Platelet aggregation
    Ristocetin, heparin

idiopathic but may be seen in association with other diseases, e.g. SLE (systemic lupus erythematosus), HIV infection, chronic lymphocytic leukaemia (CLL), Hodgkin's disease or autoimmune haemolytic anaemia.

Pathogenesis
Platelet sensitization with auto-antibodies (usually IgG) results in their premature removal from the circulation by cells of the reticuloendothelial (RE) system (Fig. 17.3). In many cases the antibody is directed against antigen sites on the glycoprotein IIb–IIIa complex. The normal lifespan of a platelet is 7–10 days but in ITP this is reduced to a few hours. Lightly sensitized platelets are mainly destroyed by macrophages in the spleen because of Fc recognition but heavily sensitized platelets or platelets coated with complement as well as IgG are destroyed throughout the RE system, mainly in the liver. Total megakaryocyte mass and platelet turnover are increased in parallel to about five times normal.

Clinical features
The onset is often insidious with petechial haemorrhage, easy bruising and, in women, menorrhagia. Mucosal bleeding occurs in severe cases but intracranial haemorrhage is rare. The severity of bleeding in ITP is less than that seen in patients with comparable degrees of thrombocytopenia from bone marrow failure; this is attributed to the circulation of predominantly young, functionally superior platelets in ITP.

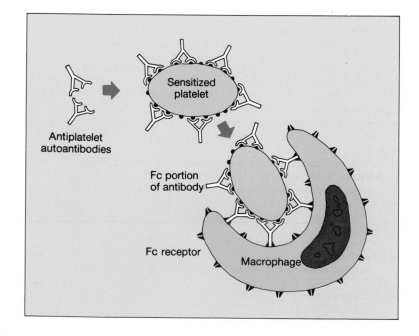

Fig. 17.3 The pathogenesis of thrombocytopenia in autoimmune thrombocytopenic purpura.

The spleen is not palpable unless there is an associated disease causing splenomegaly.

Diagnosis
1 The platelet count is usually $10-50 \times 10^9/l$. The haemoglobin concentration and white cell count are typically normal.
2 The blood film shows reduced numbers of platelets, those present often being large.
3 The bone marrow shows normal or increased numbers of megakaryocytes.
4 Sensitive tests are able to demonstrate antiplatelet IgG either alone or with complement or IgM, on the platelet surface or in the serum in most patients.
5 Antinuclear factor is present in serum in patients with underlying SLE.
6 The direct antiglobulin test is positive in cases with associated autoimmune haemolytic anaemia (Evans' syndrome).

Treatment
A spontaneous recovery occurs in less than 10% of patients with chronic ITP. Treatment is aimed at reducing the level of auto-antibody and reducing the destruction rate of sensitized platelets. A proportion of cases relapse, however, months or years after remitting with the treatment discussed below.
1 *Steroids.* 80% of patients remit on high-dose corticosteroid therapy. Prednisolone 60 mg daily is the usual initial therapy in adults and the dose is gradually reduced after a remission has been achieved. In poor responders the dose is reduced more slowly but splenectomy or immunosuppression is considered.
2 *Splenectomy* (Fig. 17.4). This operation is recommended in patients who do not recover within 3 months of steroid therapy or who require unacceptably high doses of steroids to maintain a platelet count above $30 \times 10^9/l$. Good results occur in most of the patients, but in patients with ITP refractory to steroids there may be little benefit. This is often the case in older patients.
3 *High-dose intravenous immunoglobulin therapy* is able to produce a rapid rise in platelet count in the majority of patients. A dose of 400 mg/kg/day for 5 days is recommended. This expensive therapy is particularly useful in selected patients who have life-threatening haemorrhage. It has also been used successfully in steroid-refractory ITP, during pregnancy or prior to surgery. The mechanism of action may be blockage of Fc receptors on macrophages or modification of autoantibody production.
4 *Immunosuppressive drugs*, e.g. vincristine, vinblastine, cyclophosphamide, azathioprine or cyclosporin, are usually reserved for those patients who do not respond to steroids and splenectomy.
5 *Experimental therapy* with danazol (an androgen which may

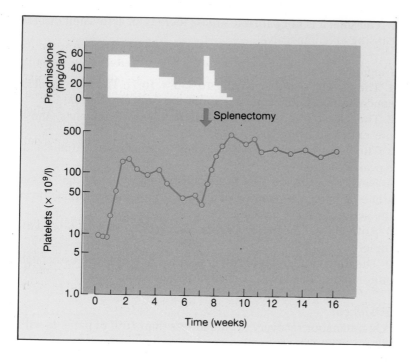

Fig. 17.4 Response to prednisolone in chronic immune thrombocytopenic purpura with subsequent relapse and response to splenectomy.

virilise in women), vitamin C in large doses, colchicine, anti-D immunoglobulin and α-interferon has been tried with limited success in refractory cases.

6 *Platelet transfusions.* Although isologous platelets do not survive longer than the patient's own (i.e. a few hours), platelet concentrates are beneficial in patients with acute, life-threatening bleeding.

Pregnancy
Since the antibody crosses the placenta, the foetus may become severely thrombocytopenic. High-dose systemic immunoglobulin and corticosteroids are used if necessary.

Acute immune thrombocytopenia

Acute thrombocytopenia is most common in children. The mechanism is not well established. In about 75% of patients, the thrombocytopenia and bleeding follows vaccination or an infection, e.g. measles, chicken pox or infectious mononucleosis, and an allergic reaction with immune complex formation and complement deposition on platelets is suspected.

Spontaneous remissions are usual but in 5–10% of cases the disease becomes chronic. Short-term steroid therapy or intravenous immunoglobulin is sometimes used in severe cases.

Infections

It seems likely that the thrombocytopenia associated with many viral and protozoal infections is immune-mediated. In malaria it has been shown that the IgG antibodies are directed against malarial antigen bound to the platelet membrane. The raised platelet-bound IgG in viral infections, including infectious mononucleosis and AIDS, probably reflects immune complex deposition on the platelet surface. In AIDS, reduced platelet production is also involved (p. 183).

Post-transfusion purpura

Thrombocytopenia occurring about 10 days after a blood transfusion has been attributed to antibodies in the recipient developing against the Pl^{A1} antigen (absent from the patient's own platelets) on transfused platelets. The reason why the patient's own platelets are also destroyed is unknown. Treatment is with steroids and high-dose immunoglobulin.

Drug-induced immune thrombocytopenia

An allergic mechanism has been demonstrated as the cause of many drug-induced thrombocytopenias. Drug-induced antibodies have been demonstrated in patients suffering from thrombocytopenia in association with therapy with quinine (also in tonic water), quinidine, heparin, *para*-aminosalicylate (PAS), sulphonamides, rifampicin, stibophen, digitoxin and other drugs. In most drug-dependent immune thrombocytopenias, the

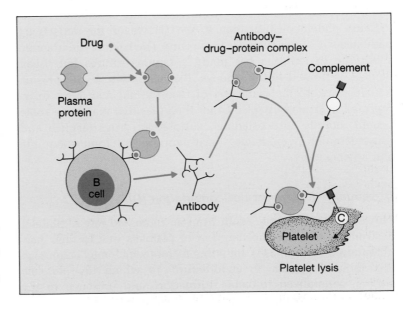

Fig. 17.5 Usual type of platelet damage caused by drugs in which an antibody–drug–protein complex is deposited on the platelet surface. If complement is attached and the sequence goes to completion, the platelet may be lysed directly. Otherwise it is removed by reticuloendothelial cells due to opsonization with immunoglobulin and/or the C3 component of complement.

antibody is directed against the drug bound to a plasma protein as antigen and circulating immune complexes are adsorbed onto the platelet (Fig. 17.5). The platelet is damaged as an 'innocent bystander' and is removed by the RE cells due to the immuno-globulin or complement coating. If the complement sequence is fully activated, the platelets are lysed directly in the circulation. Patients present with acute purpura, sometimes heralded by a chill, headache and flushing.

The platelet count is often less than $10 \times 10^9/l$, and the bone marrow shows normal or increased numbers of megakaryocytes. Drug-dependent antibodies against platelets may be demonstrated in the sera of some patients.

The immediate treatment is to stop all suspected drugs. Plate-let concentrates are given to patients with dangerous bleeding. Recovery usually occurs after a few hours or days depending on the rapidity of eliminating the drug from the body. These patients must avoid the offending drug and those structurally related to it.

Thrombotic thrombocytopenic purpura (TTP) and haemolytic uraemic syndrome (HUS)

In the sometimes fatal disorder of TTP there is severe thrombo-cytopenia, confluent purpura, fragmentation haemolysis and widespread ischaemic organ damage, e.g. of the brain and kidney. There is extensive deposition of arteriolar thrombi. Immune-mediated damage to the vessel wall and platelet hyperaggre-gatability have been suggested as pathogenetic factors. Diminished production of prostacyclin by the vessel walls has been demon-strated. The plasma from some TTP patients agglutinates normal platelets *in vitro* and there is evidence that a platelet-agglutinating factor interacts with the large multimers of von Willebrand factor to cause platelet agglutination *in vivo*. However, the underlying pathogenesis of this disorder is obscure. The haemolytic uraemic syndrome in children has many common features but organ damage is limited to the kidneys. Plasma exchange and plasma transfusions are the mainstays of therapy and may have to be repeated over many weeks. Other therapies that may have some benefit include corticosteroids, antiplatelet drugs (aspirin and dipyridamole), vincristine, azathiaprine, cyclophosphamide and splenectomy.

Disseminated intravascular coagulation (DIC)

Thrombocytopenia may result from an increased rate of platelet destruction through consumption of platelets due to their par-ticipation in DIC (p. 344). Initiating factors which may encourage this include damage to endothelium to which the platelets adhere, generalized thrombin formation, and presence in the circulation of viruses, bacteria and endotoxin—all of which

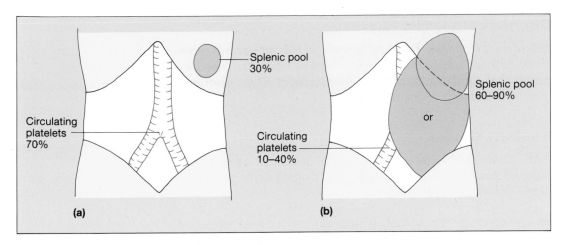

Fig. 17.6 The platelet distributioin between the circulation and spleen in normal individuals (a) and in patients with moderate or massive splenomegaly (b).

produce platelet aggregation. After aggregation, the platelets become trapped in arterioles and capillaries and their level in the circulation falls.

Increased splenic pooling

Kinetic studies using ^{51}Cr-labelled platelets indicate that the major factor responsible for thrombocytopenia in splenomegaly is platelet 'pooling' by the spleen. Normally, platelets in the general circulation exchange freely with a 'reservoir' or 'pool' of platelets in the splenic microcirculation which accounts for about a third of the total platelet mass. In splenomegaly, the fraction in the exchangeable splenic pool increases and may represent the bulk, e.g. 90% of the marrow output (Fig. 17.6). The platelet lifespan is normal since platelets, unlike red cells, tolerate splenic stasis without injury. In the absence of additional haemostatic defects, the thrombocytopenia of splenomegaly is not usually associated with bleeding.

Massive transfusion syndrome

Platelets are unstable in blood stored at 4°C and the platelet count rapidly falls in blood stored for more than 24 hours. Some clotting factors, e.g. factor VIII, also lose activity on storage.

Patients transfused with massive amounts of stored blood (more than 10 units over a 24-hour period) frequently show abnormal bleeding. The defect produced by transfusion with large volumes of stored blood can be minimized if replacement with specific screened products (e.g. fresh frozen plasma (FFP) and platelet concentrates) is used, for example 2 units FFP plus 5 units platelets for 8–10 units of blood. Established bleeding is treated by administration of fresh whole blood, supplemented by platelet transfusions and FFP.

Disorders of platelet function

Disorders of platelet function are suspected in patients who show skin and mucosal haemorrhage and in whom the bleeding time is prolonged despite a normal platelet count. These disorders may be hereditary or acquired.

Hereditary disorders

Rare inherited disorders may produce defects at each of the different phases of the platelet reactions leading to the formation of the haemostatic platelet plug.

Thrombasthenia (Glanzmann's disease). There is a failure of primary platelet aggregation due to a deficiency of membrane glycoproteins IIb and IIIa. Platelet-specific antigen $Zw^a(Pl^{A1})$ is located on this complex and is not expressed on thrombasthenic platelets.

Bernard–Soulier syndrome. In this disease the platelets are larger than normal and there is a deficiency of glycoprotein Ib. There is defective binding to von Willebrand factor, defective adherence to exposed subendothelial connective tissues and platelets do not aggregate with ristocetin. There is a variable degree of thrombocytopenia.

Other membrane defects include defects in the response to collagen and of platelet phospholipid. In the platelet-type von Willebrand's disease there is increased ristocetin-induced platelet aggregation and deficiency of von Willebrand factor in plasma.

Storage pool diseases. In the rare Grey platelet syndrome the platelets are larger than normal and there is a virtual absence of α-granules with deficiency of their proteins. In the more common δ-storage pool disease there is a deficiency of dense granules. Consequently, the secondary wave of platelet aggregation does not occur since there is no storage pool of ADP to release. Bleeding is moderate to severe. Combined with albinism, it is called the Hermansky–Pudlak syndrome. Combined α- and δ-storage pool disease has also been described.

Other rare hereditary disorders include failure of thromboxane synthesis due to either cyclooxygenase or thromboxane synthetase deficiency, and defects of response to thromboxane.

Acquired disorders

Aspirin therapy is the most common cause of defective platelet function. It produces an abnormal bleeding time and, although purpura may not be obvious, the defect may contribute to the associated gastrointestinal haemorrhage. The cause of the aspirin defect is inhibition of cyclooxygenase with impaired thromboxane A_2 synthesis (see Fig. 19.4). There is consequent impairment of the release reaction and aggregation with adrenaline and ADP. After a single dose the defect lasts 7–10 days. A similar inhibition occurs with sulphinpyrazone and indomethacin.

Hyperglobulinaemia associated with multiple myeloma or Waldenström's disease may cause interference with platelet adherence, release and aggregation.

Myeloproliferative and myelodysplastic disorders. Intrinsic abnormalities of platelet function occur in many patients with essential thrombocythaemia and other myeloproliferative and myelodysplastic diseases and in paroxysmal nocturnal haemoglobinuria.

Uraemia is associated with various abnormalities. The defects may be caused by high guanidinosuccinic acid levels or abnormal arachidonate metabolism with reduced synthesis of thromboxane.

Heparin, in high concentration, and dextrans have been found to inhibit platelet aggregation and secretion. Alcohol and radiographic contrast agents may also cause defective function.

Antiplatelet drugs

Several clinical trials have assessed the antithrombotic effect of drugs which suppress platelet function. Drugs are used to reduce the incidence of both arterial and venous thrombosis in a variety of clinical situations. Their use and mechanisms of action are discussed in Chapter 19.

Diagnosis

As thrombocytopenia is the commonest cause of abnormal bleeding, patients with suspected platelet or blood vessel abnormalities should initially have a blood count and blood film examination (see Fig. 17.7). In addition to establishing the presence of thrombocytopenia, the cause of this may be obvious, e.g. acute leukaemia. Bone marrow examination is essential in thrombocytopenic patients to determine whether or not there is a failure of platelet production. The marrow may also reveal one of the conditions associated with defective production (see Table 17.1). In patients with thrombocytopenia, a negative drug history, normal or excessive numbers of marrow megakaryocytes and no other marrow abnormality or splenomegaly, ITP is the usual diagnosis. Tests for platelet antibodies may confirm this. Screening tests for DIC are needed to establish this as a cause of consumptive thrombocytopenia.

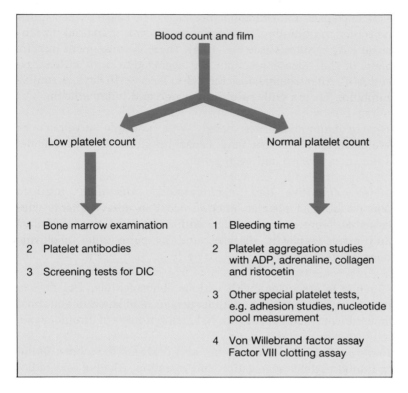

Fig. 17.7 Laboratory tests for platelet disorders. NB some intrinsic platelet functional disorders are associated with thrombocytopenia, e.g. Bernard–Soulier syndrome.

When the blood count, platelet count and film examination are all normal the bleeding time is done to detect abnormal platelet function. This test mainly measures platelet plug formation *in vivo*. Bleeding stops normally in 3–8 minutes.

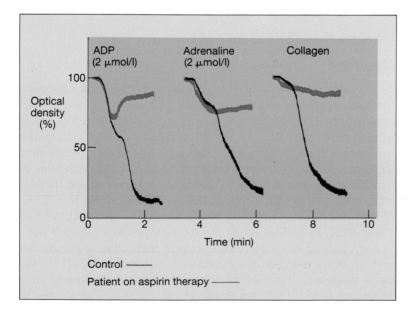

Fig. 17.8 Defective platelet aggregation in a patient on aspirin therapy. There is no secondary phase aggregation with ADP (adenosine diphosphate) and reduced responses to both adrenaline and collagen. Similar results are obtained in δ-storage granule deficiency and cyclo-oxygenase deficiency.

In most patients with abnormal platelet function demonstrated by prolonged bleeding time, the defect is acquired and associated either with systemic disease (e.g. uraemia) or with aspirin therapy. The very rare hereditary defects of platelet function require more elaborate *in vitro* tests to define the specific abnormality. These include platelet aggregation studies with ADP, adrenaline, collagen (Fig. 17.8) and ristocetin. If von Willebrand's disease is suspected, assay of von Willebrand factor and coagulation factor VIII are required.

Platelet transfusions

Platelet transfusions are indicated in the following circumstances.
1 Thrombocytopenia or abnormal platelet function when bleeding or before invasive procedures and there is no alternative therapy (e.g. steroids or high-dose immunoglobulin) available.
2 Prophylactically in patients with platelet counts of less than $5-10 \times 10^9/l$. If there is infection, potential bleeding sites or coagulopathy the count should be kept $>20 \times 10^9/l$).
3 Massive transfusion if thrombocytopenia is documented and clinical bleeding is evident.

The indications for transfusion of platelet concentrates are discussed on p. 405.

Bibliography

Abrams C. & Shattil S.J. (1991) Immunological detection of activated platelets in clinical disorders. *Thrombosis Haemostasis*, **65**, 467−473.

Berchtold P. & McMillan R. (1989) Therapy of chronic idiopathic thrombocytopenic purpura in adults. *Blood*, **74**, 2309−2317.

British Committee for Standards in Haematology, Working Party of Blood Transfusion Task Force (1992) Guidelines for platelet transfusions. *Transfusion Medicine*, **2**, 1777−1780.

Caen J.P. (1989) Platelet disorders. *Clinical Haematology*, **2**, 587−786.

Colman R.W. & Rao A.K. (eds) (1990) Platelets in health and disease. *Hematology/Oncology Clinics of North America*, **4**, 1−313.

Hutton R.W. & Ludlam C.A. (1989) Guidelines on platelet function testing. *Journal of Clinical Pathology*, **41**, 1322−1330.

Page C.P. (ed.) (1991) *The Platelet in Health and Disease*. Blackwell Scientific Publications, Oxford.

Chapter 18
Coagulation Disorders

Hereditary deficiencies of each of ten coagulation factors have been described. Haemophilia A (factor VIII deficiency), haemophilia B (Christmas disease, factor IX deficiency) and von Willebrand's disease are uncommon; the others are rare.

Haemophilia A (haemophilia)

Haemophilia is the most common hereditary disorder of blood coagulation. The inheritance is sex-linked (Fig. 18.1) but 33% of patients have no family history and presumably result from spontaneous mutation. The incidence is of the order of 30–100/10^6 population.

The defect is an absence or low level of plasma factor VIII. The gene for factor VIII is located near the tip of the long arm of the X chromosome (Xq2.8). The cDNA for factor VIII has been cloned and many genetic defects have been identified in haemophilic families. These include many deletions and different point mutations some of which are represented in Fig. 18.2.

Clinical features

Infants may suffer from profuse post-circumcision haemorrhage. Recurrent painful haemarthroses and muscle haematomas dominate the clinical course of severely affected patients with progressive deformity and crippling (Figs 18.3–18.6). Prolonged bleeding occurs after dental extractions. Haematuria is more common than gastrointestinal haemorrhage. The clinical severity of the disease correlates well with the extent of the coagulation factor deficiency (Table 18.1). Operative and post-traumatic haemorrhage are life-threatening both in severely and mildly affected patients. Although not common, spontaneous intra-cerebral haemorrhage occurs more frequently than in the general population and is an important cause of death in patients with severe disease.

Haemophilic pseudotumours may occur in the long bones, pelvis, fingers and toes. These result from repeated subperiosteal haemorrhages with bone destruction, new bone formation, expansion of the bone and pathological fractures.

It is becoming apparent that many haemophiliacs have sub-

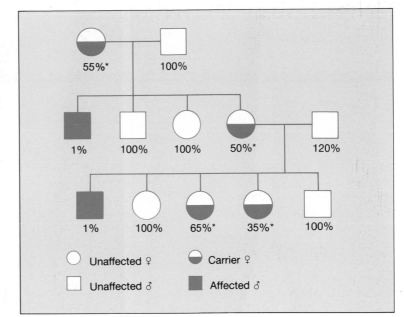

Fig. 18.1 A typical family tree in a family with haemophilia. Note the variable levels of factor VIII activity in carriers (*) due to random inactivation of X chromosome (lyonization). The percentages show the degree of factor VIII activity as a percentage of normal.

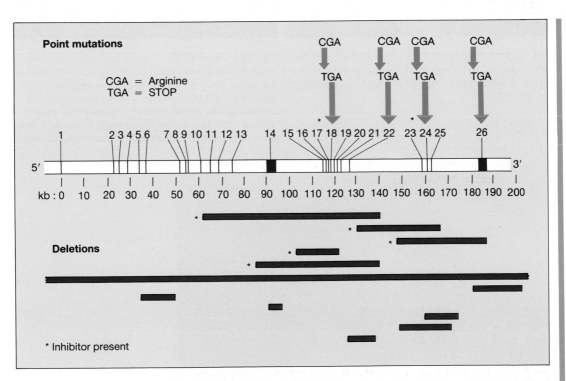

Fig. 18.2 The gene for factor VIII clotting factor showing the 26 exons separated by 25 non-coding sequences. Some of the genetic deletions and point mutations associated with haemophilia are shown.

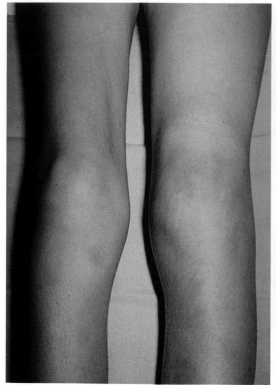 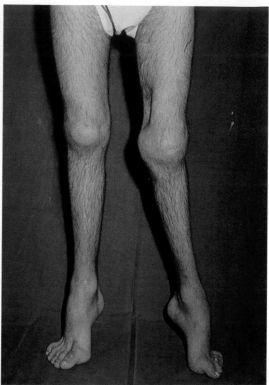

Fig. 18.3 Haemophilia A: acute haemarthrosis of the left knee joint with swelling of the suprapatellar region. There is wasting of the quadriceps muscles, particularly on the right.

Fig. 18.4 Haemophilia A: gross crippling. The right knee is swollen with posterior subluxation of the tibia on the femur. The ankles and feet show residual deformities of talipes equinus, with some cavus and associated toe clawing. There is generalized muscle wasting. The scar on the medial side of the right lower thigh is the site of a previously excised pseudotumour.

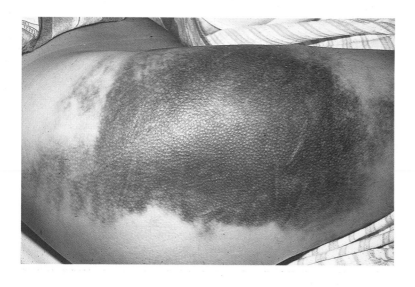

Fig. 18.5 Haemophilia A: massive haemorrhage in the area of the right buttock.

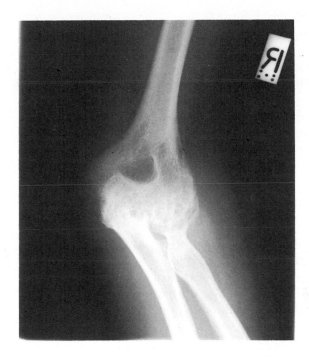

Fig. 18.6 Haemophilia A: radiographic appearances of the right elbow joint in a 25-year-old male. The joint space has been destroyed and there is bony ankylosis. Subchondral cystic areas are prominent.

clinical liver disease, and a few show clinical features of chronic hepatitis. This is largely due to the many infusions of blood products and consequent transmission of hepatitis B or more frequently hepatitis C or possibly other non-A, non-B hepatitis viruses. Hepatitis B and C screening of donors, vaccination against hepatitis B of the non-immune and viral inactivation procedures during the preparation of factor VIII concentrates have reduced or eliminated the incidence of hepatitis B, hepatitis C and HIV (human immunodeficiency virus) transmission (see below).

AIDS (acquired immune deficiency syndrome) is now the commonest cause of death in severe haemophilia. As a result of HIV present in concentrates during the early 1980s, over 50% of

Table 18.1 Correlation of coagulation factor activity and disease severity in haemophilia and factor IX deficiency.

Coagulation factor activity (% of normal)	Clinical manifestations
<1	Severe disease Frequent spontaneous bleeding episodes from early life Joint deformity and crippling if not adequately treated
1–5	Moderate disease Post-traumatic bleeding Occasional spontaneous episodes
5–20	Mild disease Post-traumatic bleeding

haemophilics treated in the USA or Western Europe show HIV antibodies in their blood. The incidence of clinical AIDS is gradually increasing. Thrombocytopenia from HIV infection may exacerbate bleeding episodes. Donor testing and viral inactivation steps during concentrate preparation now prevent HIV infection during therapy. Factor VIII made by recombinant DNA techniques is also free of infection risk.

Drug addiction due to repeated need for analgesics is a problem in some teenagers or adults with severe disease and progressive joint destruction.

Laboratory findings (see Table 18.2)

The following tests are abnormal:
1 Activated partial thromboplastin time (APTT).
2 Factor VIII clotting assay.

Immunological methods show normal von Willebrand factor (VWF) activity and platelet aggregation to ristocetin is normal. The bleeding time and prothrombin time tests are also normal.

Carrier detection and antenatal diagnosis
Until recently, carrier detection and antenatal diagnosis were limited to measuring plasma levels of factor VIII and VWF. Carrier females may be identified with reasonable confidence if their factor VIII coagulant activity is only half that expected from the level of VWF. However, the normal range of factor VIII is broad and random X chromosome inactivation makes it diffi-

	Haemophilia A	Factor IX deficiency	Von Willebrand's disease
Inheritance	Sex-linked	Sex-linked	Dominant (incomplete)
Main sites of haemorrhage	Muscle, joints post-trauma or operation	Muscle, joints post-trauma or operation	Mucous membranes, skin cuts, post-trauma and operation
Platelet count	Normal	Normal	Normal
Bleeding time	Normal	Normal	Prolonged
Prothrombin time	Normal	Normal	Normal
Partial thrombo-plastin time	Prolonged	Prolonged	Prolonged or normal
Factor VIII	Low	Normal	Low
VWF	Normal	Normal	Low
Factor IX	Normal	Low	Normal
Ristocetin-induced platelet aggregation	Normal	Normal	Impaired

Table 18.2 Main clinical and laboratory findings in haemophilia A, factor IX deficiency (haemophilia B, Christmas disease) and von Willebrand's disease.

VWF, von Willebrand factor.

cult to exclude the carrier state in many females in affected families. Carrier status is better determined with DNA probes. The discovery of restriction fragment length polymorphisms (see p. 116) within or close to the factor VIII gene now allow the mutant allele to be tracked with confidence in the majority of women carriers. Alternatively, a known specific mutation can be directly probed for. Chorionic biopsies at 8−10 weeks' gestation provide sufficient DNA from foetal cells to analyse for the characteristic defect or linked polymorphism using PCR (polymerase chain reaction) technology. Antenatal diagnosis and abortion of affected foetuses is also possible following the demonstration of low levels of factor VIII in foetal blood obtained at 18−20 weeks gestation from the umbilical vein by ultrasound-guided needle aspiration. This service is available at specialized centres.

Treatment

Most patients attend specialized haemophilia centres. Bleeding episodes are treated with factor VIII replacement therapy or by the administration of desmopressin (DDAVP). Factor VIII levels are raised most effectively with infusions of factor VIII concentrates. Spontaneous bleeding is usually controlled if the patient's factor VIII level is raised above 20% of normal. For major surgery, serious post-traumatic bleeding or when haemorrhage is occurring at a dangerous site, however, the factor VIII level should be elevated to 100% and then maintained above 60% when acute bleeding has stopped, until healing has occurred.

The units of factor VIII needed, X, can be calculated:

$$X = \frac{\% \text{ rise in factor VIII} \times \text{weight (kg)}}{K}$$

Where $K = 1.5$ for factor VIII ($K = 1.0$ for factor IX and 2.0 for factor XI); 1 unit of factor VIII = 1% of the factor VIII activity in normal plasma.

DDAVP provides an alternative means of increasing the plasma factor VIII level in milder haemophilics. Following the intravenous administration of this drug there is a moderate rise in the patient's own factor VIII which is proportional to the resting level. DDAVP may also be inhaled as snuff—this has been used as immediate treatment for mild haemophilics after accidental trauma or haemorrhage. A fibrinolytic inhibitor, e.g. tranexamic acid, is often given with DDAVP to counteract the release of tissue plasminogen activator which occurs with this agent.

Local supportive measures used in treating haemarthroses and haematomas include resting the affected part and the prevention of further trauma.

The increased availability of factor VIII concentrates which may be stored in domestic refrigerators has dramatically altered haemophilia treatment. At the earliest suggestion of bleeding the haemophilic child may be treated at home. This advance has reduced the occurrence of crippling haemarthroses and the need for inpatient care. Severely affected patients are now reaching adult life with little or no arthritis.

Haemophilics are advised to have regular conservative dental care. Haemophilic children and their parents often require extensive help with social and psychological matters. With modern treatment the lifestyle of a haemophilic child can be almost normal but certain activities such as body contact sports are to be avoided.

One of the most serious complications of haemophilia is the development of antibodies (inhibitors) to infused factor VIII which occurs in 5–10% of patients. This renders the patient refractory to further replacement therapy so that tremendous doses have to be given to achieve a significant rise in plasma factor VIII activity. Immunosuppression has been used in an attempt to reduce formation of the antibody. Some factor IX concentrates contain activated factor X which by-passes factor VIII. A special preparation known as FEIBA (factor VIII inhibitor by-passing activity) has been used successfully in the treatment of severe haemorrhage in these patients. Porcine factor VIII concentrates have also been effective in some patients and recombinant factor VIIa has been used with good effect.

Immunoaffinity purified factor VIII including monoclonal products and factor VIII prepared by recombinant DNA technology are now available for clinical use.

Factor IX deficiency

The inheritance and clinical features of factor IX deficiency (Christmas disease, haemophilia B) are identical to those of haemophilia A. Indeed the two disorders can only be distinguished by specific coagulation factor assays. The incidence is one-fifth that of haemophilia A. Factor IX is coded by a gene close to the gene for factor VIII near the tip of the long arm of the X chromosome (Xq2.6 region). The factor IX gene is about one-fifth of the size of the factor VIII gene. As in haemophilia a number of point mutations and deletions have been found in affected kindreds.

Laboratory findings (see Table 18.2)

The following tests are abnormal:
1 APTT.
2 Whole blood coagulation time (severe cases).
3 Factor IX clotting assay.

As in haemophilia A, the bleeding time and prothrombin time tests are normal.

Carrier detection and antenatal diagnosis

Restriction fragment length polymorphisms have been identified within the factor IX gene. Carrier detection and antenatal diagnosis by chorionic biopsy is possible using DNA probes and Southern blotting or PCR technology.

Treatment

The principles of replacement therapy are similar to those of haemophilia A. Bleeding episodes are treated with factor IX concentrates. Because of its longer biological half-life, infusions do not have to be given as frequently as factor VIII concentrates in haemophilia A. Trials with immunoaffinity purified factor IX have commenced.

Von Willebrand's disease

In this disorder abnormal platelet adhesion is associated with low factor VIII activity. The introduction of more reliable tests for this condition and the awareness that clinical features may be mild has changed the previous concept that the condition is rare. The true incidence may be similar to, or even exceed, that of haemophilia A ($30-100/10^6$ population). The inheritance is autosomal dominant with varying expression. The primary defect appears to be a reduced synthesis of VWF (p. 303).

This protein promotes platelet adhesion and is also the carrier molecule for factor VIII, protecting it from premature destruction. The latter property explains the reduced factor VIII levels found in von Willebrand's disease. The molecular defects that have been identified include point mutations and major deletions.

The bleeding is characterized by operative and post-traumatic haemorrhage, mucous membrane bleeding (e.g. epistaxes, menorrhagia) and excessive blood loss from superficial cuts and abrasions. Haemarthroses and muscle haematomas are rare, except in homozygous cases.

Laboratory findings (see Table 18.2)

1 Prolonged bleeding time.
2 Low levels of factor VIII activity.
3 Low levels of VWF.
4 Defective platelet aggregation with ristocetin. Ristocetin, an antibiotic which was withdrawn because of its side effect of thrombocytopenia, induces platelet aggregation in normal

platelet-rich plasma, but not in that from patients with severe von Willebrand's disease. In the majority of patients the aggregation response to other agents (ADP, collagen, thrombin or adrenaline) is normal (see Fig. 17.8).

5 Low VWF activity in patient's plasma (assay uses ristocetin-treated donor 'pool' platelets or immunological methods).

The laboratory results in mildly affected patients are variable and there is also marked variability of VWF and factor VIII levels in different members of the same family. A number of subtypes are recognized, including those with normal (type I) or abnormal (type II) multimeric structures and those with particularly severe disease (type III). At least 22 variants of type I and type II disease have been described based on phenotypic differences of the abnormal protein.

Treatment

Bleeding episodes are treated with intermediate-purity, factor VIII concentrates, which contain VWF and factor VIII, or with DDAVP. Factor VIII infusions may be associated with sustained and often delayed increases of factor VIII clotting activity (Fig. 18.7). This is because the infused VWF in the factor VIII preparation prolongs the survival of the patient's own factor VIII. Bleeding from the mouth, nose or uterus can often be alleviated with fibrinolytic inhibitors (tranexamic or aminocaproic acids).

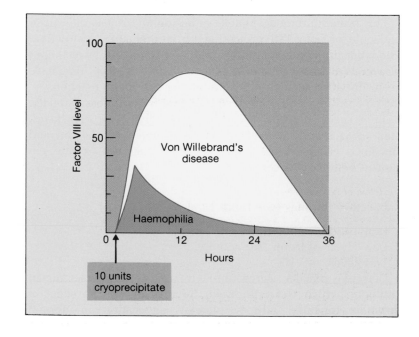

Fig. 18.7 Comparison of the activity of factor VIII in plasma following the infusion of factor VIII (as cryoprecipitate) in haemophilia and von Willebrand's disease.

Hereditary disorders of other coagulation factors

All these disorders are rare. In most the inheritance is autosomal recessive. There is usually a good correlation between the patient's symptoms and the severity of the coagulation deficiency; however, there are exceptions. Factor XII deficiency is not associated with abnormal bleeding and, although factor XI deficiency (more common in Ashkenazi Jews) produces a marked laboratory defect, the clinical symptoms are mild. Factor XIII deficiency produces a severe bleeding tendency but the usual screening tests for coagulation disorders are normal. A test of clot stability in the presence of 5 M urea is required to reveal this rare autosomal recessive defect.

Acquired coagulation disorders

The acquired coagulation disorders (Table 18.3) are more common than the inherited disorders. Unlike the inherited disorders, multiple clotting-factor deficiencies are usual.

Vitamin K deficiency

Fat-soluble vitamin K is obtained from green vegetables and bacterial synthesis in the gut. Deficiency may present in the newborn (haemorrhagic disease of the newborn) or in later life.

Deficiency of vitamin K caused by an inadequate diet, malabsorption, or drugs such as warfarin which act as vitamin K antagonists, is associated with a decrease in the functional

Table 18.3 The acquired coagulation disorders.

Deficiency of vitamin K-dependent factors
Haemorrhagic disease of the newborn
Biliary obstruction
Malabsorption of vitamin K, e.g. sprue, coeliac disease
Vitamin K-antagonist therapy, e.g. coumarins, indanediones

Liver disease

Disseminated intravascular coagulation

Inhibition of coagulation
Specific inhibitors, e.g. antibodies against factor VIII components
Non-specific inhibitors, e.g. antibodies found in systemic lupus
    erythematosus, rheumatoid arthritis

Miscellaneous
Diseases with M-protein production
L-Asparaginase
Therapy with heparin, defibrinating agents or thrombolytics
Massive transfusion syndrome

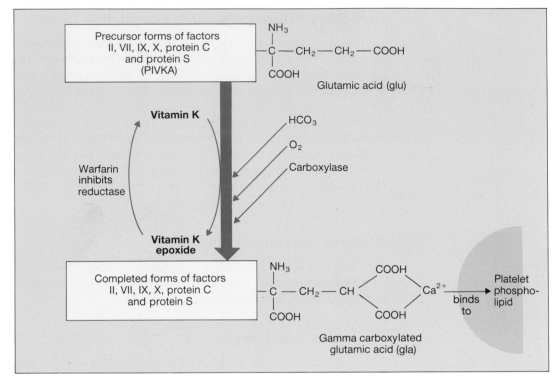

Fig. 18.8 The action of vitamin K in γ-carboxylation of glutamic acid in coagulation factors which are then able to bind Ca^{2+} and attach to the platelet phospholipid.

activity of factors II, VII, IX, X and proteins C and S, but immunological methods show normal levels of these factors. The non-functional proteins are called PIVKA—proteins formed in vitamin K absence. Conversion of PIVKA factors to their biologically active forms is a post-translational event involving carboxylation of the γ-carbon of a number of glutamic acid residues in the N-terminal region where these factors show strong sequence homology. (Fig. 18.8). Gamma-carboxylated glutamic acid binds calcium ions through which it forms a complex with phospholipid. In the process of carboxylation, vitamin K is converted to vitamin K epoxide which is cycled back to the reduced form by reductases. Warfarin is thought to interfere with the reduction of vitamin K epoxide leading to a functional vitamin K deficiency but this concept may need revision.

Haemorrhagic disease of the newborn

Vitamin K-dependent factors are low at birth and fall further in breastfed infants in the first few days of life. Liver cell immaturity, lack of gut bacterial synthesis of the vitamin and low quantities in breast milk may all contribute to a deficiency which may cause haemorrhage, usually on the second to fourth day of life.

Diagnosis

The prothrombin time and APTT are both abnormal. The platelet count and fibrinogen are normal with absent fibrin degradation products.

Treatment

1 Prophylaxis: vitamin K (phytomenadione) 1 mg intramuscularly after birth is given to all newborn babies (except those likely to be G6PD deficient).
2 In bleeding infants: vitamin K 1 mg intramuscularly is given every 6 hours with, initially, fresh frozen plasma if haemorrhage is severe.

A good response is usual in healthy full-term babies. Because of liver cell immaturity the response in premature babies is often suboptimal. If bleeding is not controlled with vitamin K, fresh blood or plasma may be necessary.

Vitamin K deficiency in children or adults

Deficiency resulting from obstructive jaundice, pancreatic or small bowel disease occasionally causes a bleeding diathesis in children or adults.

Diagnosis

Both the prothrombin time and APTT are prolonged. There are low levels of factors II, VII, IX and X in plasma.

Treatment

1 Prophylaxis: vitamin K 5 mg orally each day.
2 Active bleeding or prior to liver biopsy: vitamin K 10 mg intravenously. Some correction of prothrombin time is usual within 6 hours. The dose should be repeated on the next 2 days after which time optimal correction is usual.

Liver disease

Multiple haemostatic abnormalities contribute to a bleeding tendency and may exacerbate haemorrhage from oesophageal varices.
1 Biliary obstruction results in impaired absorption of vitamin K and therefore decreased synthesis of factors II, VII, IX and X by liver parenchymal cells.
2 With severe hepatocellular disease, in addition to a deficiency of these factors, there are often reduced levels of factor V and

fibrinogen and increased amounts of plasminogen activator.

3 Hypersplenism associated with portal hypertension frequently results in thrombocytopenia.

4 Patients with liver failure have variable platelet functional abnormalities.

5 Functional abnormality of fibrinogen (dysfibrinogenaemia) is found in many patients.

6 Disseminated intravascular coagulation (DIC, see below) may be related to release of thromboplastins from damaged liver cells and reduced concentrations of antithrombin III, protein C and α_2-antiplasmin. In addition there is impaired removal of activated clotting factors and increased fibrinolytic activity.

Disseminated intravascular coagulation

Widespread intravascular deposition of fibrin with consumption of coagulation factors and platelets occurs as a consequence of many disorders which release procoagulant material into the circulation or cause widespread endothelial damage or platelet aggregation (Table 18.4). It may be associated with a fulminant haemorrhagic syndrome or run a less severe and more chronic course.

Pathogenesis (Fig. 18.9)

1 DIC may be triggered by the entry of procoagulant material into the circulation in the following situations: amniotic fluid embolism, premature separation of the placenta, widespread mucin-secreting adenocarcinomas, acute promyelocytic leukaemia (AML M_3), liver disease, severe *Falciparum* malaria, haemolytic transfusion reaction and some snake bites.

Table 18.4 Causes of disseminated intravascular coagulation.

Infections
- Gram-negative and meningococcal septicaemia
- Septic abortion and *Clostridium welchii* septicaemia
- Severe falciparum malaria
- Viral infection (purpura fulminans)

Malignancy
- Widespread mucin-secreting adenocarcinoma
- Acute promyelocytic leukaemia

Obstetric complications
- Amniotic fluid embolism
- Premature separation of placenta
- Eclampsia; retained placenta

Hypersensitivity reactions
- Anaphylaxis
- Incompatible blood transfusion

Widespread tissue damage
- Following surgery or trauma

Miscellaneous
- Liver failure
- Snake and invertebrate venoms
- Severe burns
- Hypothermia
- Heat stroke
- Acute hypoxia
- Vascular malformations (Kasabach–Merritt syndrome)

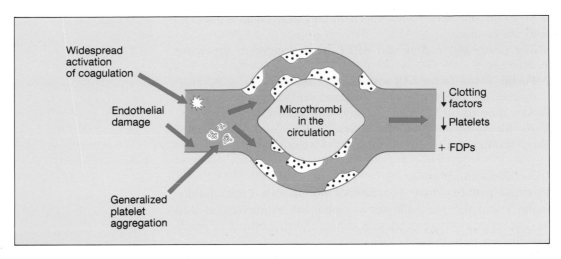

Fig. 18.9 The pathogenesis
of disseminated intravascular
coagulation and the changes
in clotting factors, platelets
and fibrin degradation
products (FDPs) that occur in
this syndrome.

2 DIC may also be initiated by widespread endothelial damage and collagen exposure (e.g. endotoxaemia, Gram-negative and meningococcal septicaemia, septic abortion), certain virus infections (e.g. purpura fulminans) and severe burns or hypothermia.

3 Widespread intravascular platelet aggregation may also precipitate DIC. Some bacteria, viruses and immune complexes may have a direct effect on platelets.

In addition to its role in the deposition of fibrin in the microcirculation, intravascular thrombin formation produces large amounts of circulating fibrin monomers which form complexes with available fibrinogen. Intense fibrinolysis is stimulated by thrombi on vascular walls and the release of split products interferes with fibrin polymerization, thus contributing to the coagulation defect. The combined action of thrombin and plasmin normally causes depletion of fibrinogen, prothrombin, factor V and factor VIII. Intravascular thrombin also causes widespread platelet aggregation, release and deposition. The bleeding problems of DIC are compounded by the inevitable thrombocytopenia due to consumption of platelets.

Laboratory findings

In many acute syndromes the blood may fail to clot because of gross fibrinogen deficiency.

Tests of haemostasis
1 The platelet count is low.
2 Fibrinogen screening tests, titres or assays indicate deficiency.
3 The thrombin time is prolonged.
4 High levels of fibrinogen (and fibrin) degradation products are found in serum and urine.

5 Tests for the fibrin—monomer complex (e.g. ethanol gelation test) are positive.
6 The prothrombin time and APTT are prolonged in the acute syndromes.
7 Factor V and factor VIII activities are reduced.

In more chronic syndromes increased synthesis of coagulation factors may result in normal assays and screening test results. Tests for systemic fibrinolysis (euglobulin clot lysis) usually show no increase in circulating plasminogen activator.

Blood film examination
In many patients there is a haemolytic anaemia ('microangiopathic') and the red cells show prominent fragmentation due to damage caused when passing through fibrin strands in small vessels (see p. 91).

Treatment

1 Treatment of the underlying cause is most important.
2 Supportive therapy with fresh blood, fresh frozen plasma, fibrinogen and platelet concentrates is indicated in patients with dangerous or extensive bleeding.

The use of heparin or antiplatelet drugs to inhibit the coagulation process is usually not indicated since bleeding may, in some cases, be aggravated. Fibrinolytic inhibitors should not be considered because failure to lyse thrombi in organs such as the kidney may have adverse effects.

Coagulation deficiency caused by antibodies

Circulating antibodies to coagulation factors are occasionally seen. Alloantibodies to factor VIII occur in 5—10% of haemophiliacs. Factor VIII autoantibodies may also result in a bleeding syndrome. These IgG antibodies occur rarely post-partum, in certain immunological disorders (e.g. rheumatoid arthritis) and in old age. Many of these antibodies combine with, and inactivate, the coagulation protein but do not lead to premature removal of the protein from the circulation.

Another protein known as the *lupus anticoagulant* interferes with lipoprotein-dependent stages in coagulation and is usually detected by prolongation of the APTT test. This inhibitor is detected in 10% of patients with SLE (systemic lupus erythematosus) and in patients with other autoimmune diseases who frequently have antibodies to other lipid-containing antigens, e.g. cardiolipin. The antibody is not usually associated with a bleeding tendency but there is an increased risk of thrombosis (see Chapter 19) and an association with recurrent abortion.

Table 18.5 Haemostasis tests: typical results in acquired bleeding disorders.

	Platelet count	Prothrombin time	Activated partial thromboplastin time	Thrombin time
Liver disease	Low	Prolonged	Prolonged	Normal (rarely prolonged)
Disseminated intravascular coagulation	Low	Prolonged	Prolonged	Grossly prolonged
Massive transfusion	Low	Prolonged	Prolonged	Normal
Oral anticoagulants	Normal	Grossly prolonged	Prolonged	Normal
Heparin	Normal (rarely low)	Mildly prolonged	Prolonged	Prolonged
Circulating anticoagulant	Normal	Normal or prolonged	Prolonged	Normal

Overdosage with anticoagulants

Anticoagulant and thrombolytic therapy is discussed in Chapter 19. Overdosage with oral anticoagulants which are vitamin K antagonists results in a severe deficiency of coagulation factors II, VII, IX and X. Patients may present with extensive skin bruising or internal bleeding. Poorly controlled heparin or systemic thrombolytic agent therapy may also produce severe derangement of blood coagulation with consequent bleeding.

Massive transfusion syndrome

Many factors may contribute to a bleeding disorder following massive transfusion. Blood loss results in reduced levels of platelets, coagulation factors and inhibitors. Further dilution of these factors occurs during replacement with stored blood. After 24 hours storage at 4°C platelets aggregate and function poorly and the platelet count falls progressively. The labile coagulation factors V and VIII are also poorly preserved after a few days storage. Minor activation of coagulation factors, microaggregates and degenerate cells may initiate or aggravate DIC. Some patients may have a pre-existing bleeding defect. Management is discussed on p. 327.

The results of haemostasis screening tests in acquired bleeding disorders are shown in Table 18.5.

Bibliography

Antonarakis S.E. & Kazazian H.H. (1988) The molecular basis of haemophilia A in man. Trends in Genetics, 4, 233–237.
Brownlee G.G. (1988) Haemophilia B: a review of patient defects, diagnosis with gene probes and prospects for gene therapy. In Recent Advances in Haematology, 5 (ed. A.V. Hoffbrand). Churchill Livingstone, Edinburgh, pp. 251–264.
Furie B. & Furie B.C. (1990) Molecular basis of haemophilia. Seminars in Hematology, 27, 270–285.
Green P.M., Montandon A.J., Bentley D.R. & Giannelli F. (1991) Genetics and molecular biology of haemophilia A and B. Blood Coagulation and Fibrinolysis, 2, 539–565.
Hemter H.C. & Sixma J.J. (eds) (1991) State of the art. Thrombosis and Haemostasis, 66, 1–189.
Joist J.H. & Bajaj S.P. (eds) (1990) Current issues in laboratory diagnosis of bleeding disorders and hypercoaguable states. Seminars in Thrombosis and Haemostasis, 16, 151–197.
Lee C.A. (1992) Coagulation factor replacement therapy. Recents Advances in Haematology, 6 (eds A.V. Hoffbrand & M.K. Brenner). Churchill Livingstone, Edinburgh pp. 73–88.
Manucci P.M. (1988) Desmopressin: a non-transfusional form of treatment for congenital and acquired bleeding disorders. Blood, 72, 1449–1455.
Muller-Berghaus G. (1989) Pathophysiologic and biochemical events in disseminated intravascular coagulation dysregulation of procoagulant and

anti-coagulant pathways. *Seminars in Thrombosis and Hemostasis*, **15**, 58–87.

Ratnoff O.D. & Forbes C.D. (1991) *Disorders of Hemostasis*, 2nd Edition. W.B. Saunders, Philadelphia.

Rodeghiero F., Castaman G. & Mannucci P.M. (1991) Clinical indications for desmopressin (DDAVP) in congenital and acquired von Willebrand's disease. *Blood Reviews*, **5**, 153–161.

Tuddenham E.G.D. (1989) Von Willebrand's factor and its disorders: an overview of recent molecular studies. *Blood Reviews*, **3**, 251–262.

Tuddenham E.G.D. (ed.) (1991) The molecular biology of coagulation. *Clinical Haematology*, **2**, 787–1042.

Vehar G.A., Lawn R.M., Tuddenham E.G.D. & Wood W.I. (1989) Factor VIII and factor V: biochemistry and pathophysiology. In *Metabolic Basis of Inherited Disease*, 6th Edition (eds C.R. Scriver, A.L. Beaudet, W.S. Sly & D. Valle). McGraw Hill, New York, pp. 2155–2170.

Warnock L.J. (1991) The application of molecular biology techniques to haemostasis and thrombosis. *Blood Coagulation and Fibrinolysis*, **2**, 529–538.

White G.C. & Shoemaker C.B. (1989) Factor VIII gene and haemophilia. *Blood*, **73**, 1–12.

Chapter 19
Thrombosis and
Antithrombotic Therapy

Thrombi are solid masses or plugs formed in the circulation
from blood constituents. Platelets and coagulated blood form the
basic structure. Their clinical significance results from ischaemia
from local vascular obstruction or from embolization and obstruction of a distal part of the circulation. If a dominant role of
thrombi is assumed in the pathogenesis of myocardial infarction,
cerebrovascular disease, peripheral arterial disease and deep
vein occlusion, thrombosis is probably the most important problem facing Western medicine.

Although the pathogenesis of thrombi formed in different parts
of the circulation is broadly similar, arterial thrombi show structural differences from their venous counterparts. In arteries,
thrombi develop in relation to platelet reaction and accumulation
in response to vessel wall damage. In veins, thrombus formation
usually follows the generation of thrombin in areas of retarded
blood flow and coagulated blood is a much more dominant
component. Multiple thrombi in the microcirculation result in
the syndrome of disseminated intravascular coagulation (DIC)
which has been discussed in Chapter 18.

Thrombosis is more common as age increases and is frequently
associated with risk factors, e.g. operations or pregnancy. Some
patients develop thrombi at a younger age in the absence of one
of these easily identified factors. The term thrombophilia is used
to describe the familial or acquired disorders of the haemostatic
mechanism which are likely to predispose to thrombosis.

Arterial thrombosis

Pathogenesis

1 Atherosclerosis of the arterial wall, plaque rupture and endothelial injury expose blood to subendothelial collagen and tissue
factor. This initiates the formation of a platelet nidus. Haemo-
dynamic stress may also produce repeated episodes of endothelial
injury. Platelets adhere to the site of endothelial damage. Collagen
activates platelet prostaglandin synthesis to produce thromboxane A_2 which causes platelet aggregation. Aggregation is enhanced by the liberation of ADP from damaged platelets and
from the vessel walls. The amount of prostacyclin produced by

the vessel wall may be critical in preventing the development and propagation of the initial thrombus.

2 The platelet aggregate is anchored on its external surface by fibrin formed following exposure of tissue factor at the vessel wall and the release of coagulant activities of platelets.

3 Reduced blood flow and increased turbulence from vessel wall stenosis are probably important in the thrombosis of coronary arteries and other medium-sized vessels.

4 Small emboli of platelets and fibrin may break away from the primary thrombus to occlude small distal arteries, e.g. carotid artery thrombi leading to cerebral thrombosis and transient ischaemic attacks (TIAs) and heart valve and chamber thrombi leading to systemic emboli and infarcts.

5 Platelet deposition and thrombus formation are important in the pathogenesis of atherosclerosis. Platelet-derived growth factor (PDGF) stimulates the migration and proliferation of smooth muscle cells and fibroblasts in the arterial intima. Regrowth of endothelium and repair at the site of arterial damage and incorporated thrombus result in thickening of the vessel wall.

Clinical risk factors

The risk factors for arterial thrombosis are related to the development of atherosclerosis and are listed in Table 19.1. The identification of patients at risk is largely based on clinical assessment. A number of epidemiological studies including those at Framingham have resulted in the construction of coronary artery risk profiles based on sex, age, elevated blood pressure, high levels of serum cholesterol, glucose intolerance, cigarette smoking and ECG (electrocardiogram) abnormalities. These profiles have allowed presymptomatic assessment of young and apparently fit subjects and are valuable in counselling a change in lifestyle or for recommending medical therapy in individuals at risk. The Northwick Park heart study showed that elevated plasma levels of factor VII and fibrinogen are the strongest independent predictors of coronary events.

Table 19.1 Risk factors in arterial thrombosis (atherosclerosis).

Positive family history
Male sex
Hyperlipidaemia
Hypertension
Diabetes mellitus
Gout
Polycythaemia
Cigarette smoking
ECG abnormalities
Elevated factor VII
Elevated fibrinogen

Venous thrombosis

Pathogenesis

1 Increased systemic coagulability is usually of major importance. Peri-operative and post-operative deep vein thrombosis follows the activation of blood coagulation by procoagulant tissue factor at the time of surgery. In many patients there may be excessive local production of thrombin in immobile leg veins. Repeated venous thromboses occur in many hereditary and acquired disorders associated with hypercoagulability (see below).

2 Stasis is also of prime importance. It allows the completion of blood coagulation with fibrin formation at the site of initiation of the thrombus, e.g. behind the valve pockets of leg veins or in the stationary blood in the sacs and sinuses of the deep veins of the calf in immobile patients.

3 Vessel wall damage is not required although it may be important in the pathogenesis of local venous thromboses in patients with sepsis or indwelling catheters.

4 Platelet adhesion and aggregation are of secondary importance. The venous thrombus has a primary structure of loosely adherent fibrin clot. However, thrombin formation results in platelet aggregation and accumulation. Platelets contribute to the expansion and propagation of the thrombus providing both phospholipid for promoting the formation of enzyme−cofactor complexes of blood coagulation and high concentrations of factor V derived from platelet granules.

5 Propagation of the thrombus is enhanced by blood stagnation or sluggish flow. Increased blood viscosity due to polycythaemia or increases in plasma fibrinogen or globulins encourage growth of the thrombus.

Propagation is inhibited by rapid blood flow which may wash away the initial fibrin−platelet nidus, cause dispersion of thrombin and the activated coagulation factors and allows a more effective neutralization by physiological inhibitors, such as antithrombin III and protein C. The other major protective mechanism is the natural fibrinolytic activity of blood and the vessel wall.

Clinical risk factors

Major factors in the pathogenesis of venous thromboses are reduced blood flow and hypercoagulability. Changes in the vessel wall usually play a less significant role. Table 19.2 lists a number of recognized risk factors.

Hereditary disorders of haemostasis

The prevalence of inherited disorders associated with increased risk of thrombosis is, at least, as high as that of hereditary bleeding disorders. A hereditary 'thrombophilia' should be suspected when young patients suffer from spontaneous thrombosis or recurrent deep vein thromboses. In most cases, however, no cause can be identified. Five abnormalities are now well characterized: deficiency or functional abnormality of antithrombin III, protein C, protein S, fibrinogen and plasminogen.

1 *Antithrombin III deficiency.* This deficiency was first recognized in 1965. Inheritance is autosomal dominant. There are recurrent venous thromboses usually starting in early adult life. Arterial thrombi occur occasionally. Antithrombin III concentrates are

Table 19.2 Risk factors in venous thrombosis.

Related to coagulation abnormality	*Related to stasis*
Hereditary haemostatic disorders	Cardiac failure
● Antithrombin III deficiency	Stroke
● Protein C deficiency	Prolonged immobility
● Factor V Leiden	Pelvic obstruction
● Protein S deficiency	Nephrotic syndrome
● Abnormal fibrinogen	Dehydration
● Abnormal plasminogen	Hyperviscosity, polycythaemia
Hereditary or acquired haemostatic disorders	Varicose veins
● Raised levels of factor VII	
● Raised levels of fibrinogen	*Related to unknown factors*
Coagulation factor IX concentrates	Age
Lupus anticoagulant	Obesity
Oestrogen therapy	Sepsis
Pregnancy and puerperium	Paroxysmal nocturnal
Surgery—especially abdominal and hip	haemoglobinuria
Major trauma	
Malignancy	
Myocardial infarct	
Thrombocythaemia and thrombocytosis	

available and are used to prevent thombosis during surgery or childbirth. Many molecular variants of antithrombin III have been categorized in different affected families.

2 *Protein C deficiency.* This is the commonest form of hereditary thrombophilia. Inheritance is autosomal dominant with variable penetrance and occasional homozygous patients have presented with severe DIC or purpura fulminans in infancy. Many patients developed skin necrosis when treated with warfarin, thought to be due to reduction of protein C levels even further in the first day or two of warfarin therapy before reduction in the levels of the vitamin K-dependent clotting factors.

3 *Factor V Leiden gene mutation* (activated protein C co-factor deficiency). This is the commonest inherited cause of an increased risk of thrombosis (responsible for about 20% of all cases). The mutation is in the factor V gene which results in activated factor V being resistant to inactivation by protein C.

4 *Protein S deficiency.* Protein S deficiency has been found in a number of families with thrombotic tendency. The inheritance is autosomal dominant.

5 *Defects of fibrinogen and plasminogen.* Abnormal fibrinogens and defects of plasminogen are rare causes of familial thrombotic tendency.

6 *Hereditary or acquired disorders of haemostasis.* High factor VII or fibrinogen levels are associated with venous and arterial thrombosis.

Treatment. The patients with all these inherited defects usually need life-long warfarin therapy.

Acquired risk factors

1 *Post-operative venous thrombosis.* This is more likely to occur in the aged, obese, those with a previous or family history of venous thrombosis, and in those in whom major abdominal or hip operations are performed.

2 *Venous stasis and immobility.* These factors are probably responsible for the high incidence of post-operative venous thrombosis and for venous thrombosis associated with congestive cardiac failure, myocardial infarction and varicose veins. The use of muscle relaxants during anaesthesia may also contribute to venous stasis.

3 *Malignancy.* Patients with carcinoma of the breast, lung, prostate, pancreas or bowel have an increased risk of venous thrombosis. Mucin from adenocarcinomas and proteases from bowel and breast cancers are capable of activating factor X.

4 *Blood disorders.* Increased viscosity, thrombocytosis, altered platelet membrane receptors and responses are possible factors for the high incidence of thrombosis in patients with polycythaemia vera and essential thrombocythaemia. There is a high incidence of venous thrombosis, including thrombi in large veins, e.g. the hepatic vein, in patients with paroxysmal nocturnal haemoglobinuria. An increased tendency to venous thrombosis has been observed in patients with sickle cell disease and patients with post-splenectomy thrombocytosis, particularly those with continuing anaemia.

5 *Oestrogen therapy.* Oestrogen therapy, particularly high-dose therapy, is associated with increased plasma levels of factors II, VII, VIII, IX and X and depressed levels of antithrombin III and tissue plasminogen activator in the vessel wall. There is a high incidence of post-operative venous thrombosis in women on high-dose oestrogen therapy and full-dose oestrogen-containing oral contraceptives. The risk is much less with low-dose oestrogen contraceptive preparations.

6 *The 'lupus anticoagulant'.* This factor, initially found in plasma in patients with systemic lupus erythematosus, is identified by finding a prolonged plasma APTT (activated partial thromboplastin time) which does not correct with a 50:50 mixture of normal plasma. It is also found in patients with other autoimmune disorders, lymphoproliferative diseases, post-viral infections, with certain drugs including phenothiazines, and as an 'idiopathic' phenomenon. Paradoxically, it is associated with venous and arterial thrombosis and recurrent abortion due to placental infarction (Table 19.3). The plasma factor appears to be an antibody directed against membrane phospholipids and it

Table 19.3 Clinical associations of lupus anticoagulant and anticardiolipin antibodies.

Venous thrombosis
  Deep venous thrombosis/
    pulmonary embolism
  Renal, hepatic,
    retinal veins
Arterial thrombosis
Recurrent foetal loss
Thrombocytopenia

is only associated with classical systemic lupus erythematosus in a minority of patients.

7 *Factor IX concentrates.* Venous thrombosis may complicate the use of factor IX concentrates which contain trace amounts of activated coagulation factors. Patients with liver disease who are unable to clear these activated factors are especially at risk.

Laboratory evaluation of increased thrombotic risk

Many of the conditions associated with an increased thrombotic risk are obvious following clinical examination. A haematological assessment is indicated in patients who have recurrent deep vein thrombosis or pulmonary emboli especially while taking oral anticoagulant therapy, in patients who have recurrent thrombosis at a young age and in those patients with an apparent familial tendency to thrombosis. The following laboratory tests are used in diagnosis.

Screening tests

1 Blood count and ESR (erythrocyte sedimentation rate) — to detect elevation in haematocrit, white count, platelet count, fibrinogen and globulins.

2 Blood film examination — may provide evidence of myeloproliferative disorder; leuco-erythroblastic features may indicate malignant disease.

3 Prothrombin time and APTT. A shortened APPT is often seen in thrombotic states and may indicate the presence of activated clotting factors. A prolonged APPT test, not corrected by the addition of normal plasma, suggests a 'lupus anticoagulant'.

4 Thrombin time and reptilase time — prolongation suggests an abnormal fibrinogen.

5 Fibrinogen assay.

6 Antithrombin III — immunological and functional assays.

7 Protein C and protein S — immunological and functional assays.

8 DNA analysis for Factor V Leiden.

Further tests

1 Plasminogen — immunological and functional assays.

2 Euglobulin lysis time, with or without venous occlusion.

3 Other tests for fibrinolysis.

4 Acid lysis test for paroxysmal nocturnal haemoglobinuria.

Results

A positive haematological diagnosis is made in only a third or less of the total patients investigated. In most patients, even full investigation yields no abnormalities and, usually, treatment with oral anticoagulants remains empirical.

Anticoagulant drugs

Anticoagulant drugs are used widely in the treatment of venous thromboembolic disease. Their value in the treatment of arterial thrombosis is less well established.

Heparin

This acidic mucopolysaccharide of average molecular weight 15 000–18 000 is an inhibitor of blood coagulation due to its interaction with antithrombin III (see below). As it is not absorbed from the gastrointestinal tract, it must be given by injection. It is inactivated by the liver and excreted in the urine. The effective biological half-life is about 1 hour.

Mode of action
Heparin dramatically potentiates the formation of complexes between antithrombin III and activated serine protease coagulation factors, thrombin (IIa) and factors IXa, Xa, and XIa (Fig. 19.1). This complex formation inactivates these factors irreversibly. In addition, heparin impairs platelet function. Low-molecular-weight preparations (4000–8000) have a greater ability to inhibit factor Xa than to inhibit thrombin and interact less with platelets compared with standard heparin, and so may have a lesser tendency to cause bleeding.

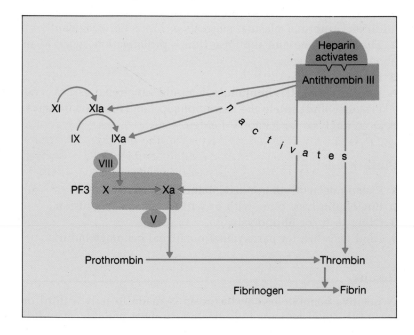

Fig. 19.1 The action of heparin. This activates antithrombin III which then forms complexes with activated serine protease coagulation factors (thrombin, Xa, IXa and XIa) and so inactivates them.

Indications

Heparin is given to treat deep vein thrombosis, pulmonary embolism, myocardial infarct, unstable angina pectoris and acute peripheral arterial occlusion. It is also used in disseminated intravascular coagulation if the manifestations are predominantly vaso-occlusive. It is the drug of choice for women requiring anticoagulation in pregnancy since it doses not cross the placenta. It is also used during cardio-pulmonary by-pass surgery and for maintaining in-dwelling venous lines patent.

Administration and laboratory control

1 *Continuous intravenous infusion* provides the smoothest control of heparin therapy and is the recommended method of administration in treatment of acute deep venous thrombosis (DVT) or pulmonary embolus. In an adult, doses of 30 000–40 000 units over 24 hours (1000–2000 units/hour with a loading dose of 5000 units) are usually satisfactory. Therapy is monitored by maintaining the APPT at between 1.5 and 2 times the normal time. It is usual to start warfain therapy after 2–7 days of heparin therapy and overlap for 3 days before stopping heparin because of the delay in warfarin effect.

2 *Subcutaneous heparin* 15 000 units 12-hourly can be used as an alternative to the intravenous route. Intermittent subcutaneous injections are preferred when heparin is given as prophylaxis against venous thrombosis, e.g. for surgical procedures. The usual dose is 5000 units 12-hourly pre-operatively followed by this dose 8–12 hourly for 7 days or until the patient is mobile. Low MW heparin is given once daily, 5000 units. It is monitored by factor Xa assay. Graduated elastic stockings are also used.

Complications

Bleeding during heparin therapy

This may be due to prolonged coagulation, to an antiplatelet functional effect of heparin or to heparin-induced thrombocytopenia. Intravenous heparin has a half-life of less than 1 hour and it is usually only necessary to stop the infusion. Protamine is able to inactivate heparin immediately, and for severe bleeding a dose of 1 mg/100 units of heparin provides effective neutralization. However, protamine itself may in excess act as an anticoagulant.

Osteoporosis

This occur with long-term (>2 months) heparin therapy, especially in pregnancy. The drug complexes minerals from the bones but the exact pathogenesis is unknown.

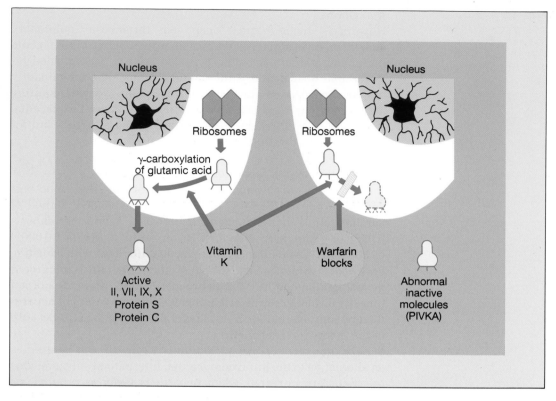

Fig. 19.2 The action of vitamin K in γ-carboxylation of factors II (prothrombin), VII, IX and X. Oral anticoagulants (e.g. warfarin) are vitamin K antagonists and lead to accumulation in plasma of inactive molecules (PIVKA).

Direct thrombin inhibitors

Hirudins, hirudin fragments and other low-molecular-weight direct inhibitors of thrombin have potential as antithrombotic agents, but are not yet in routine clinical use.

Oral anticoagulants

These are derivatives of coumarin or indanedione. Warfarin, a coumarin, is most widely used. It is well absorbed from the gut, and it is usual to start treatment with 10 mg, 10 mg, 5 mg or 5 mg, 5 mg, 5 mg on the first three days and then to alter the dose according to the results of the prothrombin time. The usual maintenance dose of warfarin is 3–9 mg daily but individual responses vary greatly. The indications for warfarin are summarized in Table 19.4.

Mode of action

These drugs are vitamin K antagonists. Therapy results in decreased biological activity of the vitamin K-dependent factors II, VII, IX and X. Oral anticoagulants block the post-ribosomal γ-carboxylation of glutamic acid residues of these proteins (Fig. 19.2) and the resulting abnormal molecules—known as PIVKA (proteins formed by vitamin K absence)—are released

Table 19.4 Oral anticoagulant control tests. Therapeutic ranges recommended by the British Socieŧ for Haematology.

INR	Clinical state
2.0−2.5	Prophylaxis of DVT, including high-risk surgery
2.0−3.0	Hip surgery, repair of fractures of femur
	Treatment of DVT, pulmonary embolism, systemic embolism, prevention of venous thromboembolism after myocardial infarction, mitral stenosis with embolism, atrial fibrillation, transient ischaemic attacks
3.0−4.5	Recurrent DVT, pulmonary embolism, arterial disease including myocardial infarction, arterial grafts, prosthetic valves and grafts

DVT, deep venous thrombosis; INR, international normalized ratio.

into the circulation (Fig. 19.2). After warfarin is given, factor VII levels fall considerably within 24 hours but prothrombin has a longer plasma half-life and only falls to 50% of normal at 3 days; the patient is fully anticoagulated only after this period. Warfarin crosses the placenta and is teratogenic. Heparin is preferred in pregnancy since it does not cross the placenta and its action is short-lived.

Indications and laboratory control
The effect of oral anticoagulants is monitored by the prothrombin time. The World Health Organization has recommended a calibration scheme for reporting prothrombin time results in terms of an international normalized ratio (INR). The INR is based on the patient's prothrombin time and the mean normal plasma prothrombin time corrected for the 'sensitivity' of the thromboplastin used. This is accomplished by using the reagent's

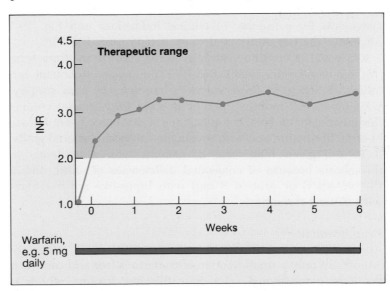

Fig. 19.3 The laboratory control of oral anticoagulant therapy using the international normalized ratio (INR).

Table 19.5 Drugs and other factors which interfere with the control of anticoagulant therapy.

Potentiation of oral anticoagulants	Inhibition of oral anticoagulants
DRUGS WHICH INCREASE THE EFFECT OF COUMARINS	DRUGS WHICH DEPRESS THE ACTION OF COUMARINS
Reduced coumarin binding to serum albumin	*Acceleration of hepatic microsomal degradation of coumarin*
• Phenylbutazone	• Barbiturates
• Sulphonamides	• Rifampicin
Inhibition of hepatic microsomal degradation of coumarin	*Enhanced synthesis of clotting factors*
• Cimetidine	• Oral contraceptives
• Allopurinol	
• Tricyclic antidepressants	HEREDITARY RESISTANCE TO ORAL ANTICOAGULANTS
• Metronidazole	
• Sulphonamides	PREGNANCY
Alteration of hepatic receptor site for drug	
• Thyroxine	
• Quinidine	
Decreased synthesis of vitamin K factors	
• High doses of salicylates	
• Some cephalosporins	
LIVER DISEASE Decreased synthesis of vitamin K factors	
DECREASED ABSORPTION OF VITAMIN K For example malabsorption, antibiotic therapy, laxatives	

NB Patients are also more likely to bleed if taking antiplatelet agents (e.g. NSAIDs, dipyridamole or aspirin).

calibration value or international sensitivity index (ISI). Reporting results in terms of the INR allows more accurate control of anticoagulant therapy and improves interlaboratory correlation. Table 19.4 lists the recommended therapeutic ranges of anticoagulants for a number of clinical indications and Fig. 19.3 illustrates the laboratory control of therapy using the INR.

It is usual to continue warfarin in the short to medium term (up to 6 months) for established DVT, pulmonary embolism and following xenograft heart valves or coronary by-pass surgery. Long-term (>12 months) therapy is given for recurrent venous thrombosis, for embolic complications of rheumatic heart disease or atrial fibrillation and with prosthetic valves and arterial grafts. It is also given long term in patients with a tendency to thrombosis because of congenital deficiencies of antithrombin III, protein C or protein S and with lupus-like anticoagulant with clinical thrombosis.

Drug interactions

About 97% of warfarin in the circulation is albumin-bound and only a small fraction of warfarin is free and can enter the liver parenchymal cells. It is this free fraction which is

Table 19.6 Recommendations on the reversal of oral anticoagulant treatment by the British Society for Haematology.

1 *Life-threatening haemorrhage* Immediately give vitamin K (5.0 mg) intravenously and either a concentrate of factors II, IX, X with factor VII (if available) or fresh frozen plasma
2 *Less severe haemorrhage, e.g. haematuria or epistaxis* Withhold warfarin for 1 or more days and consider giving vitamin K, (0.5−2.0 mg) intravenously
3 *INR >4.5 with no haemorrhage* Withhold warfarin for 1 or 2 days, then review
4 *Unexpected bleeding at therapeutic levels* Investigate for underlying cause, e.g. renal or alimentary tract abnormality

INR, international normalized ratio.

Table 19.7 Fibrinolytic agents — plasminogen activators.

1 Streptokinase (SK)
2 Urokinase (UK)
3 Tissue plasminogen activator (tPA)
4 Single chain urokinase-type plasminogen activator (SCU-PA)
5 Acylated plasminogen streptokinase activator complex (APSAC)

active. In the liver cells, warfarin is degraded in microsomes to an inactive water-soluble metabolite which is conjugated and excreted in the bile and partially re-absorbed to be also excreted in urine. Drugs which affect the albumin-binding or excretion of warfarin (or of other oral anticoagulants) or those which decrease the absorption of vitamin K will interfere with the control of therapy (Table 19.5).

Bleeding during warfarin therapy
Mild bleeding usually only needs a prothrombin ratio assessment, drug withdrawal and subsequent dosage adjustment (Table 19.6). More serious bleeding may need cessation of therapy, vitamin K therapy and the infusion of fresh frozen plasma or factor concentrates. The latter, however, carry the risks of DIC and both may transmit viruses. Vitamin K is the specific antidote; an intravenous injection of 2.5 mg is effective but will result in resistance to further warfarin therapy for 2−3 weeks.

Fibrinolytic agents

A number of fibrinolytic agents are able to lyse fresh thrombi (Table 19.7). They have been used systemically for patients with acute major pulmonary embolism or iliofemoral thrombosis, and locally in patients with acute peripheral arterial occlusion.

Most studies indicate that the majority of cases of acute myocardial infarction are associated with an acute thrombus complicating a stenosing atherosclerotic lesion in the coronary artery.

Absolute contraindications	Relative contraindications
Active gastrointestinal bleeding	Traumatic cardiopulmonary
Aortic dissection	resuscitation
Head injury or cerebrovascular	Major surgery in the past 10 days
accident in the past 2 months	Past history of gastrointestinal bleeding
Neurosurgery in the past 2 months	Recent obstetric delivery
Intracranial aneurysm or neoplasm	Prior arterial puncture
Proliferative diabetic retinopathy	Prior organ biopsy
	Serious trauma
	Severe arterial hypertension
	(systolic pressure >200 mmHg,
	diastolic pressure >110 mmHg)
	Bleeding diathesis

Table 19.8 Contraindications to thrombolytic therapy.

Natural lysis occurs in 25–35% of patients within 24 hours but is too slow to prevent infarction in most patients. Recent clinical trials of thrombolytic therapy in acute myocardial infarction have shown a reduction in acute mortality of 20–25%.

Administration of thrombolytic agents has been simplified with standardized dosage regimens. The therapy is most effective in the first 6 hours after symptoms begin but is still of benefit up to 24 hours. Streptokinase and urokinase are given in a loading dose (250 000 units and 350 000 units, respectively) followed by a maintenance dose (100 000 units and 300 000 units, respectively) hourly for 12–48 hours. In acute myocardial infarction, streptokinase is given as a single dose of 1 500 000 units over 60 minutes. Aspirin therapy is also given and the value of additional heparin therapy is under study.

The use of laboratory tests for monitoring and control of short-term thrombolytic therapy is now considered unnecessary. However, certain clinical complications exclude the use of thrombolytic agents (Table 19.8).

DNA technology may offer advantages. Recombinant tissue plasminogen activator (tPA) has a particularly high affinity for fibrin and this allows lysis of thrombi with less systemic activation of fibrinolysis. Trials in patients following myocardial infarction, however have not shown any definite advantages of tPA over streptokinase and it is far more expensive.

Acylated plasminogen streptokinase activator complex (APSAC) and single chain urokinase-type plasminogen activator (SCU-PA) are two other recently introduced fibrinolytic agents which are being evaluated in clinical trials.

Phenformin, ethyloestrenol and stanozolol have been used to enhance fibrinolysis in patients with arterial disease, retinal vein occlusion and recurrent DVT. The action of these orally administered drugs is weak and there is no firm evidence that they have significant antithrombotic activity.

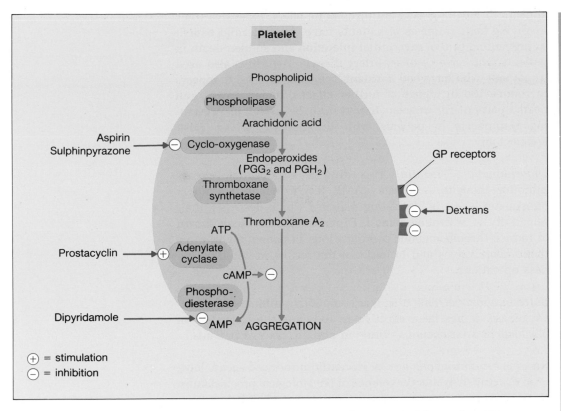

Fig. 19.4 Sites of action of antiplatelet drugs. Aspirin acetylates the enzyme cyclo-oxygenase irreversibly. Sulphinpyrazone inhibits cyclo-oxygenase reversibly. Dipyridamole inhibits phosphodiesterase, increases cAMP levels and inhibits aggregation. Inhibition of adenosine uptake by red cells allows adenosine accumulation in plasma which stimulates platelet adenylate cyclase. Prostacyclin (epoprostenol) stimulates adenylate cyclase. The lipid soluble β-blockers inhibit phospholipase. Calcium channel antagonists block the influx of free calcium ions across the platelet membrane. Dextrans coat the surface interfering with adhesion and aggregation.

Antiplatelet drugs

Several major clinical trials have assessed the antithrombotic effect of drugs which suppress platelet function. The evidence suggests that these drugs are of only moderate benefit in preventing major thrombotic disease. The site of action of the antiplatelet drugs are illustrated in Fig. 19.4.

Aspirin. Aspirin inhibits platelet cyclo-oxygenase irreversibly, thus reducing the production of platelet thromboxane A_2. It has been suggested that vascular endothelial cyclo-oxygenase is less sensitive to aspirin than platelet cyclo-oxygenase. Low-dose therapy (40 or 80 mg daily) is more effective than standard doses at enhancing the prostacyclin:thromboxane A_2 ratio and appears to have a greater antithrombotic effect. Extensive trials involving large numbers of patients have shown a mild benefit in preventing further myocardial infarction and sudden death in patients who have coronary artery disease. Aspirin is also used in patients who have had transient ischaemic attacks. It appears to reduce the incidence of further attacks, major strokes and death, particularly in men. It may also be useful in preventing thrombosis in patients with thrombocytosis, e.g. post-splenectomy.

Dipyridamole (Persantin). This drug is a phosphodiesterase inhibitor thought to elevate cAMP (cyclic adenosine monophosphate) levels in circulating platelets which decreases their sensitivity to activating stimuli. Dipyridamole has been shown to reduce thromboembolic complications in patients with prosthetic heart valves and to improve the results in coronary by-pass operations.

Sulphinpyrazone. This drug is a competitive inhibitor of cyclo-oxygenase. It has been effective in reducing the frequency of blockage in arteriovenous shunts in chronic dialysis patients.

Specific antithrombotic agents. Recently introduced agents have been developed to alter the balance of physiological prostaglandin metabolism. Intravenous epoprostenol (prostacyclin) has been used in clinical trials in patients with peripheral vascular disease and thrombotic thrombocytopenic purpura. It has also reduced arteriovenous shunt blockage in haemodialysis patients. Analogues that are active following oral therapy are under evaluation. Other drugs being used in trials include those which inhibit the synthesis or activity of thromboxane A_2 and drugs such as nafazantrom which both stimulate prostacyclin synthesis and retard its degradation. Eicosapentaenoic acid extracted from fish oils is a precursor of PGI_2 (prostacyclin), one of the antithrombotic prostaglandin metabolites.

Other drugs with non-specific actions. It is uncertain whether the antiplatelet actions of propanolol, other β-adrenoceptor antagonists or the calcium channel antagonists (nifedipine, diltiazem) are of clinical importance. When used in combination with aspirin or other antiplatelet drugs, these agents may have synergestic or additive effects.

Bibliography

British Committee for Standards in Haematology (1990a) Guidelines on oral anticoagulation. *Journal of Clinical Pathology*, **43**, 177–183.
British Committee for Standards in Haematology (1990b) Guidelines on the

investigation and management of thrombophilia. *Journal of Clinical Pathology*, **43**, 703−709.

British Society for Haematology (1992) Guidelines on the use and monitoring of heparin: second revision. *Journal of Clinical Pathology*, **46**, 97−103.

Cade J.D. (1989) Thrombolytic therapy. *Blood Reviews*, **3**, 5−10.

Fareed J., Kwaan H.C., Ganguley P., Walenga J.M., Breddin H.K. & Strano A. (eds) (1991) Thrombosis and fibrinolysis: current clinical and therapeutic aspects. *Seminars in Thrombosis and Hemostasis*, **17**, 317−470.

Hirsh J. (ed.) (1990) Anti-thrombotic therapy. *Clinical Haematology*, **3**, 483−830.

Hirsh J. (1991) Heparin. *New England Journal of Medicine*, **324**, 1565−1574.

Kwaan H.C. & Kazama M. (eds) (1990) Clinical aspects of fibrinolysis. *Seminars in Thrombosis and Hemostasis*, **16**, 207−273.

Lane D.A. & Lindahl U. (eds) (1989) *Heparin: Chemical and Biological Properties, Clinical Application*. Edward Arnold, London.

Ljinen H.R. & Collen D. (1989) Congenital and acquired deficiencies of components of the fibrinolytic system and their relation to bleeding or thrombosis. *Fibrinolysis*, **3**, 67−77.

Machin S.J., Giddings J.S., Greaves M. *et al.* (1990) Detection of lupus-like anticoagulant. *Journal of Clinical Pathology*, **43**, 73−76.

Markwardt F. (1991) Past, present and future of hirudin. *Haemostasis*, **21** (Suppl. 1), 11−26.

Ofosu F.A., Agnelli G. & Hirsh J. (1992) New thrombin inhibitors: mode of action, experimental findings and clinical potential. *Recent Advances in Haematology*, 6 (eds A.V. Hoffbrand & M.K. Brenner). Churchill Livingstone, Edinburgh, pp. 45−72.

Triplett D.A. (1990) Laboratory diagnosis of lupus anti-coagulants. *Seminars in Thrombosis and Hemostasis*, **16**, 182−192.

Chapter 20
Haematological Changes in Systemic Disease

Anaemia of chronic disorders

Many of the anaemias seen in clinical practice occur in patients with systemic disorders and are the result of a number of contributing factors. The anaemia of chronic disorders is of central importance and occurs in patients with a variety of chronic inflammatory and malignant diseases (Table 20.1). It may be complicated by additional features which may be due to disease affecting particularly one or other system.

The characteristic features are:

1 Normochromic, normocytic or mildly hypochromic indices and red cell morphology.

2 Mild and non-progressive anaemia (haemoglobin rarely less than 9.0 g/dl) — the severity being related to the severity of the disease.

3 Both the serum iron and TIBC (total iron-binding capacity) are reduced.

4 The serum ferritin is normal or raised.

5 Bone marrow (reticuloendothelial) storage iron is normal but incorporation of iron into erythroblasts is reduced.

The pathogenesis of this anaemia appears to be related to the decreased release of iron from macrophages to plasma and so to erythroblasts, reduced red cell lifespan and an inadequate erythropoietin response to anaemia. The anaemia is corrected by the successful treatment of the underlying disease but does not respond to iron therapy despite the low serum iron. Responses to recombinant erythropoietin therapy may be obtained, e.g. in rheumatoid arthritis or myeloma, but this alone does not correct

Table 20.1 Causes of anaemia of chronic disorders.

Chronic inflammatory diseases
- Infectious, e.g. pulmonary abscess, tuberculosis, osteomyelitis, pneumonia, bacterial endocarditis

- Non-infectious, e.g. rheumatoid arthritis, SLE and other connective tissue diseases, sarcoid, Crohn's disease, cirrhosis

Malignant disease
- For example carcinoma, lymphoma, sarcoma, myeloma

the anaemia completely. In many conditions this anaemia is complicated by anaemia due to other causes, e.g. iron or folate deficiency, renal failure, bone marrow infiltration, hypersplenism or endocrine abnormality.

Malignant diseases (other than primary bone marrow diseases)

Anaemia

Contributing factors include anaemia of chronic disorders, blood loss and iron deficiency, marrow infiltration (Fig. 20.1) often associated with a leuco-erythroblastic blood film, folate deficiency, haemolysis and marrow suppression from radiotherapy or chemotherapy (Table 20.2).

Microangiopathic haemolytic anaemia (p. 91 and Fig. 20.2) occurs with mucin-secreting adenocarcinoma, particularly of the stomach, lung and breast. Less common forms of anaemia with malignant disease include autoimmune haemolytic anaemia with malignant lymphoma and, rarely, with other tumours; primary red cell aplasia with thymoma; and myelodysplastic syndromes secondary to chemotherapy. There is also an association of pernicious anaemia with carcinoma of the stomach.

The anaemia of malignant disease may respond partly to erythropoietin. Folic acid should only be given if there is definite megaloblastic anaemia due to the deficiency; it might 'feed' the tumour.

Polycythaemia

Secondary polycythaemia is occasionally associated with renal, hepatic, cerebellar and uterine tumours (p. 292).

White cell changes

Leukaemoid reactions (p. 155) may occur with tumours showing widespread necrosis and inflammation. Hodgkin's disease is associated with a variety of white cell abnormalities including eosinophilia, monocytosis and leucopenia. In non-Hodgkin's lymphoma, malignant cells may circulate in the blood (p. 263).

Platelet and blood coagulation abnormalities

Patients with malignant disease may show either thrombocytosis or thrombocytopenia. Disseminated tumours, particularly mucin-secreting adenocarcinomas are associated with disseminated intravascular coagulation (DIC) (p. 344) and generalized haemo-

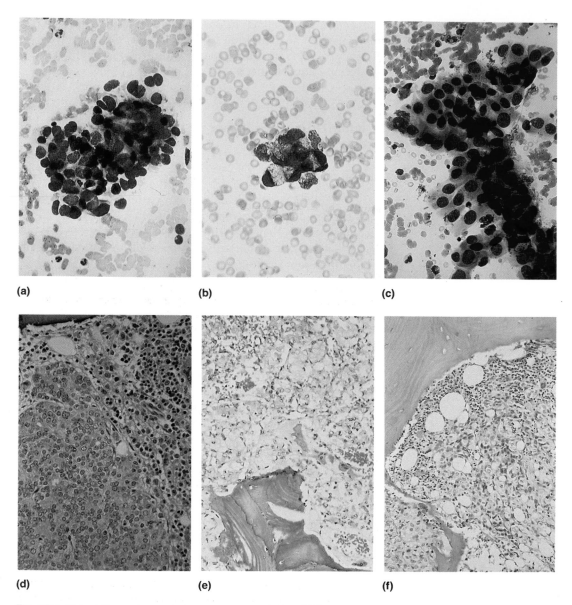

Fig. 20.1 Metastatic carcinoma in bone marrow aspirates: (a) breast;
(b) stomach; (c) colon and bone marrow trephine biopsies; (d) prostate;
(e) stomach; (f) kidney.

static failure. Activation of fibrinolysis occurs in some patients
with carcinoma of the prostate. Occasional patients with malignant disease have spontaneous bruising or bleeding due to
an acquired inhibitor of one or other coagulation factor, most
frequently factor VIII.

Table 20.2 Haematological abnormalities in malignant disease.

Haematological abnormality	Tumour or treatment associated
Pancytopenia	
● Marrow hypoplasia	● Chemotherapy, radiotherapy
● Myelodysplasia	● Chemotherapy, radiotherapy
● Leuco-erythroblastic	● Metastases in marrow
● Megaloblastic	● Folate deficiency
	● B_{12} deficiency (carcinoma of stomach)
Red cells	
● Anaemia of chronic disorders	● Most forms
● Iron deficiency anaemia	● Especially gastrointestinal, uterine
● Pure red cell aplasia	● Thymoma
● Immune haemolytic anaemia	● Lymphoma, ovary, other tumours
● Microangiopathic haemolytic anaemia	● Mucin-secreting carcinoma
● Polycythaemia	● Kidney, liver, cerebellum, uterus
White cells	
● Neutrophil leucocytosis	● Most forms
● Leukaemoid reaction	● Disseminated tumours, those with necrosis
● Eosinophilia	● Hodgkin's disease, others
● Monocytosis	● Various tumours
Platelets and coagulation	
● Thrombocytosis	● Gastrointestinal tumours with bleeding, others
● Disseminated intravascular coagulation (DIC)	● Mucin-secreting carcinoma, prostate
● Activation of fibrinolysis	● Prostate
● Acquired inhibitors of coagulation	● Most forms

Rheumatoid arthritis (and other connective tissue disorders)

In patients with rheumatoid arthritis, the anaemia of chronic disorders is proportional to the severity of the disease. It is complicated in some patients by iron deficiency due to gastrointestinal bleeding related to therapy with salicylates, non-steroidal anti-inflammatory agents or corticosteroids. Bleeding into inflamed joints may also be a factor. Marrow hypoplasia may follow therapy with gold or phenylbutazone. In Felty's syndrome splenomegaly is associated with neutropenia. Anaemia and thrombocytopenia may also be present.

In SLE (systemic lupus erythematosus) there may be anaemia of chronic disorders and 50% of patients are leucopenic with reduced neutrophil and lymphocyte counts often associated with circulating immune complexes. Renal impairment and drug-

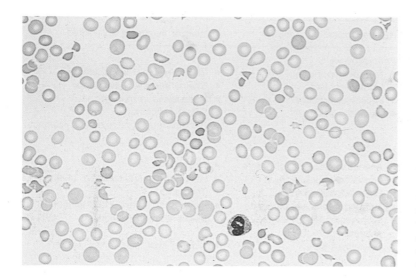

Fig. 20.2 Peripheral blood film in metastatic mucin-secreting adrenocarcinoma of the stomach showing red cell polychromasia and fragmentation and thrombocytopenia. The patient had disseminated intravascular coagulation.

induced gastrointestinal blood loss also contribute to the anaemia. Autoimmune haemolytic anaemia (typically with IgG and the C3 component of complement on the surface of the red cells) occurs in 5% of patients and may be the presenting feature of the syndrome. There may be autoimmune thrombocytopenia in 5% of patients. The lupus anticoagulant has been described on p. 354. This circulating anticardiolipin interferes with blood coagulation by altering the binding of coagulation factors to platelet phospholipid and predisposes to both arterial and venous thrombosis and recurrent abortions. The antibody may be responsible for a false positive Wassermann reaction. Tests for antinuclear factor (ANF) and antiDNA antibodies (Fig. 20.3) are positive.

Patients with temporal arteritis and polymyalgia rheumatica have a markedly elevated ESR (erythrocyte sedimentation rate), pronounced red cell rouleaux in the blood film and a polyclonal immunoglobulin response. These and other collagen vascular disorders are associated with anaemia of chronic disorders.

Renal failure

Anaemia

A normochronic anaemia is present in most patients with chronic renal failure. Generally there is a 2 g/dl fall in haemoglobin level for every 10 mmol/l rise in blood urea. There is impaired red cell production due to defective erythropoietin

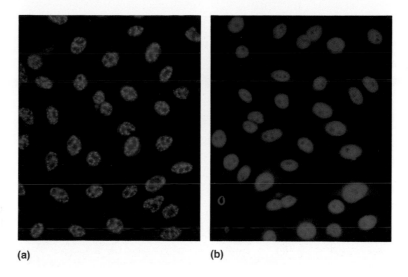

Fig. 20.3 Antinuclear factor test by indirect immunofluorescence on human epithelial carcinoma cell line HEP-2. (a) Mixed connective tissue disease showing a positive speckled pattern; (b) systemic lupus erythematosus showing a homogeneous pattern. (Courtesy of Dept of Immunology, Royal Free School of Medicine.)

(a)   **(b)**

production (see Fig. 2.5). Uraemic serum has also been shown to contain factors which inhibit proliferation of erythroid progenitors but, in view of the excellent response to erythropoietin in most patients, the clinical relevance of these is doubtful. Variable shortening of red cell lifespan occurs and in severe uraemia the red cells show abnormalities including spicules (spurs) and 'burr' cells (Fig. 20.4). Increased red cell 2,3-DPG levels in response to the anaemia and hyperphosphataemia result in decreased oxygen affinity and a shift of the haemoglobin oxygen-dissociation curve to the right (p. 20), which is augmented by uraemic acidosis. The patient's symptoms are therefore relatively mild for the degree of anaemia.

Other factors may complicate the anaemia of chronic renal failure (Table 20.3). These include the anaemia of chronic disorders, iron deficiency from blood loss during dialysis or due to bleeding because of defective platelet function, and folate deficiency in some chronic dialysis patients. Aluminium excess in patients on chronic dialysis also inhibits erythropoiesis. Patients with polycystic kidneys usually have retained erythropoietin production and may have less severe anaemia for the degree of renal failure.

Treatment

Erythropoietin therapy has been found to correct the anaemia in patients on dialysis or in chronic renal failure, providing that iron and folate deficiency, aluminium excess and infections have been corrected. The dose of erythropoietin usually required

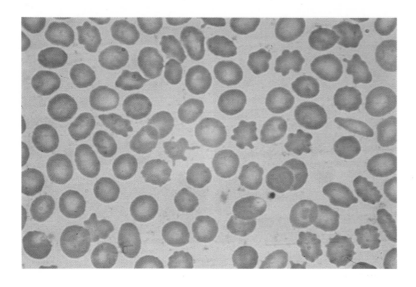

Fig. 20.4 Peripheral blood film in chronic renal failure showing red cell acanthocytosis and numerous 'burr' cells.

Table 20.3 Haematological abnormalities in renal failure.

Anaemia
- Reduced erythropoietin production
- Aluminium excess in dialysis patients
- Anaemia of chronic disorders
- Iron deficiency
    Blood loss, e.g. dialysis, venesection, defective platelet function
- Folate deficiency
    Chronic haemodialysis without replacement therapy

Abnormal platelet function

Thrombocytopenia
- Immune complex-mediated, e.g. SLE, polyarteritis nodosa
- Some cases of acute nephritis and following allograft
- Haemolytic uraemic syndrome and thrombotic thrombocytopenic purpura

Thrombosis
- Some cases of the nephrotic syndrome

Polycythemia
- In renal allograft recipients

is 50–150 units/kg three times a week intravenously or by subcutaneous infusion. The response is faster after intravenous administration, but greater with the subcutaneous route. Maintenance by 75 units/kg/week subcutaneously is typical. Complications of therapy have been initial transient 'flu-like symptoms, hypertension, clotting of the dialysis lines and, rarely, fits.

Platelet and coagulation abnormalities

A bleeding tendency with purpura, gastrointestinal or uterine bleeding occurs in 30–50% of patients with chronic renal failure and is marked in patients with acute renal failure. The bleeding is out of proportion to the degree of thrombocytopenia and has been associated with abnormal platelet or vascular function which can be reversed by dialysis. Correction of the anaemia with erythropoietin also improves the bleeding tendency. Immune complex-mediated thrombocytopenia occurs in some patients with acute nephritis, SLE and polyarteritis nodosa and also following renal allografts. Renal allografts may also lead to polycythemia in 10–15% of patients.

The haemolytic uraemic syndrome and thrombotic thrombocytopenic purpura have been discussed on p. 326. Patients with the nephrotic syndrome have an increased risk of thrombosis.

Liver disease

The haematological abnormalities in liver disease are noted in Table 20.4. Chronic liver disease is associated with anaemia which is mildly macrocytic and often accompanied by target cells mainly due to increased cholesterol in the membrane (Fig. 20.5). Contributing factors to the anaemia may include blood loss (e.g. bleeding varices) with iron deficiency, dietary folate

Table 20.4 Haematological abnormalities in liver disease.

Liver failure ± obstructive jaundice ± portal hypertension

Refractory anaemia—usually mildly macrocytic, often with target cells; may be associated with:
- blood loss and iron deficiency
- alcohol (± ring sideroblastic change)
- folate deficiency
- haemolysis, e.g. Zieve's syndrome, Wilson's disease, immune
- hypersplenism from portal hypertension

Bleeding tendency
- deficiency of vitamin K-dependent factors; also of factor V and fibrinogen
- thrombocytopenia—hypersplenism, immune
- platelet function defects
- functional abnormalities of fibrinogen
- increased fibrinolysis
- portal hypertension — haemorrhage from varices

Virus hepatitis
Aplastic anaemia

Tumours
Polycythaemia
Neutrophil leucocytosis and leukaemoid reactions

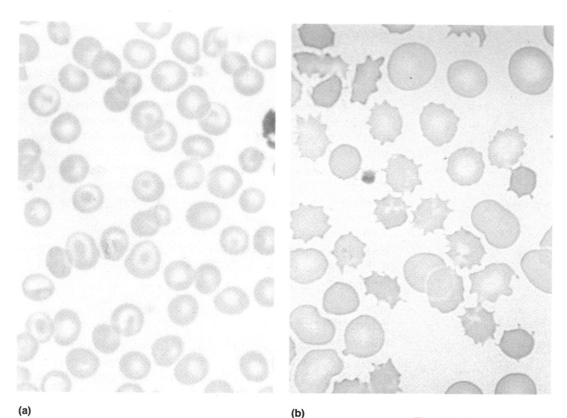

(a)   **(b)**

Fig. 20.5 Liver disease: peripheral blood film showing (a) macrocytosis and target cells; and (b) marked acanthocytosis in Zieve's syndrome.

deficiency and direct suppression of haemopoiesis by alcohol. Alcohol may have an inhibiting effect on folate metabolism and is occasionally associated with (ring) sideroblastic changes which disappear when alcohol is withdrawn (see Fig. 3.10b).

Haemolytic anaemia may occur in patients with alcohol intoxication (Zieve's syndrome) (Fig. 20.5) and in Wilson's disease (due to copper oxidation of red cell membranes) and autoimmune haemolytic anaemia is found in some patients with chronic immune hepatitis. Viral hepatitis (usually non-A, non-B, non-C) is rarely associated with aplastic anaemia.

The acquired coagulation abnormalities associated with liver disease have been described on p. 343. There are deficiencies of vitamin K-dependent factors (II, VII, IX and X) and, in severe disease, of factor V and fibrinogen. Thrombocytopenia may occur from hypersplenism or from immune complex-mediated platelet destruction. Abnormalities of platelet function may also be present. Dysfibrinogenaemia with abnormal fibrin polymerization may occur due to excess sialic acid in the fibrinogen molecules. A consumptive coagulopathy may be superimposed. These haemostatic defects may contribute to major blood loss from bleeding varices caused by portal hypertension.

Hypothyroidism

A moderate anaemia is usual and may be due to lack of thyroxine. T_3 and T_4 potentiate the action of erythropoietin. There is also a reduced oxygen need and thus reduced erythropoietin secretion. The anaemia is often macrocytic and the MCV (mean corpuscular volume) falls with thyroxine therapy. Autoimmune thyroid disease, especially myxoedema or Hashimoto's disease, is associated with pernicious anaemia. Iron deficiency may also be present, particularly in women with menorrhagia.

Infections

Haematological abnormality is usually present in patients with infections of all types (Table 20.5).

Bacterial infections

Acute bacterial infections are the most common cause of neutrophil leucocytosis. Toxic granulation, Döhle bodies and metamyelocytes may be present in the blood. Leukaemoid reactions with a white cell count $>50 \times 10^9/l$ and granulocyte precursors in the blood may occur in severe infections, particularly in infants and young children. The LAP (leucocyte alkaline phosphatase) score is raised in contrast to the low LAP score in chronic myeloid leukaemia. Mild anaemia is common if the infection is prolonged. Severe haemolytic anaemia occurs in bacterial septicaemias particularly due to Gram-negative organisms, where there is usually associated DIC (p. 344).

Clostridium welchii organisms produce an α-toxin, a lecithinase acting directly on the circulating red cells (Fig. 20.6). Haemo-

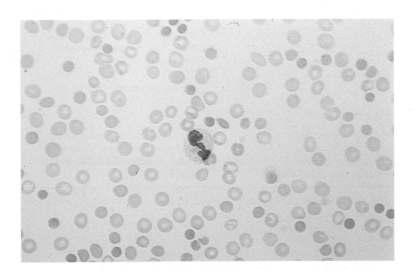

Fig. 20.6 Peripheral blood film in patient with haemolytic anaemia in clostridial septicaemia showing red cell contraction and spherocytosis.

Haematological abnormality	Infection associated
Anaemia	
Anaemia of chronic disorders	Chronic infections especially tuberculosis
Hypoplastic anaemia	Viral hepatitis
Transient red cell aplasia	Human parvovirus
Marrow fibrosis	Tuberculosis
Immune haemolytic anaemia	Infectious mononucleosis, *Mycoplasma pneumoniae*
Direct red cell damage or microangiopathic	Bacterial septicaemia (associated DIC), *Clostridium welchii*, malaria, bartonellosis Viruses—haemolytic uraemic syndrome and TTP
Sideroblastic	Antituberculosis therapy: isoniazid cycloserine
Hypersplenism	Chronic malaria, tropical splenomegaly syndrome, leishmaniasis, schistosomiasis
White cell changes	
Neutrophil leucocytosis	Acute bacterial infections
Leukaemoid reactions	Severe bacterial infections particularly in infants Tuberculosis
Eosinophilia	Parasitic diseases, e.g. hookworm, filariasis, schistosomiasis, trichinosis, etc. Recovery from acute infections
Monocytosis	Chronic bacterial infections: tuberculosis, brucellosis, bacterial endocarditis, typhoid
Neutropenia	Viral infections: HIV, hepatitis, influenza Fulminant bacterial infections, e.g. typhoid, miliary tuberculosis
Lymphocytosis	Infectious mononucleosis, toxoplasmosis, cytomegalovirus, rubella, viral hepatitis, pertussis, tuberculosis, brucellosis
Lymphopenia	AIDS *Legionella pneumonophilia*
Thrombocytopenia	
Megakaryocytic depression, immune complex-mediated and direct interaction with platelets	Acute viral infections particularly in children, e.g. measles, varicella, rubella; malaria; severe bacterial infection

Table 20.5 Blood abnormalities associated with infections.

DIC, disseminated intravascular coagulation; HIV, human immunodeficiency virus; TTP, thrombotic thrombocytopenic purpura.

lysis in bartonellosis (Oroya fever) is caused by direct red cell infection. With severe acute bacterial infections there may be thrombocytopenia. *Mycoplasma pneumoniae* infections are associated with autoimmune haemolytic anaemia of the 'cold' type (p. 89).

Chronic bacterial infections are associated with the anaemia of chronic disorders. In tuberculosis, additional factors in the pathogenesis of anaemia include marrow replacement and fibrosis associated with miliary disease and reactions to anti-tuberculous therapy (e.g. isoniazid is a pyridoxine antagonist and may cause sideroblastic anaemia). Disseminated tuberculosis is associated with leukaemoid reactions and patients with involvement of bone marrow may show leuco-erythroblastic changes in the peripheral blood film.

Viral infections

Acute viral diseases are often associated with a mild anaemia. An immune haemolytic anaemia with an anti-i autoantibody is associated with infectious mononucleosis (p. 89). Viral infections, as well as syphilis, have been associated with paroxysmal cold haemoglobinuria (p. 89). Viruses have also been linked to the pathogenesis of the haemolytic uraemic syndrome and thrombotic thrombocytopenic purpura (p. 91 and p. 326). Aplastic anaemia may occur with viral A or more usually non-A, non-B, non-C hepatitis. Transient red cell aplasia is associated with human parvovirus infection and this may result in severe anaemia in patients with a haemolytic anaemia because of the shortened red cell survival, e.g. in hereditary spherocytosis, pyruvate kinase deficiency or sickle cell disease.

Acute thrombocytopenia is not uncommon in rubella, morbilli and varicella infections. Rubella and cytomegalovirus (CMV) infections may cause a reactive lymphocytosis similar to that found in infectious mononucleosis. CMV may be responsible for a post-transfusion mononucleosis-like syndrome, CMV being transmitted by leucocytes. CMV infections in infants are associated with massive hepatosplenomaly. In bone marrow transplant recipients or other immunosuppressed patients CMV infections may cause pancytopenia as well as other severe disorders, e.g. pneumonitis or hepatitis (see p. 136). Haematological abnormalities associated with HIV infection and AIDS are dealt within Chapter 9.

Malaria

Some degree of haemolysis is seen in all types of malarial infection. The most severe abnormalities are found in *Plasmodium falciparum* infections (Fig. 20.7). In the worst cases intravascular

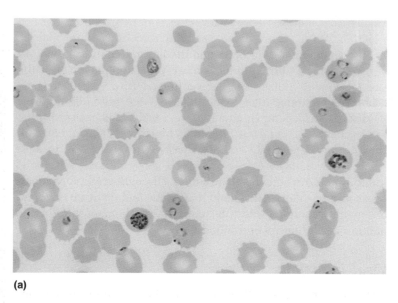

(a)

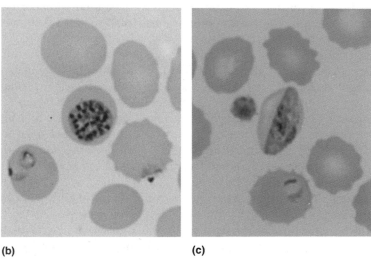

(b)   (c)

Fig. 20.7 Malaria: peripheral blood in severe *Plasmodium falciparum* infection showing: (a) many ring forms and a meront; and at higher magnification: (b) a meront, and (c) a gametocyte.

haemolysis is marked with haemoglobinuria. This may be associated with quinine therapy ('Blackwater fever'). Thrombocytopenia is commonly found in acute malaria. Patients with chronic malaria have an anaemia of chronic disorders; hypersplenism may contribute to the anaemia and result in moderate thrombocytopenia and neutropenia. Dyserythopoiesis in the marrow, folate deficiency and protein−calorie malnutrition may contribute to the anaemia.

Toxoplasmosis

Toxoplasmosis in children and adults is associated with lymph-adenopathy and large numbers of atypical lymphocytes in the blood. Congenital disease may be confused with hydrops foetalis in a severely anaemic hydropic infant with gross hepatospleno-megaly, thrombocytopenia or a leuco-erythroblastic blood film.

Kala-azar (visceral leishmaniasis)

The visceral form of leishmaniasis is associated with pancyto-penia, hepatosplenomegaly and lymphadenopathy. Bone marrow or splenic aspirates may show large numbers of parasitized macrophages (Fig. 20.8).

Other parasitic diseases

In the acute phase of both African and South American trypano-somiasis, organisms are found in the peripheral blood (Fig. 20.9). Microfilaria of Bancroftian filariasis and loiasis are also detected

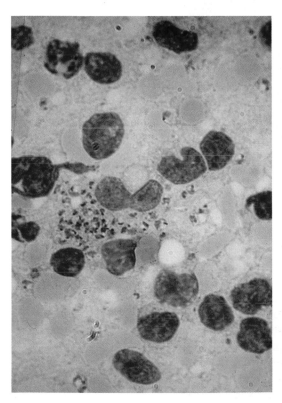

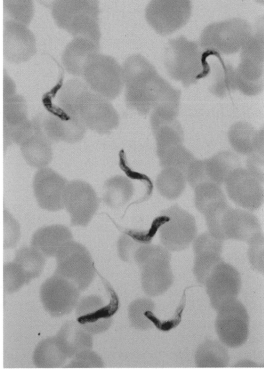

Fig. 20.8 Kala-azar: spleen aspirate showing macrophages containing Leishman–Donovan bodies.

Fig. 20.9 African trypanosomiasis: blood film showing *Trypanosoma brucei*.

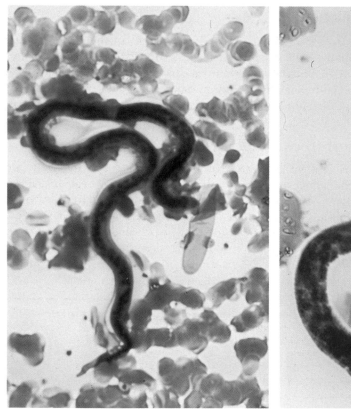

(a)

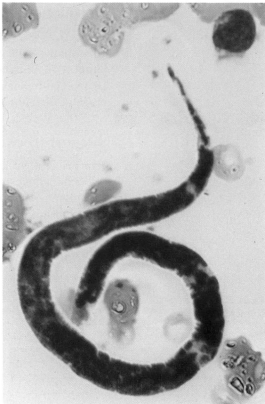

(b)

Fig. 20.10 Peripheral blood films showing microfilariae of (a) *Wuchereria bancrofti* and (b) *Loa loa*.

during blood film examination (Fig. 20.10). In chronic schistosomiasis, hypersplenism follows the splenic enlargement associated with portal hypertension. In many parasitic diseases there is eosinophilia (see Table 20.5).

Pulmonary eosinophilia

Eosinophilia associated with pulmonary infiltrates (Loeffler's syndrome) occurs in a number of conditions. In most cases Loeffler's syndrome is a relatively mild condition, probably due to either hypersensitivity to parasites or parasitic passage through the lungs, e.g. in ascariasis, ankylostomiasis, filariasis or *Toxocara* infestations. The syndrome occasionally occurs with hypersensitivity to drugs, e.g. penicillin, nitrofurantoin or sulphonamides. Severe forms of pulmonary eosinophilia may occur in polyarteritis nodosa. The syndrome is seen in the allergic alveolitis group of disorders including farmer's lung, bird fancier's lung and hypersensitivity to fungi, e.g. *Aspergillus fumigatus*.

Splenomegaly

With few exceptions disease involvement of the spleen results in its enlargement. Splenomegaly is consequently a frequent and important clinical sign and a palpable spleen is at least twice its normal size. Table 20.6 presents a simple classification of splenomegaly. In some of the diseases listed splenic enlargement is only found occasionally and when it occurs it is seldom marked, e.g. in acute septicaemias, the megaloblastic anaemias, most collagen disorders and amyloidosis.

The relative incidence of the causes of splenomegaly are subject to enormous geographical variation. In Great Britain the leukaemias, malignant lymphomas, myeloproliferative disorders, haemolytic anaemias and portal hypertension account for most cases. Infective endocarditis is also relatively frequent. In tropical countries, the incidence of these haematological causes of splenomegaly is far exceeded by the frequency of splenic

Table 20.6 Causes of splenomegaly.

Haematological
Chronic myeloid leukaemia
Chronic lymphocytic leukaemia
Acute leukaemia
Malignant lymphoma
Chronic myelosclerosis
Polycythaemia vera
Hairy cell leukaemia
Thalassaemia major or intermedia
Sickle cell anaemia (before splenic infarction)
Haemolytic anaemias
Megaloblastic anaemia

Portal hypertension
Cirrhosis
Hepatic, portal, splenic vein thrombosis

Storage diseases
Gaucher's
Niemann—Pick
Histiocytosis X

Systemic diseases
Sarcoidosis
Amyloidosis
Collagen diseases—systemic lupus erythematosus, rheumatoid arthritis
Systemic mastocytosis

Infections
Acute
   Septicaemia, bacterial endocarditis, typhoid, infectious mononucleosis
Chronic
   Tuberculosis, brucellosis, syphilis, tropical: malaria, leishmaniasis, schistosomiasis

enlargement caused by the parasitic tropical infections: malaria, leishmaniasis and schistosomiasis. Portal hypertension remains an important cause of splenomegaly in most tropical countries but is especially prevalent in northeastern India and southern China. The 'tropical splenomegaly syndrome' is seen in large numbers of patients in New Guinea and Central Africa. Among the causes of splenomegaly due to blood disorders the haemoglobinopathies become relatively more important in some countries. Haemoglobin C disease in West Africa and haemoglobin E disease in the Far East are associated with splenomegaly and the thalassaemia syndromes have a wide distribution throughout the tropics. Because of the multiplicity of factors responsible for splenomegaly in such countries, more than one pathology may contribute to splenomegaly in a particular patient.

Hypersplenism: haematological effects of splenomegaly

Splenic enlargement is asociated with anaemia, leucopenia and thrombocytopenia (pancytopenia) caused by an enhanced capacity of the enlarged spleen for pooling, sequestering and destroying blood cells and also leading to an increased plasma volume. The term 'hypersplenism' is used to describe this reduction in blood cell counts. In many conditions causing splenomegaly factors other than the enlarged spleen may also contribute to the pancytopenia. Many haemolytic anaemias and myeloproliferative or lymphoproliferative disorders are associated with splenic enlargement. Although intrinsic red cell defects, immunological abnormalities or bone marrow failure are the primary causes of the reduction of blood elements in these disorders the associated splenomegaly (*per se*) may also contribute to the observed cytopenias.

Gaucher's disease

In the course of normal cell growth, development and ageing, cells are being replaced in all tissues. Breakdown of complex components of the cells requires sequential enzymatic degradation which takes place in secondary lysosomes. The glycolipids, globosides and gangliosides (Fig. 20.11) are first degraded by cleavage of the carbohydrate residues and then the ceramide is hydrolysed. Hereditary deficiency of the enzymes required for glycolipid breakdown results in Gaucher's, Tay−Sachs and Niemann−Pick diseases (Fig. 20.11).

Gaucher's disease is an uncommon familial disorder characterized by an accumulation of glucocerebroside in reticuloendothelial (RE) cells. Like Niemann−Pick and Tay−Sachs diseases it is more common in Ashkenazi Jews. There is a deficiency of lysosomal β-glucocerebrosidase. Three types occur:

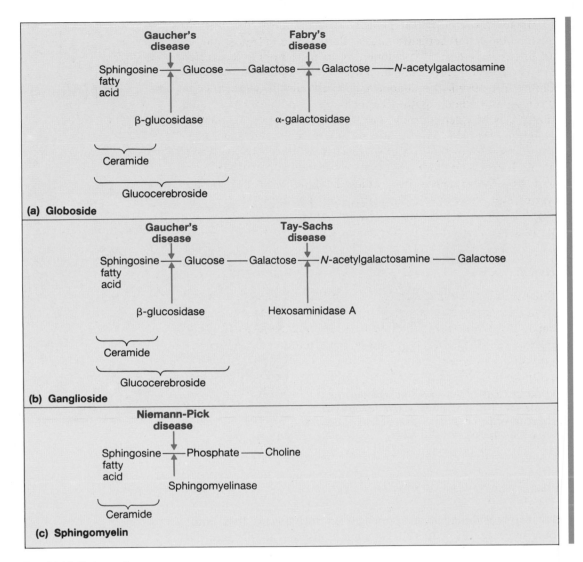

Gaucher's disease   Fabry's disease

Sphingosine fatty acid ——— Glucose ——— Galactose ——— Galactose ——— *N*-acetylgalactosamine

β-glucosidase   α-galactosidase

Ceramide

Glucocerebroside

(a) Globoside

Gaucher's disease   Tay-Sachs disease

Sphingosine fatty acid ——— Glucose ——— Galactose ——— *N*-acetylgalactosamine ——— Galactose

β-glucosidase   Hexosaminidase A

Ceramide

Glucocerebroside

(b) Ganglioside

Niemann-Pick disease

Sphingosine fatty acid ——— Phosphate ——— Choline

Sphingomyelinase

Ceramide

(c) Sphingomyelin

Fig. 20.11 Defects of glycolipid cleavage enzymes in Gaucher's, Niemann–Pick, Fabry's and Tay–Sachs diseases.

(I) a chronic adult type; (II) an acute infantile neuronopathic type (not particularly common in Jews); and (III) a subacute neuronopathic type with onset in childhood or adolescence and a better prognosis than type II. In type II, the course is usually malignant with neurological as well as RE involvement. In type I presenting in childhood or in adults a chronic disease is the rule. The outstanding physical sign is splenomegaly. Moderate liver enlargement and pingueculae are other characteristic findings. In many cases bone deposits cause bone pain and pathological fractures. Expansion of the lower end of the femur may produce the 'Erlenmeyer flask deformity'.

The clinical manifestations are due to the accumulation of

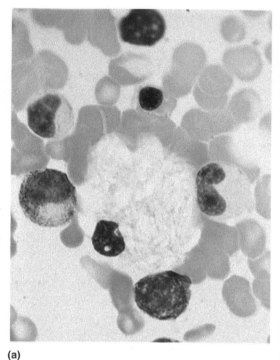

(a)

Fig. 20.12 Gaucher's disease: (a) bone marrow
aspirate—a Gaucher cell with 'fibrillar' cytoplasmic
pattern; (b) spleen histology—pale clusters of Gaucher
cells in the reticuloendothelial cords.

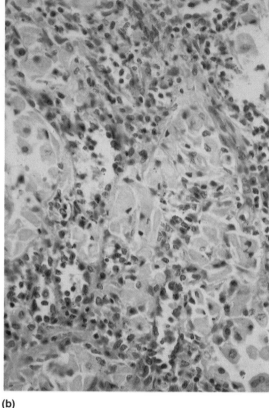

(b)

glucocerebroside-laden macrophages in the spleen, liver and
bone marrow (Fig. 20.12). Gaucher's disease at all ages is
commonly associated with marked anaemia, leucopenia
and thrombocytopenia occurring singly or in combination.
The thrombocytopenia may be sufficiently severe to cause
spontaneous bruising or bleeding.

Genetic aspects

The inheritance is autosomal recessive. The glucocerebrosidase
gene is on chromosome 1 region q2.1. The defect is due to either
a point mutation or unequal crossing-over between the glucuro-
cerebrosidase gene and its pseudogene which occurs 3′ to the
functional gene. In rare cases the defect is in a sphingolipid-
activator protein which activates glucocerebrosidase. DNA
technology (e.g. the ARMS technique, p. 118) can now be used
for carrier detection and antenatal diagnosis.

Treatment

Splenectomy can result in haematological improvement but following this operation there is often increased deposition of cerebroside in extrasplenic tissue, particularly bones. Trials of enzyme replacement therapy with Ceredase, glucocerebrosidase purified from human placenta, are encouraging. Bone marrow transplantation has been carried out successfully in 20 or so severly affected patients.

Niemann–Pick disease

Niemann–Pick disease shows certain clinical and pathological similarities to Gaucher's disease. The majority of patients are infants who die in the first few years of life although occasional patients survive to adult life. Massive hepatosplenomegaly occurs and there is usually lung and nervous system involvement with retarded physical and mental development. A 'cherry-red' spot is commonly seen in the retina of affected infants. Pancytopenia is a regular feature and in marrow aspirates 'foam cells' of similar size to Gaucher cells are seen. Chemical analysis of the tissues reveals that the disorder is caused by an accumulation of sphingomyelin and cholesterol.

Tropical splenomegaly syndrome

A syndrome of massive splenomegaly of uncertain aetiology has been frequently found in many malarious zones of the tropics including Uganda, Nigeria, New Guinea and the Congo. Smaller numbers of patients with this disorder are seen in Southern Arabia, the Sudan and Zambia. In the past such titles as 'big spleen disease', 'cryptogenic splenomegaly' and 'African macroglobulinaemia' have been used to describe this syndrome.

While it seems probable that malaria is the fundamental cause of the tropical splenomegaly syndrome, this disease is not the result of active malarial infection as parasitaemia is usually scanty and malarial pigment is not found in biopsy material from the liver and spleen. The available evidence suggests that an abnormal host response to the continual presence of malarial antigen results in a reactive and relatively benign lymphoproliferative disorder which predominantly affects the liver and spleen.

Splenomegaly is usually gross and the liver is also enlarged. Portal hypertension may be a feature. The anaemia is often severe and the lowest haemoglobin levels are found in subjects with the largest spleens. While leucopenia is usual, some patients develop a marked lymphocytosis. The moderate degree of thrombocytopenia present does not often cause spontaneous bleeding. Serum IgM levels are high and fluorescent techniques reveal high titres of malarial antibody.

Although splenectomy corrects the pancytopenia there is an increased risk of fulminant malarial infection. Trials of anti-malarial prophylaxis, e.g. proguanil and other antimalarial drugs, have proved successful in the management of many affected patients supporting the view that a continuing presence of malarial antigen is needed for the perpetuation of the lympho-proliferation associated with this syndrome. Resistant cases have also been treated successfully with chemotherapy.

Systemic mast cell syndrome

In systemic mastocytosis in adults there is a confluent macular urticaria which often evolves into a chronic lichenified derma-titis. Splenomegaly, hepatomegaly and generalized lymph-adenopathy occur with advanced disease and the bone marrow contains increased numbers of mast cells. Splenomegaly may be associated with pancytopenia but some patients have a 'leukaemoid' blood film appearance with monocytosis, lympho-cytosis or eosinophilia. Rarely there is mast cell leukaemia with large numbers of mast cells in the blood.

Effects of splenectomy

Splenectomy is undertaken in a number of disorders (Table 20.7) and the effects often depend on the underlying disease. However, certain changes in the blood occur irrespective of the underlying pathology.

Haematological effects

Red cell changes
The changes in red cell morphology include the presence of Howell—Jolly bodies (Fig. 20.13 and Table 20.8) and Pappenheimer (siderotic) granules (p. 30) in some of the cells and the appearance of target cells. In a proportion of subjects

---

Chronic immune thrombocytopenia (failed steroids)
Haemolytic anaemia
  Hereditary spherocytosis
  Autoimmune haemolytic anaemia (failed steroids)
  Thalassaemia major or intermedia
Chronic lymphocytic leukaemia
Lymphoma
Myelosclerosis
Tropical splenomegaly
Systemic mast cell syndrome

Table 20.7 Indications for elective splenectomy (some cases only).

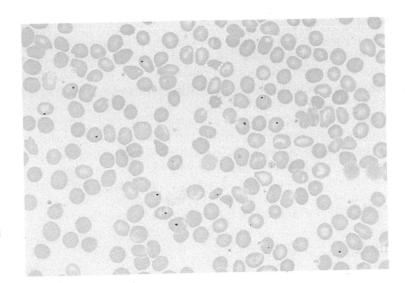

Fig. 20.13 Splenic atrophy: peripheral blood film showing Howell—Jolly bodies, Pappenheimer bodies and misshapen cells.

irregularly contracted or crenated, acanthocytic forms are also a feature. Occasional erythroblasts may be seen. These red cell changes are often referred to as hyposplenism (Table 20.8). The presence of red cell inclusions reflects the absence of the splenic 'pitting' function.

Leucocyte changes
After splenectomy there is a rise in the total leucocyte count. A neutrophil leucocytosis in the immediate post-operative period is, in the majority of subjects, later replaced by a small but significant and permanent increase in both lymphocytes and monocytes.

In response to infection, splenectomized subjects produce a greater leucocytosis than persons with intact spleens and often there is a marked left shift in the differential leucocyte count with myelocytes and occasional more primitive cells.

Table 20.8 Causes of hyposplenism and blood film features.

Causes	Blood film features
Splenectomy	*Red cells*
Sickle cell disease	Target cells
Essential	Acanthocytes
thrombocythaemia	Irregularly contracted or crenated cells
Adult coeliac disease	Howell—Jolly bodies (DNA remnants)
Dermatitis herpetiformis	Siderotic (iron) granules (Pappenheimer)
Rarely:	bodies
Ulcerative colitis	
Crohn's disease	*White cells*
	± Mild lymphocytosis, monocytosis
	Platelets
	± Thrombocytosis

Platelet changes

The spleen normally pools a third of the circulating platelets. In the immediate post-operative period in uncomplicated splenectomized patients, the platelet count rises steeply to a maximum of usually less than $1000 \times 10^9/l$ with a peak at $7-12$ days. The thrombocytosis is usually transitory and a fall to a level a third higher than in normal subjects over the following $1-2$ months is the rule. Occasional large and bizarre platelets can be seen in the blood films of many splenectomized subjects; their presence suggests that these particular platelets are normally removed by the spleen. In a number of patients thrombocytosis persists indefinitely after splenectomy and this appears to be usually a consequence of continuing anaemia with a hypercellular marrow.

Immunological effects

The spleen is assumed to play an important role in immunoglobulin synthesis and, indeed, a fall in the IgM fraction of the serum immunoglobulins is commonly found post-splenectomy.

In temperate climates, splenectomy in adults without complicating disease is associated with a slight increased incidence of infection with capsulated bacteria. However, splenectomized individuals have a definite increased susceptibility to severe malaria including cerebral malaria, and in the tropics dramatic reactivation of latent malarial infection is seen after splenectomy.

In the very young, splenectomy is associated with a substantial increase in fatal and life-threatening bacterial infections. This is particularly noticeable in infants during the first year of life. Septicaemias and meningitis are the usual documented causes of death and there is a predominance of pneumococcal infections, although there is also an increased risk of infection with *Haemophilus influenzae* and *Neisseria meningitidis*. Accordingly, at any age it is usual to give pneumococcal vaccination 1 month before splenectomy and to give regular penicillin prophylaxis following the operation which, if possible, is delayed until after the age of 6 years. Therapy with penicillin (or erythromycin in penicillin-allergic individuals) is continued in children until adulthood or even for life. It would also seem prudent to give Hib vaccine which has been shown to be effective in preventing *H. influenzae* infections in immunocompetent children, and to consider meningococcal vaccine, particularly for patients travelling, or residing outside the UK.

Causes of splenic atrophy

The appearance of hyposplenism in the blood film may be acquired as a result of splenic atrophy. Sickle cell disease, adult coeliac disease and essential thrombocythaemia (see Fig. 20.13) are the commonest causes of splenic atrophy but it has also been reported in tropical sprue and in intestinal malabsorption associated with dermatitis herpetiformis, ulcerative colitis and Crohn's disease (Table 20.8).

General indicators of systemic disease: tests for monitoring the acute phase response

The inflammatory response to tissue injury includes changes in plasma concentrations of proteins known as acute phase proteins. These proteins include fibrinogen and other clotting factors, complement components and C-reactive protein (CRP) (see p. 390), haptoglobin, serum amyloid A (SAA) protein, serum ferritin and others. The rise in these liver-derived proteins is part of a wider response which includes fever, leucocytosis and increased immune reactivity. The acute phase response is mediated by cytokines, e.g. interleukin-1 (IL-1) (see Fig. 8.5) and TNF, released from macrophages and possibly other cells. Patients with chronic disease may show periodic or continuous evidence of the acute phase response depending upon the extent of inflammation. Quantitative measurements of acute phase proteins are valuable indicators of the presence and extent of inflammation and of its response to treatment. When short-term (less than 24-hour) changes in the inflammatory response are expected CRP is the test choice. Long-term changes in the acute phase proteins are monitored by either the ESR or plasma viscosity. These tests are influenced by plasma proteins that are either slowly responding acute phase reactants, e.g. fibrinogen, or are not acute phase proteins, e.g. immunoglobulins.

Erythrocyte sedimentation rate

This commonly used but non-specific test measures the speed of sedimentation of red cells in plasma over a period of 1 hour. The speed is mainly dependent on the plasma concentration of large proteins, e.g. fibrinogen and immunoglobulins. The normal range in men is 1–5 mm/hour and in women 5–15 mm/hour and there is a progressive increase in old age. The ESR is raised in a wide variety of systemic inflammatory and neoplastic diseases and in pregnancy. The highest values (>100 mm/hour) are found in chronic infections, including tuberculosis and leishmaniasis, myeloma and macroglobulinaemia, connective tissue disorders and disseminated cancer. A raised ESR is associated with marked rouleaux formation of red cells in the peripheral blood film (see Fig. 14.5). Changes in the ESR can be used to monitor the response to therapy.

Lower than expected readings occur in polycythaemia vera due to the high red cell concentration. Higher than expected values may occur in severe anaemia due to the low red cell concentration.

Plasma viscosity

In many laboratories measurement of ESR has been replaced by plasma viscosity measurement. Plasma viscosity is affected by the concentration of plasma proteins of large molecular size, especially those with pronounced axial asymmetry — fibrinogen and some immunoglobulins. Normal values at room temperature are usually in the range of 1.50–1.70 mPa/s. Lower levels are formed in neonates because of lower levels of proteins particularly fibrinogen. Viscosity increases only slightly in the elderly as fibrinogen increases. There is no difference in values between men and women. Other advantages over the ESR test include independence from the effects of anaemia and results that are available within 15 minutes.

C-reactive protein

Phylogenetically CRP is a crude 'early' immunoglobulin which initiates the inflammatory reaction. CRP — antigen complexes can substitute for antibody in the fixation of C1q and trigger the complement cascade initiating the inflammatory response to antigens or tissue damage. Subsequent binding of C3b on the surface of microorganisms opsonizes them for phagocytosis.

After tissue injury, an increase in CRP, SAA protein and other acute-phase reactants may be detected within 6–10 hours. In-

Advantages	Disadvantages
C-reactive protein (CRP)	
Specific test of acute phase protein	More than one protein required to measure acute (CRP) and chronic inflammation
Fast response (6 hours) to change in disease activity	Costly when assayed in small numbers
High sensitivity — owing to large incremental change	Sophistocated equipment and antisera required
Can be measured on stored serum	
Small sample volumes	
Automated analysis	
Erythrocyte sedimentation rate (ESR) and plasma viscosity	
Useful in chronic disease	Not sensitive to acute changes (< 24 hours)
ESR inexpensive, easy, no electrical power required	Not specific for acute phase response
Plasma viscosity — result obtained quickly (15 min)	Slow to change with alteration in disease activity and insensitive to small changes in activity
Plasma viscosity not affected by anaemia	Fresh samples (<2 hours) required for ESR

Table 20.9 Advantages and disadvantages of the tests used to monitor the acute phase response.

crease in fibrinogen may not occur until 24—48 hours following injury. Immunoassays of CRP are now widely used for early detection of acute inflammation or tissue injury and for the monitoring of remission, e.g. response of infection to an antibiotic.

CRP is normally present in low concentrations (<8 mg/l). Levels are not influenced by anaemia, pregnancy or heart failure. During severe acute infection the plasma concentration may rise 1000-fold.

Table 20.9 lists the advantages and disadvantages of the tests used to assess the acute phase response.

Bibliography

Adamson J.W. & Eschbach J.W. (1989) Management of the anaemia of chronic renal failure with recombinant erythropoietin. *Quarterly Journal of Medicine, New Series*, **73**, 1093—1101.

Bagby G.C. (ed.) (1987) Hematologic aspects of systemic disease. *Hematology/Oncology Clinics of North America*, **1**, 167—350.

Bain B.J., Clark D.M. & Lampert I.A. (1992) *Diagnostic Bone Marrow Pathology*. Blackwell Scientific Publications, Oxford.

Beutler E. (1991) Gaucher's disease. *New England Journal of Medicine*, **325**, 1354—1360.

Bowdler A.J. (ed.) (1990) *The Spleen: Structure, Function and Clinical Significance*. Chapman & Hall, London.

Delamore I.W. & Liu Yin J.A. (1990) *Haematological Aspects of Systemic Disease*. Baillière Tindall, London.

Hamblin T.J. (1987) Haematological problems in the elderly. *Clinical Haematology*, **1**, 271—593.

International Committee for Standardisation in Haematology (1988) Guidelines on selection of laboratory tests for monitoring the acute phase response. *Journal of Clinical Pathology*, **41**, 1203—1212.

Knox-Macaulay H.H.M. (1992) Tuberculosis and the haemopoietic system. *Clinical Haematology*, **5**, 101—130.

Mistry P.K., Smith S.J., Ali M., Hatton C.S.R., McIntyre N. & Cox T.M. (1992) Genetic diagnosis of Gaucher's disease. *Lancet*, **339**, 889—992.

Phillips R.E. & Pavsol G. (1992) Anaemia of *Plasmodium falciparum* malaria. *Clinical Haematology*, **5**, 315—330.

Chapter 21
Blood Transfusion

Blood transfusion involves the infusion of whole blood or a blood component from one individual (the donor) to another (the recipient). The major clinical aspect is the transfusion of red cells. Compatibility between donor red cell antigens and the recipient's plasma antibodies must be ensured, otherwise potentially fatal haemolytic reactions may occur. Whole blood is also a source of other important components needed in therapy including platelets, haemostatic agents, plasma protein colloids and immunoglobulins.

Red cell antigens

Approximately 400 red blood cell group antigens have been described. The vast majority are inherited in a simple Mendelian fashion and are stable characteristics which are therefore useful in paternity testing. The significance of blood groups in blood transfusion is that individuals who lack a particular blood group antigen may produce antibodies reacting with that antigen. These may lead to a transfusion reaction if red cells bearing the antigen are transfused. Different blood group antigens have different potential for immunizing. The ABO and rhesus (Rh) groups are of major clinical significance. Some other systems of less overall importance are listed in Table 21.1.

Blood group antibodies

Naturally occurring antibodies occur in the plasma of subjects who lack the corresponding antigen and who have not been transfused or been pregnant. The most important are anti-A and anti-B. They are usually IgM, and react optimally at cold temperatures (4°C) and, although reactive at 37°C, are called cold antibodies.

Immune antibodies develop in response to the introduction — by transfusion or by transplacental passage during pregnancy — of red cells possessing antigens which the subject lacks. These antibodies are commonly IgG, although some IgM antibodies may also develop — usually in the early phase of an immune response. Immune antibodies react optimally at 37°C (warm

Table 21.1 Clinically important blood group systems.

Systems	Frequency of antibodies	Cause of haemolytic transfusion reaction	Cause of haemolytic disease of newborn
ABO	Very common	Yes (common)	Yes
Rh	Common	Yes (common)	Yes
Kell	Occasional	Yes (occasional)	Yes
Duffy	Occasional	Yes (occasional)	Yes
Kidd	Occasional	Yes (occasional)	Yes
Lutheran	Rare	Yes (rare)	No
Lewis	Occasional	Yes (rare)	No
P	Occasional	Yes (rare)	Yes (rare)
MN	Rare	Yes (rare)	Yes (rare)
Ii	Rare	Unlikely	No

antibodies). Only IgG antibodies are capable of transplacental passage from mother to foetus. The most important immune antibody is the Rh antibody, anti-D.

ABO system

This consists of three allelic genes: A, B and O. The A and B genes control the synthesis of specific enzymes responsible for the addition of single carbohydrate residues (N-acetyl galactosamine for group A and D-galactose for group B) to a basic antigenic glycoprotein or glycolipid with a terminal sugar L-fucose on the red cell, known as the H substance (Fig. 21.1). The O gene is an amorph and does not transform the H substance. Although there are six possible genotypes, the absence of a specific anti-O prevents the serological recognition of more than four phenotypes (Table 21.2). Subgroups of A complicate the

Fig. 21.1 Structure of ABO blood group antigens. Each consists of a chain of sugars attached to lipids or proteins which are an integral part of the cell membrane. The H antigen of the O blood group has a terminal fucose (fuc). The A antigen has an additional N-acetyl galactosamine (galnac), and the B antigen has an additional galactose (gal). glu, glucose; gnac, N-acetyl glucosamine.

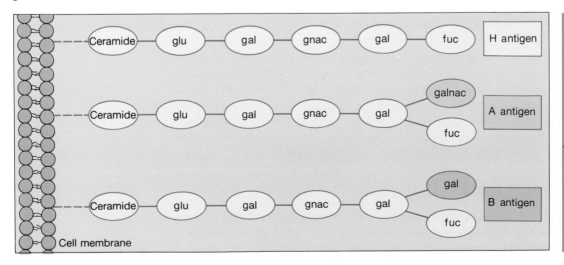

Phenotype	Genotype	Antigens	Naturally occurring antibodies	Frequency (UK) (%)
O	OO	O	Anti-A, anti-B	46
A	AA or AO	A	Anti-B	42
B	BB or BO	B	Anti-A	9
AB	AB	AB	None	3

Table 21.2 The ABO blood group system.

issue but are of minor clinical significance. A_1 and A_2 are commonly distinguished using specific anti-A_1 reagents. A_2 cells react more weakly than A_1 cells with anti-A and patients who are A_2B can be wrongly grouped as B.

The A, B and H antigens are present in most body cells including white cells and platelets. In the 80% of the population who possess secretor genes, these antigens are also found in soluble form in secretions and body fluids, e.g. plasma, saliva, semen and sweat. The stability of ABO antigens allows their detection on dried blood stains and semen and this is important in forensic medicine.

Naturally occurring antibodies to A and/or B antigens are found in the plasma of subjects whose red cells lack the corresponding antigens (Table 21.2, Fig. 21.2).

Rh system

This complex system is coded by allelic genes at three closely linked loci; alternative antigens Cc, Ee together with D or no D (termed 'd') exist. Thus a person may inherit CDe from the mother and cde from the father to have a genotype CDe/cde. There is a shortened nomenclature for these linked sets of genes shown in Table 21.3.

Rh antibodies rarely occur naturally; most are *immune*, i.e. they result from previous transfusion or pregnancy. Anti-D is responsible for most of the clinical problems associated with the system and a simple subdivision of subjects into Rh D positive and Rh D negative using anti-D is sufficient for routine clinical purposes. Anti-C, anti-c, anti-E and anti-e are occasionally seen and may cause both transfusion reactions and haemolytic disease of the newborn. Anti-d does not exist. Rh haemolytic disease of the newborn is described later in this chapter.

Other blood group systems

Other blood group systems are less frequently of clinical importance. Although naturally occurring antibodies of the P, Lewis and MN system are not uncommon they usually only react at

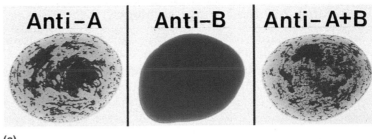

(a)

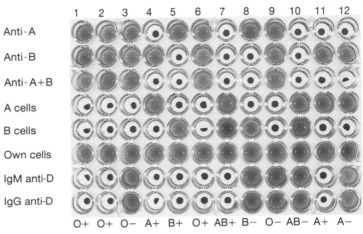

(b)

Fig. 21.2 (a) The ABO grouping in a group A patient. The red cells suspended in saline agglutinate in the presence of anti-A or anti-A+B (serum from a group O patient). (b) Routine grouping in a 96-well microplate. Positive reactions show as sharp agglutinates; in negative reactions the cells are dispersed. Rows 1–3, patient cells against antisera; rows 4–6, patient sera against known cells; rows 7–8, anti-D against patient cells.

low temperatures and hence are of no clinical consequence. Immune antibodies against antigens of these systems are detected infrequently. Many of the antigens are of low antigenicity and others (e.g. Kell), although comparatively immunogenic, are of relatively low frequency and therefore provide few opportunities for iso-immunization except in multiply-transfused patients.

Table 21.3 The Rh system — genotypes.

CDE nomenclature	Short symbol	Caucasian frequency (%)	Rh D status
cde/cde	rr	15	Negative
CDe/cde	R_1r	32	Positive
CDe/CDe	R_1R_1	17	Positive
cDE/cde	R_2r	13	Positive
CDe/cDE	R_1R_2	14	Positive
cDE/cDE	R_2R_2	4	Positive
Other genotypes		5	Positive (almost all)

Techniques in blood group serology

The following techniques are used. They rely on the identification, visually or microscopically, of the agglutination of red cells.

1 *Saline agglutination.* This is important in detecting mainly IgM antibodies, usually at room temperature and 4°C, e.g. anti-A, anti-B (Fig. 21.2). Antibodies are referred to as saline or complete agglutinins.

2 *Addition of colloid*, e.g. albumin, polyvinylpyrrolidone. Both are used to enhance agglutination, usually for IgG antibodies at 37°C.

3 *Proteolytic enzyme treatment of red cells*, e.g. papain (most commonly), bromelin, ficin, trypsin. These can be combined with the indirect antiglobulin test for extra sensitivity or used on their own in a two-stage method.

4 *Low ionic strength saline (LISS).* Incubation times can be shortened and some antibodies may be enhanced by allowing the reaction to occur in low ionic strength conditions. LISS-suspended red cells or LISS additive is now common practice as the demand for group and save procedures, and rapid supply of compatible blood, is increasing. LISS can be combined with polybrene in a manual or automated test to provide rapid but sensitive methods to detect most blood group antibodies.

5 *The antiglobulin (Coombs) test.* This is a fundamental and widely used test in both blood group serology and general immunology. Antihuman globulin (AHG) may be produced in various animals (e.g. rabbits, goats and sheep) following the injection of human globulin, purified complement or specific immunoglobulin (e.g. IgG, IgA or IgM). When AHG is added to human red cells coated with immunoglobulin or complement components, agglutination of the red cells indicates a positive test (Fig. 21.3). Polyspecific antiglobulin reagent, mainly anti-IgG and anti-C3d, is routinely used in either conventional liquid-phase methods, or more recently in solid-phase methods. Mono-specific reagents include anti-IgG, anti-IgM, anti-IgA, anti-C3c, anti-C3d and anti-C4. These are used mainly to investigate auto-immune haemolytic anaemias.

Direct antiglobulin test

This is used for detecting antibody or complement on the red cell surface where sensitization has occurred *in vivo*. The AHG reagent is added to washed red cells and agglutination indicates a positive test.

A positive direct antiglobulin test occurs in the following.

1 Haemolytic disease of the newborn, usually Rh.

2 Autoimmune haemolytic anaemia.

3 Drug-induced immune haemolytic anaemia.

4 Haemolytic transfusion reactions.

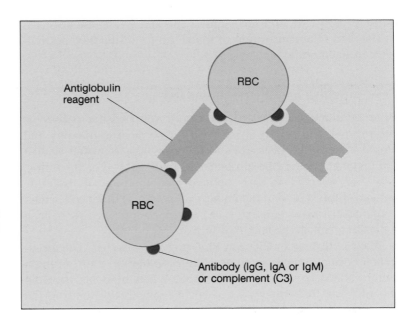

Fig. 21.3 The antiglobulin test for antibody or complement on the surface of red blood cells (RBC). The antihuman globulin (Coombs) reagent may be broad spectrum or specific for IgG, IgM, IgA or complement (C3).

Indirect antiglobulin test

This is used to detect antibodies that have coated the red cells *in vitro*. It is a two-stage procedure: the first step involves the incubation of test red cells with serum; in the second step, the red cells are thoroughly washed with saline to remove free globulins. The AHG reagent is then added to the washed red cells. Agglutination in the test implies that the original serum contained antibody which has coated the red cells *in vitro*. This test is used in the following situations.

1 As part of the routine cross-matching procedure for detecting antibodies in the patient's serum against donor red cells.

2 For detecting atypical blood group antibodies in serum during screening procedures.

3 For detecting blood group antibodies in a pregnant woman.

4 For detecting antibodies in serum in autoimmune haemolytic anaemia.

Most of the above methods were originally developed for tube techniques but 96-well microplates have found favour as costs are reduced and sensitivity enhanced in some situations. U- or V-shaped well methods are employed and the plates can be read manually (Fig. 21.2) or agitated and read using a plate reader.

Specificity of AHG

A broad-spectrum reagent is usually preferred in normal blood transfusion procedures as it detects both antibodies and complement components. Monospecific AHG reagents include anti-IgG, anti-IgM, anti-IgA, anti-C3 and anti-C4. These are used in detailed characterization of blood group antibodies, particularly in haemolytic anaemias.

Cross-matching and pretransfusion tests

Prior to blood transfusion, the blood group of the patient is determined, the serum is screened for atypical antibodies and stored frozen. Red cells from each donor unit are tested against the patient's serum (the cross-match, Table 21.4). For screening, cells are selected to give optimal combinations of desirable antigens represented in the homozygous state. A three-cell screen containing homozygous D, C, E, c, e, Fy^a, Fy^b, JK^a, JK^b and a K-positive cell is the standard format.

   Blood of the same ABO and Rh D group is selected. The cross-match normally takes about 40 minutes in normal ionic strength saline (NISS) or 20 minutes in LISS. When blood is required urgently, the tests may be carried out quickly by limiting the tests performed and modifying the techniques. This reduces test sensitivity but will detect all gross incompatibilities. Transfusion of un-cross-matched blood in emergencies carries considerable risk and should be avoided when possible. When the urgency of a clinical situation does not allow time for grouping the patient, group O Rh-negative blood should be transfused. Two units of group-checked blood are kept for emergency situations.

Donor cells tested against recipient serum and agglutination detected visually or microscopically after mixing and incubation at the appropriate temperature

For detecting clinically significant IgM antibodies
Saline 37°C

For detecting immune antibodies (mainly IgG)
Enzyme-treated red cells at 37°C
Low ionic strength saline at 37°C
Indirect antiglobulin test at 37°C

Table 21.4 Techniques used in compatibility testing.

Complications of blood transfusion (Table 21.5)

Haemolytic transfusion reactions

Haemolytic transfusion reactions may be immediate or delayed. Immediate life-threatening reactions associated with massive intravascular haemolysis are the result of complement-activating antibodies of IgM or IgG classes (e.g. ABO antibodies). The severity of the reaction depends on the recipient's titre of antibody; severe reactions are rare with other antibodies. Reactions associated with extravascular haemolysis (e.g. immune antibodies

Table 21.5 Complications of blood transfusion.

Early	Late

Haemolytic reactions
  Immediate
  Delayed
Reactions due to infected blood
Allergic reactions to white cells,
  platelets or proteins
Pyrogenic reactions (to plasma
  proteins or due to HLA
  antibodies)
Circulatory overload
Air embolism
Thrombophlebitis
Citrate toxicity
Hyperkalaemia
Clotting abnormalities (after massive
  transfusion)
	Transmission of disease, e.g.
	  Virus
	    hepatitis A, B, C and others
	    HIV
	    CMV
	  Bacteria
	    Treponema pallidum
	    Brucella
	    Salmonella
	  Parasites
	    malaria
	    Toxoplasma
	    microfilaria
	Transfusional iron overload
	Immune sensitization, e.g. to Rh
	  D antigen

CMV, cytomegalovirus; HIV, human immunodeficiency virus; HLA, human leucocyte antigen.

of the Rh system which are unable to activate complement) are generally less severe but may still be life-threatening. The cells become coated with IgG and are removed in the reticulo-endothelial (RE) system. In mild cases, the only signs of a transfusion reaction may be a progressive unexplained anaemia with or without jaundice. In some cases where the pretransfusion level of an antibody was too low to be detected in a cross-match, a patient may be reimmunized by transfusion of incompatible red cells and this will lead to a delayed transfusion reaction with accelerated clearance of the red cells. There may be rapid appearance of anaemia with mild jaundice.

Clinical features of a major haemolytic transfusion reaction

1 *Haemolytic shock phase.* This may occur after only a few millilitres of blood have been transfused or up to 1−2 hours after the end of the transfusion. Clinical features include urticaria, pain in the lumbar region, flushing, headache, precordial pain, shortness of breath, vomiting, rigours, pyrexia and a fall in blood pressure. If the patient is anaesthetized this shock phase is masked. There is increasing evidence of blood destruction and haemoglobinuria, jaundice and disseminated intravascular coagulation (DIC) may occur. Moderate leucocytosis, e.g. $15−20 \times 10^9/l$ is usual.

2 *The oliguric phase.* In some patients with a haemolytic reaction there is renal tubular necrosis with acute renal failure.

3 *Diuretic phase.* Fluid and electrolyte imbalance may occur during the recovery from acute renal failure.

Investigation of an immediate transfusion reaction

If a patient develops features suggesting a severe transfusion reaction, the transfusion should be stopped and investigations for blood group incompatibility and bacterial contamination of the blood must be initiated.

1 Most severe reactions occur because of clerical errors in the handling of donor or recipient blood specimens. Therefore it must be established that the identity of the recipient is the same as that stated on the compatibility label and that this corresponds with the actual unit being transfused.

2 The unit of donor blood and post-transfusion samples of the patient's blood should be sent to the 'laboratory' who will:

   (a) repeat the group on pre- and post-transfusion samples and on the donor blood, and repeat the cross-match;

   (b) perform a direct antiglobulin test on the post-transfusion sample;

   (c) check the plasma for haemoglobinaemia;

   (d) perform tests for DIC;

   (e) examine the donor sample directly for evidence of gross bacterial contamination and set up blood cultures from it at 20°C and 37°C.

3 A post-transfusion sample of urine must be examined for haemoglobinuria.

4 Further samples of blood are taken 6 and/or 24 hours after transfusion for a blood count and bilirubin, free haemoglobin and methaemalbumin estimations.

5 In the absence of positive findings, the patient's serum is examined 5–10 days later for red cell or white cell antibodies.

Management of patients with major haemolysis

The principal object of initial therapy is to maintain the blood pressure and renal perfusion. Intravenous dextran, plasma or saline and frusemide are usually given. Hydrocortisone 100 mg intravenously and an antihistamine may help to alleviate shock. In the event of severe shock, support with intravenous adrenaline 1:10 000 in small incremental doses may be required. Further compatible transfusions may be required in severely affected patients. If acute renal failure occurs, this is managed in the usual way, if necessary with dialysis until recovery occurs.

Management of patients with infected blood

Fortunately these reactions are rare. Treatment includes measures to combat shock. Antibiotic therapy, as appropriate, should be commenced as soon as the diagnosis is made and before culture results are known.

Other transfusion reactions

1 *Febrile reactions due to white cell antibodies.* HLA (human leucocyte antigen) antibodies (see below) are usually the result of sensitization by pregnancy or a previous transfusion. They produce rigours, pyrexia and, in severe cases, pulmonary infiltrates. They may be minimized by giving leucocyte-depleted (i.e. filtered) packed cells. Patients with, for example, thalassaemia major, commencing regular transfusions should be given filtered red cells. Leucocyte depletion also reduces the risk of transmission of CMV (cytomegalovirus) and of HLA sensitization.

2 *Febrile or non-febrile non-haemolytic allergic reactions.* These are usually due to hypersensitivity to donor plasma proteins and if severe can result in anaphylactic shock. The clinical features are urticaria, pyrexia and, in severe cases, dyspnoea, facial oedema and rigours. Immediate treatment is with antihistamines and hydrocortisone. Adrenaline is also useful. Washed red cells or frozen red cells may be needed for further transfusions if the majority of plasma-removed blood (e.g. SAG-M, p. 403) causes reactions.

It is not possible to differentiate from the clinical symptoms the cause of many transfusion reactions. Laboratory tests are required and even these may fail to identify the mechanism for many allergic reactions.

3 *Post-transfusion circulatory overload.* The features include those of pulmonary oedema, fullness in the head and dry cough. The management is that of cardiac failure. These reactions are prevented by a slow transfusion of packed red cells or of the blood component required, accompanied by diuretic therapy.

4 *Post-transfusion hepatitis.* This may be due to one of the hepatitis viruses, i.e. types B and C and other types of non-A, non-B, non-C, and occasionally CMV and Epstein−Barr virus (EBV) have been implicated. Post-transfusion hepatitis B is seen less frequently now because of routine HB_SAg (hepatitis B surface antigen) testing of all blood donations. Donors are also tested for antibody to HCV (hepatitis C virus). Most patients developing post-transfusion hepatitis become anti-HCV positive about 3 months post-transfusion. The incidence of anti-HCV positivity is high in haemophiliacs, patients with thalassaemia major, in drug abusers, renal dialysis patients and in patients with chronic post-transfusion hepatitis. It is likely that other, as yet unidentified viruses are also responsible for some cases of non-A, non-B hepatitis.

Transmission of CMV is likely to cause problems in the newborn, bone marrow and renal transplant patients, and post-cardiac by-pass surgery. Transfusion of CMV-negative blood products or leucocyte-depleted blood to CMV-negative recipients reduces the risk.

5 HIV, the cause of AIDS and related syndromes is transmitted both in cellular and plasma components of blood. HIV infection was an unfortunate complication following the transfusion of factor VIII concentrate collected during the late 1970s and early 1980s to haemophiliacs. Heat treatment of plasma concentrates now prevents transmission of HIV. Albumin solutions are pasteurized and intramuscular immunoglobulin preparations are rendered safe from HIV contamination by the manufacturing process. Donor education and encouragement of high-risk groups (homosexuals, bisexuals, intravenous drug abusers, their sexual partners and prostitutes) to self exclude themselves from blood donation has been successful. All blood units taken are tested for anti-HIV by enzyme-linked immunoabsorbent assay (ELISA).

6 *Other infections.* CMV, infectious mononucleosis, toxoplasmosis, malaria and syphilis may all be transmitted by blood transfusion.

7 *Post-transfusional iron overload.* Repeated red cell transfusions over many years, in the absence of blood loss, cause deposition of iron initially in RE tissue at the rate of 200−250 mg/unit (450 ml) of whole blood. After 50 units in adults, and lesser amounts in children, the liver, myocardium and endocrine glands are damaged with clinical consequences. This is a major problem in thalassemia major and other severe chronic refractory anaemias (see Chapter 6).

Bank blood and blood products for transfusion

Donor blood is taken by an aseptic technique into plastic bags containing an appropriate amount of anticoagulant — usually citrate, phosphate, dextrose (CPD). The citrate anticoagulates the blood by combining with the blood calcium. Before issue the following tests are carried out: ABO and Rh D blood groups and antibody screens, serological tests to exclude syphilis, and HB_sAg and anti-HCV tests to exclude hepatitis B and C.

Blood is stored at 4−6°C; many blood transfusion centres now use a red cell preservative fluid containing adenine−CPD which increases red cell storage to 35 days. After the first 48 hours there is a slow progressive K^+ loss from the red cells into the plasma. In cases where infusion of K^+ could be dangerous, fresh blood should be used, e.g. for exchange transfusion in haemolytic disease of the new-born. During red cell storage there is a fall in 2,3-diphosphoglycerate (2,3-DPG) and levels of this glycolytic pathway metabolite are significantly reduced or negligible after 28 days. Following transfusion, 2,3-DPG levels return to normal within 24 hours. The limiting factor in determining blood bank storage of red cells is the ability of the cells to survive normally following transfusion. As the storage time increases, some red cells become spherical due to changes in energy metabolism. This is associated with an increase in red cell rigidity and after a period the cell injury becomes irreversible. If red cells are transfused at the time of maximum storage, up to 20–30% of the red cells may be destroyed within 24 hours, the remainder showing a survival close to normal.

Optimum additive solutions have been developed to increase the shelf life of plasma-depleted red cells by maintaining both ATP and 2,3-DPG levels. Saline, adenine, glucose, mannitol (SAG-M and ADSOL) medium allow red cells to be used up to 35 days after donation.

Blood may be given whole or separated into its components. It is preferable to infuse only the necessary component, e.g. packed red cells for chronically anaemic patients. A scheme for the preparation of blood components is shown in Fig. 21.4.

Whole blood

This is usually reserved for treating acute blood loss, e.g. traumatic or surgical blood loss, or severe gastrointestinal or uterine haemorrhage. For small transfusions following acute blood loss (e.g. up to 2 units in adults) the use of packed cells plus electrolyte solution is often recommended rather than whole blood, in order to conserve plasma for other clinical uses.

Packed red cells

These are the treatment of choice in chronically anaemic patients

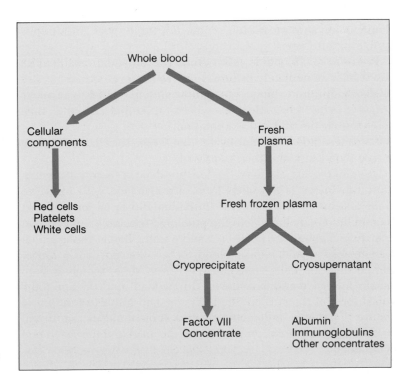

Fig. 21.4 The preparation of blood components from whole blood.

who require transfusion. In older subjects, a diuretic is often
given simultaneously and the infusion should be sufficiently
slow to avoid circulatory overload. In the majority of patients
with deficiency anaemias appropriate therapy with iron, folate
or vitamin B_{12} is sufficient and red cell transfusions are seldom
required. In chronic anaemias which do not respond to haema-
tinics, transfusion should be avoided unless the patient is at risk
from, or incapacitated by, the anaemia. The haemoglobin level
alone is not a good guide to transfusion need in view of the
wide variation in cardiovascular adaptation and shift in the
oxygen-dissociation curve between different individuals and
different types of anaemia. Once regular transfusions have
begun, iron chelation therapy should also be considered in an
attempt to avoid iron overload.

Red cell substitutes

Many types of synthetic oxygen-carrying substitutes are undergoing experimental and clinical investigation. These are fluori-
nated hydrocarbons and stromal-free pyridoxylated and poly-
merized haemoglobin solutions. Further extensive animal and
human trials are necessary before any type of solution can be
considered safe for widespread clinical use.

Autotransfusion

Anxiety over AIDS and other infections has increased the
demand for autotransfusion. There are three ways of administering an autologous transfusion.
1 Pre-deposit—blood is taken from the potential recipient in
the weeks immediately prior to elective surgery.
2 Haemodilution—blood is removed immediately prior to
surgery once the patient has been anaesthetized and then
reinfused at the end of the operation.
3 Salvage—blood lost during the operation is collected during
heavy blood loss and then reinfused.
   The increasing demand is for pre-deposit autotransfusion.
Autotransfusion is the safest form of transfusion with regard to
transmission of disease. The individual involved must be fit
enough to donate blood and the predicted operative replacement
transfusion should be between 2 and 4 units. Larger replacement
transfusions would require blood to be collected over a longer
period and red cells stored in the frozen state, which is both
labour intensive and expensive. Although autotransfusion is the
safest form of transfusion, the high cost and initial restriction of
its use to patients undergoing elective surgery means that it will
benefit only a minor proportion of the total number of blood
recipients.

Granulocyte concentrates

These are prepared as buffy coats or on blood cell separators from normal healthy donors or from patients with chronic myeloid leukaemia. They have been used in patients with severe neutropenia ($<0.5 \times 10^9/l$) who are not responding to antibiotic therapy but it is not usually possible to give sufficient. They may transmit CMV infection.

Platelet concentrates

These are harvested by cell separators or from individual donor units of blood. These concentrates are indicated in severely thrombocytopenic patients with established haemorrhage or prophylactically, e.g. during intensive myelotoxic chemotherapy to keep the platelet count $>5-10 \times 10^9/l$. Their most important use is therefore in the support of patients with severe bone marrow failure, e.g. due to acute leukaemia, aplastic anaemia, myelodysplasia, myelotoxic chemotherapy or bone marrow transplantation. If fever, infection or concurrent coagulopathy is present or the platelet count is falling rapidly or potential bleeding sites, e.g. surgical wounds are present, the platelet count should be kept $>20 \times 10^9/l$. Platelets may also be needed for patients with platelet functional disorders, following massive blood transfusion during cardiopulmonary by-pass surgery with bleeding not due to surgically correctable disorders and for patients with disseminated intravascular coagulation and bleeding. Platelets are not usually used in immune thrombocytopenias but may be given in auto-immune thrombocytopenia with major haemorrhage and in neonatal alloimmune thrombocytopenia. Platelets may be needed as prophylaxis before surgery, e.g. liver biopsy, lumbar puncture, insertion of in-dwelling lines to raise the count to $>50 \times 10^9/l$ (see also p. 331).

Platelets express only HLA class I antigens. HLA antibodies develop only when the RE system is stimulated by both class I and class II antigens, e.g. on leucocytes. Once formed, however, these HLA antibodies may destroy platelets. ABO and Rh-compatible platelets are usually used but HLA-identical platelets are needed for patients with HLA antibodies.

Human plasma preparations

Plasma is a useful volume expander. The risk of hepatitis has been reduced due to the introduction of more sensitive tests for hepatitis B and C. Frozen plasma is usually prepared from single donor units.

Fresh frozen plasma. Rapidly frozen plasma separated from fresh blood is stored at less than −30°C. Its main use is for the replacement of coagulation factors, e.g. when specific concentrates are unavailable or after massive transfusions, in liver disease, DIC or after cardiopulmonary bypass surgery, or to reverse a warfarin effect. It is also indicated in thrombotic thrombocytopenic purpura (TTP) (p. 326).

Human albumin solution (4.5%)

This contains human albumin and is free from risk. Its main use is in the treatment of shock. It is recommended as the main general purpose plasma volume expander, where a sustained osmotic effect is required prior to the administration of blood. It is also used for plasma replacement in patients undergoing plasmapheresis and sometimes for protein replacement in selected patients with hypoalbuminaemia.

Human albumin solution (20%) (salt-poor albumin)

This expensive purified preparation is not recommended as a general plasma volume expander although its usefulness for this purpose is undoubted. It may be used in severe hypoalbuminaemia when it is necessary to use a product with minimal electrolyte content. Principal indications for its use are patients with the nephrotic syndrome or liver failure.

Cryoprecipitate

This is obtained by thawing fresh frozen plasma at 4°C and contains concentrated factor VIII and fibrinogen. It is stored at less than −30°C or, if lyophylized, at 4−6°C, and was used widely as replacement therapy in haemophilia A and von Willebrand's disease before more purified preparations of factor VIII became available.

Freeze-dried factor VIII concentrates

These are also used for treating haemophilia A or von Willebrand's disease. The small volume makes them ideal for children, surgical cases, patients at risk from circulatory overload and for those on home treatment.

Freeze-dried factor IX — prothrombin complex concentrates

A number of preparations are available which contain variable amounts of factors II, VII, IX and X. They are mainly used for treating factor IX deficiency (Christmas disease) but are also used occasionally in patients with liver disease or in life-threatening haemorrhage following overdose with oral anticoagulants or in patients with factor VIII inhibitors. There is a risk of thrombosis.

Immunoglobulin

Pooled immunoglobulin is a valuable source of antibodies against common viruses. It is used in hypogammaglobulinaemia for protection against viral and bacterial disease. It may also be used in immune thrombocytopenia and other acquired immune disorders, e.g. post-transfusion purpura, alloimmune neonatal thrombocytopenia.

Specific immunoglobulin
This may be obtained from donors with high titres of antibody, e.g. anti-Rh D, anti-hepatitis B, anti-herpes zoster, anti-rubella.

Acute blood loss

This is the commonest indication for whole blood transfusion. As mentioned on p. 25, until 3−4 hours after a single episode of blood loss, the haemoglobin and PCV (packed cell volume) remain normal, since there is initial vasoconstriction with a reduction in total blood volume. After 3−4 hours, however, the plasma volume begins to expand and the haemoglobin and PCV fall and there is a rise in neutrophils and platelets. The reticulocyte response begins on the second or third day and reaches a maximum of 10−15%, lasting 8−10 days. The haemoglobin begins to rise by about the seventh day but, if iron stores have become depleted, the haemoglobin may not rise subsequently to normal. Clinical assessment is needed to gauge whether blood transfusion is needed, but this is usually unnecessary in adults with losses of 500 ml or less unless haemorrhage is continuing. Blood transfusion is not without risks and should not be undertaken lightly. The problems of massive blood loss and massive transfusion are considered on p. 348.

Haemolytic disease of the newborn

Haemolytic disease of the newborn (HDN) is the result of the passage of IgG antibodies from the maternal circulation across the placenta into the circulation of the foetus where they react with foetal red cells and mediate destruction by the foetal RE system.

Before 1967 and the introduction of prophylactic use of IgG, anti-D Rh HDN was responsible for about 800 stillbirths and neonatal deaths each year in the UK. Anti-D was responsible for 94% of Rh HDN; other cases were usually due to anti-c and anti-E, with a wide range of antibodies found in occasional cases (for examples see Table 21.1). The incidence of Rh HDN is now dramatically lower and the proportion of cases due to anti-c and anti-E has increased substantially.

The most frequent causes of HDN are now immune antibodies of the ABO blood group system — most commonly anti-A produced by a group O mother against a group A foetus. However, this form of HDN is usually mild. Occasional cases of HDN are caused by antibodies of other blood group systems, e.g. anti-Kell.

Rh HDN

Pathogenesis

A Rh D-negative (Rh d/d or rr) woman has a pregnancy with a Rh D-positive foetus. Rh D-positive foetal red cells cross into the maternal circulation (usually at parturition) and sensitize the mother to form anti-D. Sensitization is more likely if the mother and foetus are ABO compatible. The mother could also be sensitized by a previous miscarriage, amniocentesis or other trauma to the placenta or by blood transfusion.

Anti-D crosses the placenta to the foetus during the next pregnancy with a Rh D-positive foetus, coats the foetal red cells with antibody and results in RE system destruction of these cells, causing anaemia and jaundice. If the father is heterozygous for D antigen (D/d) there is a 50% probability that the foetus will be D positive.

Clinical features

1 *Severe disease*: intrauterine death from hydrops foetalis.
2 *Moderate disease*: the baby is born with severe anaemia and jaundice and may show pallor, tachycardia, oedema and hepato-splenomegaly. When the unconjugated bilirubin level exceeds 250 μmol/l, bile pigment deposition in the basal ganglia may lead to kernicterus — central nervous system damage with generalized spasticity and possible subsequent mental deficiency, deafness and epilepsy. This problem becomes acute after birth as maternal clearance of foetal bilirubin ceases and conjugation of bilirubin by the neonatal liver has to be induced to reach full activity.
3 *Mild disease*: mild anaemia with or without jaundice.

Laboratory findings at birth

1 *Cord blood.* Variable anaemia (haemoglobin <16/dl) with a high reticulocyte count; the baby is Rh D positive, the direct antiglobulin test is positive and the serum bilirubin raised. In moderate and severe cases many erythroblasts are seen in the blood film (Fig. 21.5) — erythroblastosis foetalis.

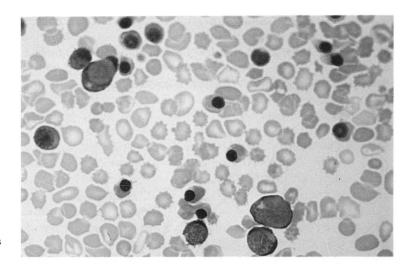

Fig. 21.5 Rh haemolytic disease of the newborn (erythroblastosis foetalis): peripheral blood film showing large numbers of erythroblasts and microspherocytes.

2 *The mother is Rh D negative* with a high plasma level of anti-D.

Treatment

Exchange transfusion may be necessary; the indications for this include:

1 *Clinical features*: obvious pallor, jaundice and signs of heart failure.

2 *Laboratory findings*: haemoglobin <14.0 g/dl with a positive direct antiglobulin test; a cord serum bilirubin >60 μmol/l or infant serum bilirubin >300 μmol/l or bilirubin level rising rapidly and positive antiglobulin test. Premature babies are more liable to kernicterus and should be exchange transfused at lower bilirubin levels (e.g. >200 μmol/l).

In infants with moderate disease, more than one exchange transfusion may be required. Exchange transfusions performed soon after birth are used to replace the infant's red cells and reduce the rate of bilirubin rise. Subsequent exchange transfusions may be required to remove unconjugated bilirubin. The procedure of removing and replacing one equivalent blood volume will remove 60% of the pre-existing constituents in the blood. The blood for the exchange transfusion should be <7 days old Rh D negative and ABO compatible with the baby and with the mother's serum by cross-match. Normally, 500 ml is sufficient for each exchange. Phototherapy (exposure of the infant to bright light of appropriate wavelength) has been used to photodegrade the bilirubin to permit urinary excretion, thus reducing the likelihood of kernicterus.

Management of pregnant women

1 At the time of booking all pregnant women should have their

ABO and Rh group determined and serum screened for antibodies at least twice during the pregnancy. Rh D-negative women
should have serum rechecked for antibodies in each trimester
(e.g. at initial presentation, 28 weeks and 36 weeks). If antibodies
are detected, they should be identified and quantitated at regular
intervals (e.g. 2–3-weekly, and more often in late pregnancy or
if antibody levels are rising or high). The strength of anti-D
present in maternal serum is related to the clinical severity of
HDN but this is also affected by such factors as the IgG subclass,
rate of rise of antibody and past history. As a rough guide levels
below 1.0 i.u./ml (0.2 μg/ml) require no action. A level of
10 i.u./ml (2.0 μg/ml) usually reflects a seriously affected infant
as does a level of 5 i.u./ml (1.0 μg/ml) which is rising rapidly.
These latter two situations and any history of a previously affected infant are indications for amniocentesis.

Other antibodies are monitored by serological titration using
the antiglobulin method. As a rough guide, titres in excess of
1/20 involving anti-c or anti-Kell are causes for concern.

2 The severity of the haemolytic disease can be assessed by
spectroscopic estimation of bile pigment derivatives in the
amniotic fluid obtained by amniocentesis. If this shows severe
haemolysis the foetus can be kept alive by intrauterine transfusion of fresh (<7 days old) Rh D-negative blood after 24 weeks
and by premature delivery after 35 weeks.

3 Suitable fresh blood should be available at the time of
induction in preparation for exchange transfusion.

4 At birth, the babies of Rh D-negative women who do not have
antibodies must have their cord blood grouped for ABO and
Rh. If the baby's blood is Rh D negative the mother will require
no further treatment. If the baby is Rh D positive, prophylactic
anti-D should be administered.

5 *Prevention of Rh immunization.* Passively administered IgG
anti-D suppresses primary immunization in the majority of Rh

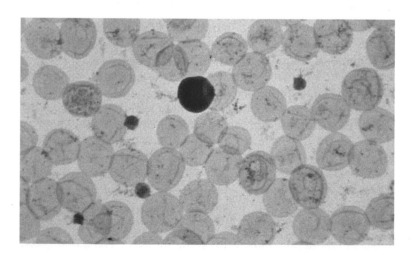

Fig. 21.6 Kleihauer test for
foetal red cells; a deeply
eosin-staining cell containing
foetal haemoglobin is seen at
the centre. Haemoglobin has
been eluted from the other red
cells by an incubation at acid
pH and these appear as
colourless ghosts.

D-negative women. Anti-D is now given to every Rh D-negative woman giving birth to an Rh D-positive child providing the woman has not been previously sensitized. The routine dose is 500 i.u. intramuscularly within 72 hours of delivery.

A Kleihauer test may be performed to estimate the severity of the foeto-maternal bleed. This uses differential staining to estimate the number of foetal cells in the maternal circulation (Fig. 21.6). The chance of developing antibodies is related to the number of foetal cells found. The dose of anti-D is increased if the Kleihauer test shows greater than 4 ml transplacental haemorrhage. To women having an abortion at under 20 weeks of pregnancy, 250 i.u. anti-D is given and, in those after 20 weeks, the usual dose of 500 i.u. is given. Similar treatment should also be given in threatened abortion and in the case of amniocentesis performed on Rh D-negative women. Some national variation exists in the size of doses employed, and depends partly on the availability of therapeutic anti-D.

ABO haemolytic disease of the newborn

In 20% of births, a mother is ABO incompatible with the foetus. Group A and group B mothers usually have only IgM ABO antibodies. The majority of cases of ABO HDN are caused by 'immune' IgG antibodies in group O mothers. Although 15% of pregnancies in Caucasians involve a group O mother with a group A or group B foetus, most mothers do not produce IgG anti-A or anti-B and very few babies have severe enough haemolytic disease to require treatment. Exchange transfusions are needed in only one in 3000 infants. The mildness of ABO HDN is partly explained by the A and B antigens not being fully developed at birth and by partial neutralization of maternal IgG antibodies by A and B antigens on other cells, in the plasma and tissue fluids.

In contrast to Rh HDN, ABO disease may be found in the first pregnancy and may or may not affect subsequent pregnancies. The direct antiglobulin test on the infant's cells may be negative or only weakly positive. Examination of the blood film shows autoagglutination and spherocytosis, polychromasia and erythroblastosis.

The human leucocyte antigen system

The short arm of chromosome 6 contains a cluster of genes known as the major histocompatibility complex (MHC) or the HLA region (Fig. 21.7). Among the genes in this region are those that determine the structure of the HLA antigens. These are present on the membrane surface of most nucleated cells, and are known to play a major role in transplant rejection as well as being involved in many aspects of immune recognition and

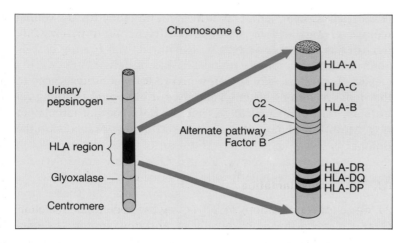

Fig. 21.7 The human leucocyte antigen (HLA) gene complex. HLA-A, -B and -C antigens are termed class I and HLA-D antigens (now divided into DP, DQ and DR) are termed class II.

reaction (see p. 165). It is now known that this region codes not only for the HLA antigens, but also for several components of the complement cascade. The gene cluster is adjacent to the loci occupied by the genes for several enzymes and this information has been used in gene mapping studies.

There are two classes of HLA antigens (Table 21.6). Class I antigens comprise two polypeptides, the larger of which is encoded by the genes on the MHC locus. The small component is a β_2-microglobulin which is encoded outside this region. Class II antigens comprise α- and β-chains both encoded by genes in the MHC locus.

The class I antigens (HLA-A, -B and -C) are usually detected on peripheral blood lymphocytes by serological tests. They may also be detected by a two-stage lymphocytotoxicity test. Mixed lymphocyte culture (MLC) is used to assess compatibility between bone marrow donor and recipient of class II (DR, DQ and DP) antigens which can also be detected serologically.

Use of RFLP (restriction fragment length polymorphism) analysis (see p. 116) and other molecular techniques reveal

Table 21.6 The human leucocyte antigens.

	Class I	Class II
Antigens	HLA-A, -B, -C	HLA-DR, -DP, -DQ
Distribution	All nucleated cells, platelets	B lymphocytes Monocytes Macrophages Activated T cells
Structure	Large polypeptide chain (MHC coded) and a β_2-microglobulin	Two polypeptide chains (α and β) both MHC coded
Interacts with	CD8 lymphocytes	CD4 lymphocytes Mixed lymphocyte reaction

MHC, major histocompatibility complex.

additional heterogeneity both inside and outside the coding regions of the HLA region and are being used to establish donor–recipient compatibility.

The inheritance of the four loci (HLA-A, -B, -C and -DR) is closely linked, one set of loci is inherited from each parent so that there is approximately a one in four chance of two siblings having identical HLA antigens (see Fig. 7.5). Crossing-over of genes during meiosis accounts for occasional unexpected disparities.

HLA and transplantation

An important application of HLA typing has been in the selection of donor–recipient pairs for renal and bone marrow transplantation. The severity of immunological rejection is influenced by the degree of compatibility between the tissue of the donor and the recipient.

The HLA matching required for successful bone marrow transplantation is fairly rigid, for added to the problems of acute graft rejection are those of graft-vs-host disease (GVHD) (see p. 137). Even when the marrow donor is an HLA-A, -B and -DR identical sibling to the recipient and there is no reactivity in the MLC test, GVHD may still occur. This may be due to histocompatibility systems not tested. Poorer results with unrelated donors, however well-matched, probably reflect genetic differences which are inaccessible to present typing techniques.

HLA and blood transfusion

Since the HLA-A, -B and -C antigens are carried by leucocytes and platelets, each transfusion of whole blood, platelet or leucocyte concentrate carries the risk of immunizing the patient to these antigens; immunization may also follow pregnancy. Immunization against HLA antigens may cause febrile, non-haemolytic transfusion reactions (see p. 401). These may be minimized by removing with filters most of the white cells and platelets from the red cells prior to transfusion. Immunization may also result in failure of patients to respond to transfusion of platelet concentrates with the expected rise in platelet count. Once immunization has occurred, concentrates should be prepared from HLA-identical or compatible donors using, if necessary, cell separators.

HLA and disease

Since the initial report in 1973 that 96% of patients suffering from ankylosing spondylitis carry the HLA-B27 antigen, more than 100 diseases have been shown to have an association with HLA. Some of the most important associations are shown in

Disease	HLA*
Rheumatoid arthritis	DR4
Ankylosing spondylitis	B27
Juvenile diabetes	DR3 or DR4
Narcolepsy	DR2
Other diseases	
Graves' disease	DR3
Myasthenia gravis	DR3
Multiple sclerosis	DR2
Psoriasis	CW6
Coeliac disease	DR3
Haemochromatosis	A3

Table 21.7 Some human leucocyte antigens and disease associations (from Bodmer, 1987b).

* The listed antigens are those with the strongest disease association.

Table 21.7. They clearly relate to the central role of the HLA gene complex and immunological responsiveness, and imply that HLA type is relevant to susceptibility or resistance to specific diseases. Recently HLA type has been shown to be relevant to susceptibility to death from cerebral malaria.

Other human leucocyte antigens

Human leucocytes carry a variety of antigens that are recognized by both monoclonal and polyclonal antibodies. These various antigens are listed in Appendix 2, p. 417. The use of antibodies to these CD antigens to define normal and malignant haemopoietic cell populations has been described in previous chapters.

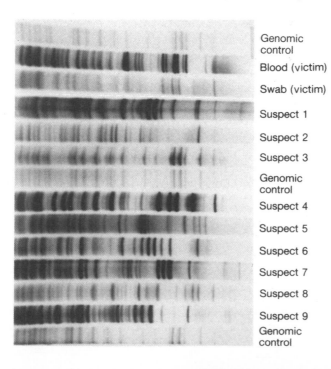

Genomic control
Blood (victim)
Swab (victim)
Suspect 1
Suspect 2
Suspect 3
Genomic control
Suspect 4
Suspect 5
Suspect 6
Suspect 7
Suspect 8
Suspect 9
Genomic control

Fig. 21.8 DNA fingerprints (Southern blotting) from a semen-contaminated vaginal swab and the blood of a murder victim compared with DNA from the blood of nine males suspected of committing the crime. The profile of the swab matches the blood profile from suspect 4. The three genomic controls are control samples for the gel. The bands are autoradiographs after use of a radioactive DNA probe. (Courtesy of Dr Stephen Cordiner.)

DNA fingerprinting

Chromosomes contain areas known as hypervariable random repeat DNA — long stretches where a simple pattern of 10–40 bases is repeated up to hundreds of times. The technique of fingerprinting relies on the use of DNA probes to detect sequences of bases in one of the families of these repetitive sequences. DNA from human cells is cut with a restriction enzyme which recognizes a 4-base sequence within the repetitive sequence. The fragments produced are separated by agarose gel electrophoresis and analysed by Southern blotting (Fig. 21.8) or PCR methods. These techniques provide patterns unique to the individual, except for monozygotic twins who are, of course, genetically identical.

DNA fingerprinting is particularly useful in paternity testing and in the examination of cellular material during forensic investigation. In the latter, genetic identity may be established from small quantities of blood (either fresh or from stains many years old), skin, hair roots and semen.

Bibliography

Bodmer W.F. (1987a) HLA, immune response and disease. In *Human Genetics* (eds F. Vogel & K. Sperling). Springer-Verlag, Berlin, pp. 107–113.

Bodmer W.F. (1987b) The HLA system: structure and function. *Journal of Clinical Pathology*, **40**, 948–958.

British Committee for Standards in Haematology, Working Party of the Blood Transfusion Task Force (1992) Guidelines for platelet transfusions. *Transfusion Medicine*, **2**, 311–318.

Contreras M. (ed.) (1990a) *The ABC of Transfusion*. British Medical Journal, London.

Contreras M. (ed.) (1990b) Blood transfusion: the impact of new technologies. *Clinical Haematology*, **3**, 219–478.

Hann I.M., Gibson B.E.S. & Letsky E.A. (eds) (1991) *Fetal and Neonatal Haematology*. Baillière Tindall, London.

Issitt P. (1993) *Applied Blood Group Serology*, 3rd Edition. Montgomery Scientific, Miami, Florida.

Mollison P.L., Engelfriet C.P. & Contreras M. (1993) *Blood Transfusion in Clinical Medicine*, 9th Edition. Blackwell Scientific Publications, Oxford.

Petz L.D. & Swisher S.N. (eds) (1989) *Clinical Practice of Transfusion Medicine*, 2nd Edition. Churchill Livingstone, Edinburgh.

Roisi E.C., Simon T.L. & Moss G.S. (eds) (1991) *Principles of Transfusion Medicine*, 2nd Edition. Williams & Watkins, Baltimore.

Rosse W.F. (1990) *Clinical Immunohaematology: Basic Concepts and Clinical Applications*. Blackwell Scientific Publications, Boston.

Taswell H.F. & Pureda A.A. (eds) (1991) *Autologous Transfusion and Hematology*. Blackwell Scientific Publications, Oxford.

Tiercy J.M., Jeannet M. & Mach B. (1990) A new approach for the analysis of HLA Class II polymorphisms: HLA oligotyping. *Blood Reviews*, **4**, 9–15.

Turgeon M.L. (1989) *Fundamentals of Immunohematology — Theory and Technique*. Lea & Febiger, Philadelphia.

Von dem Borne A.E.G.Kr. (ed.) (1991) Molecular immunohaematology. *Clinical Haematology*, **4**, 793–1014.

Widman F.K. (1991) *Standards for Blood Banks and Transfusion Services*, 14th Edition. American Association of Blood Banks, Arlington, Virginia.

Appendix 1
Recognized HLA Specificities

A	B		C	D	DR	DQ	DP
A1	B5	B50(21)	Cw1	Dw1	DR1	DQ1	DPw1
A2	B7	B51(5)	Cw2	Dw2	DR103	DQ2	DPw2
A203	B703	B5102	Cw3	Dw3	DR2	DQ3	DPw3
A210	B8	B5103	Cw4	Dw4	DR3	DQ4	DPw4
A3	B12	B52(5)	Cw5	Dw5	DR4	DQ5(1)	DPw5
A9	B13	B53	Cw6	Dw6	DR5	DQ6(1)	DPw6
A10	B14	B54(22)	Cw7	Dw7	DR6	DQ7(3)	
A11	B15	B55(22)	Cw8	Dw8	DR7	DQ8(3)	
A19	B16	B56(22)	Cw9(w3)	Dw9	DR8	DQ9(3)	
A23(9)	B17	B57(17)	Cw10(w3)	Dw10	DR9		
A24(9)	B18	B58(17)		Dw11(w7)	DR10		
A2403	B21	B59		Dw12	DR11(5)		
A25(10)	B22	B60(40)		Dw13	DR12(5)		
A26(10)	B27	B61(40)		Dw14	DR13(6)		
A28	B35	B62(15)		Dw15	DR14(6)		
A29(19)	B37	B63(15)		Dw16	DR1403		
A30(19)	B38(16)	B64(14)		Dw17(w7)	DR1404		
A31(19)	B39(16)	B65(14)		Dw18(w6)	DR15(2)		
A32(19)	B3901	B67		Dw19(w6)	DR16(2)		
A33(19)	B3902	B70		Dw20	DR17(3)		
A34(10)	B40	B71(70)		Dw21	DR18(3)		
A36	B4005	B72(70)		Dw22			
A43	B41	B73		Dw23	DR51		
A66(10)	B42	B75(15)					
A68(28)	B44(12)	B76(15)		Dw24	DR52		
A69(28)	B45(12)	B77(15)		Dw25			
A74(19)	B46	B7801		Dw26	DR53		
	B47						
	B48	Bw4					
	B49(21)	Bw6					

Established specificities are denoted by a number; and those not fully confirmed are prefixed by a 'w' (workshop). More restricted specificities are included in a broader group ('splits') shown in parentheses following the firmer specificity. Antigens Bw4 and Bw6 are very broad ('public') and include splits which have been further subdivided. Extracted from Bodmer J.G. *et. al.* (1992) Nomenclature for Factors of the HLA System 1991, *European Journal of Immunogenetics*, **19**, 35–120; *Immunogenetics*, **36**, 135–148; *Tissue Antigens*, **39**, 161–173.

Appendix 2
Principal Features of Known Cluster Differentiation (CD) Molecules

Cluster	Main cellular distribution	Comments/function/diagnostic value
CD1a	Thymocytes, dendritic cells	Ligand for some $\gamma\,\delta$ T cells
CD1b	Thymocytes, dendritic cells	Ligand for some $\gamma\,\delta$ T cells
CD1c	Thymocytes, dendritic cells	Ligand for some $\gamma\,\delta$ T cells
CD2	Pan T cell, NK cells	SRBC receptor, adhesion (LFA-2) binds LFA-3
CD3	Pan T cell	Signal transdution from the T-cell receptor
CD4	T helper subset	Adhesion (binds class II MHC)
CD5	Pan T cell, B-cell subset	B-CLL expresses
CD6	Subset of T cells	
CD7	Subset of T cells	
CD8	T-suppressor cell	Adhesion (binds class I MHC),
CD9	Pre-B cells, monocytes, platelets	
CD10	Precursor B and some mature B cells	Expressed in c-ALL, kidney, intestine, neural tissue
CD11a	Leucocytes	Adhesion (combines with CD18 to form LFA-1 integrin)
CD11b	Granulocytes, monocytes, NK cells	Adhesion (combines with CD18 to form Mac-I integrin)
CD11c	Granulocytes, monocytes, NK cells	Adhesion (combines with CD18 to form P.150.95 integrin)
CD12	Monocytes, granulocytes	
CD13	Monocytes, granulocytes	
CD14	Monocytes	
CD15	Granulocytes	x hapten (carbohydrate epitope)
CD16	NK cells, granulocytes, macrophages	FcR III
CD17	Granulocytes, monocytes, platelets	
CD18	Leucocytes	Adhesion (β chain of LFA-1 integrin family)
CD19	B cells	
CD20	B cells	
CD21	Mature B cells	C3dR, receptor for EBV
CD22	B cells	
CD23	Activated B cells, macrophages, FDC	IgE$-$FcR
CD24	B cells, granulocytes	
CD25	Activated T cells, B cells, macrophages	IL-2 receptor
CD26	Activated T cells, B cells, macrophages	
CD27	T cells, plasma cells	
CD28	T cells	
CD29	Broad	Adhesion (VLA-integrin β chain) associates with CDw49
CD30	Activated T and B cells	Reed$-$Sternberg cells express; Ki detects
CD31	Monocytes, platelets, B cells, endothelium	GPIIa
CDw32	Monocytes, platelets	FcR II (receptor for aggregated Ig)
CD33	Monocytes, myeloid progenitors	
CD34	Precursors of haemopoietic cells	Marrow progenitors
CD35	Granulocytes, monocytes, B cells	C3b receptor

CD36	Monocytes, platelets	Platelet GPIIIb
CD37	Pan-B, some T cells, FDC	
CD38	Thymocytes, activated T cells, plasma cells	Plasma cell tumours
CD39	B cells	
CD40	B cells	
CD41	Platelets	Platelet GPIIb (forms complex with GPIIIa=CD61)
CD42a&b	Platelets	Form GPIb (platelet adhesion to von Willebrand factor)
CD43	Leucocytes	
CD44	Leucocytes, erythrocytes	
CD45	Leucocytes	Leucocyte common antigen (LCA)
CD46	Leucocytes, epithelial cells, fibroblasts	Regulates complement activation
CD47	Broad	
CD48	Leucocytes	Adhesion (associates with CD29 to form VLA-1)
CDw49a	T cells, monocytes, platelets	Adhesion (associates with CD29 to form VLA-2)
CDw49b	Platelets, cultured T cells	
CDw49c	Leucocytes	Adhesion (associates with CD29 to form VLA-3)
CDw49d	T cells, monocytes, B cells	Adhesion (associates with CD29 to form VLA-4)
CDw49e	T cells, monocytes, some B cells	Adhesion (associates with CD29 to form VLA-5)
CDw49f	Platelets, megakaryocytes, activated T cells	Adhesion (associates with CD29 to form VLA-6
CDw50	Leucocytes	
CD51	Platelets	α chain of vitronectin receptor, adhesion (associates with CD61)
CDw52	Leucocytes	
CD53	Leucocytes, plasma cells	
CD54	Broad	Adhesion (ICAM-1 ligand for LFA-1)
CD55	Broad	Decay acceleration factor (DAF)
CD56	NK cells, activated lymphocytes	
CD57	NK cells, subset of T cells	
CD58	Leucocytes, epithelial cells	Adhesion (LFA-3) ligand for CD2
CD59	Broad	Membrane inhibitor of reactive lysis (MIRL)
CDw60	T subset, platelets	
CD61	Platelets, megakaryocytes	Adhesion (associates with CD51 to form GPIIIa)
CD62	Activated platelets, megakaryocytes, endothelial cells	Neutrophil, monocyte adhesion to endothelium, platelets
CD63	Activated platelets, monocytes	
CD64	Monocytes, macrophages	FcR I (high-affinity Fcγ receptor)
CDw65	Granulocytes	
CD66	Granulocytes	
CD67	Granulocytes	
CD68	Monocytes, macrophages	
CD69	Activated B, T cells, macrophages, NK cells	
CDw70	Activated B, T cells	
CD71	Proliferating cells	Transferrin receptor
CD72	B cells	
CD73	B subset, T subset	Ecto 5'-nucleotidase
CD74	B cells, monocytes	Class II, MHC invariant (γ) chain
CDw75	Mature B cells	
CD76	Mature B cells,	
CD77	Follicular centre, B cells	
CDw78	B cells	

B-CLL, B-chronic lymphocytic leukaemia; c-ALL, common (CD10+) acute lymphoblastic leukaemia; CD, cluster differentiation; C3dR, complement 3d receptor; EBV, Epstein–Barr virus; FcR, immunoglobulin Fc fragment receptor; FDC, follicular dendritic cell; GP, glycoprotein; ICAM, intercellular adhesion molecule; Ig, immunoglobulin; IL, interleukin; Ki, antibody to CD30; LFA, leucocyte function-associated antigen; Mac-I, integrin molecule; MHC, major histocompatibility complex; NK, natural killer; SRBC, sheep red cell receptor; VLA, very late antigens; w, workshop. (Footnote continued on p. 419.)

Appendix 3
Normal Values

	Males	Females	Males and females
Haemoglobin	13.5–17.5 g/dl	11.5–15.5 g/dl	
Red cells (erythrocytes)	4.5–6.5 × 10^{12}/l	3.9–5.6 × 10^{12}/l	
PCV (haematocrit)	40–52%	36–48%	
MCV			80–95 fl
MCH			27–34 pg
MCHC			20–35 g/dl
White cells (leucocytes)			
total			4.0–11.0 × 10^9/l
neutrophils			2.5–7.5 × 10^9/l
lymphocytes			1.5–3.5 × 10^9/l
monocytes			0.2–0.8 × 10^9/l
eosinophils			0.04–0.44 × 10^9/l
basophils			0.01–0.1 × 10^9/l
Platelets			150–400 × 10^9/l
Red cells mass	30±5 ml/kg	25±5 ml/kg	
Plasma volume	45±5 ml/kg	45±5 ml/kg	
Serum iron			10–30 µmol/l
Total iron-binding capacity			40–75 µmol/l (2.0–4.0 g/l as transferrin)
Serum ferritin*	40–340 µg/l	14–150 µg/l	
Serum vitamin B$_{12}$*			160–925 ng/l
Serum folate*			3.0–15.0 µg/l
Red cell folate*			160–640 µg/l

* Normal ranges differ with different commercial kits.
MCH, mean corpuscular haemoglobin; MCHC, mean corpuscular haemoglobin concentration; MCV, mean corpuscular volume; PCV, packed cell volume.

Footnote to Appendix 2 contd. For an updated CD list up to CD$_w$ 130 see Schlossman *et al.* (1994) CD antigens 1993. *Blood* , **83**, 879–880; and Pinto, A. *et al.* (1994) New molecules burst at the leucocyte surface; a comprehensive review based on the Fifth International Workshop on Leucocyte Differentiation Antigens, Boston, USA, 3–7 November 1993. *Leukaemia*, **8**, 347–358.

Glossary of
Molecular Genetics

Written in conjunction with
Professor Lucio Luzzatto

alleles Alternative forms of the gene found at a particular locus (e.g. β^A, β^S, β^E, β^{thal}, etc.). There may be many different alleles in a population, but two at the most in one individual.

amplification Production of additional copies of a particular DNA sequence, which may be extrachromosomal or become integrated in a chromosome.

anticodon A triplet of nucleotides in a special position in the structure of tRNA that is complementary to the codon(s) in mRNA to which that tRNA binds.

base pair (bp) A partnership of A with T or of C with G in a DNA double helix; in RNA, A pairs with U.

cell-specific genes Genes coding for proteins involved in specialized functions and synthesized sometimes in large amounts in particular cells types. Also sometimes referred to as luxury genes.

cDNA A single-stranded DNA molecule complementary to an RNA molecule; usually synthesized from it *in vitro* by the use of the enzyme reverse transcriptase.

cDNA clone A molecular clone in which a cDNA has been copied from a molecule of mature mRNA. It may differ from a *genomic clone* (q.v.) corresponding to the same region, because of the processing that takes place in the pathway from the primary transcript to mature mRNA.

chromosome walking The sequential isolation of clones carrying overlapping sequences of DNA to span large regions of the chromosome (often in order to reach a particular locus).

***cis*-acting** A DNA sequence that affects the expression of a gene on the same chromosome but not on the homologous chromosome.

clone, cellular The progeny of a single cell. Cells belonging to the same clone are often referred to as a *monoclonal population*. Because a neoplastic growth is mostly monoclonal, the two terms are often regarded as synonymous. This is not the case; for instance, all the cells proceeding from a single haemopoietic stem cell are a normal clone; all the cells proceeding from the proliferation of a single antibody-producing lymphocyte are also a normal clone. An individual is a clone of her/his mother's egg fertilized by her/his father's sperm cell.

clone, molecular A large number of identical DNA molecules.

The term is most commonly used to describe a sequence (for instance a gene or a portion of a gene) obtained by recombinant DNA methods. In this case the large number of identical DNA molecules is obtained by growing up a culture from a single bacterial cell or from a single bacteriophage containing that molecule. Hence a molecular clone is derived from a cellular clone.

codon A triplet of nucleotides that specifies an amino acid or a termination signal.

consensus sequence This is an idealized DNA sequence serving a particular function in which each position represents the base most often found when many actual sequences are compared.

degeneracy In the genetic code, this refers to the fact that several codons specify the same amino acid. Therefore, certain mutations in a gene may not affect the respective amino acid in the protein encoded.

deletion This constitutes removal of a sequence of DNA, the regions on either side being joined together.

domain A discrete continuous part of the amino acid sequence of a protein to which a particular function can be attributed.

dominant Allele which determines the phenotye displayed in a heterozygote, the other allele being recessive.

enhancer A DNA sequence that increases the expression of a gene in *cis*-configuration. It can function in many locations, upstream or downstream, relative to the promoter.

eukaryocytes More complex organisms, e.g. fungi, plants, animals. Eukaryocyte cells have a nucleus.

exon A segment of an interrupted gene present in its respective messenger RNA (mRNA).

footprinting A technique for identifying the site on DNA to which some protein binds, based on the protection exerted by the protein against attack by nucleases in this region.

gene The unit of inheritance. In biochemical terms, a gene specifies the structure of a polypeptide chain, or protein, which can be regarded as its product. In molecular terms, the gene is a stretch of DNA that is transcribed in one block, and therefore it can be regarded usually as a *transcription unit*.

genetic code The dictionary whereby a certain triplet of bases, called a *codon*, calls for a particular amino acid during the process of *translation*. Because in many cases several triplets call for the same amino acid, the genetic code is said to be *degenerate*.

genomic clone A molecular clone consisting of a portion of cellular DNA (as opposed to cDNA).

genotype The genetic constitution of an individual. With respect to a particular locus, the two genes present at that locus in that individual (for instance, β^A/β^S is the genotype, at the β-globin locus on chromosome 11 of a person with sickle cell trait).

haplotype A set of closely linked allelic genes or sites within a short region of one chromosome. Because they are closely linked they are almost invariably inherited as a single block. Examples are antigenic determinants of the Rh (rhesus) system, such as cDe; HLA genes, such as A10-B12; or numerous restriction sites in and around a globin gene or any other gene.

heterozygote An individual with two different alleles on homologous chromosomes at a particular locus.

housekeeping genes Genes expressed in all cells because they provide basic functions needed for sustenance of essential functions, such as cell structure, cell division and intermediary metabolism.

hybridization The pairing of complementary RNA or DNA strands to give an RNA–DNA hybrid or a DNA duplex.

intron A segment of DNA that is transcribed, but is removed from within the primary transcript by splicing together the sequences (exons) on either side of it.

kb Abbreviation for 1000 base pairs of DNA or 1000 bases of RNA.

leader The non-translated sequence at the 5′ end of mRNA that precedes the initiation codon.

library A set of cloned DNA fragments representing together the entire genome, or a portion thereof, or a population of RNA molecules. It is important to distinguish genomic libraries from cDNA libraries (*see* cDNA clone; genomic clone). Gene libraries are also referred to as gene banks.

linkage The property of genes to be inherited together as a result of their neighbouring location on the same chromosome; it is measured by percent recombination between loci.

linkage disequilibrium A situation whereby two linked alleles are found in a population to be in *cis*, or in tandem to each other, more frequently than would be expected by chance. At least two explanations are possible: (1) the mutation giving rise to one of the alleles is rather recent (therefore recombination has not yet had the time to cause equilibration with other linked genes); (2) the arrangement in tandem of the two alleles is favoured by selection.

locus The position on a chromosome where a particular gene is located. In diploid organism, like humans, there are at each locus two genes (one on each of the two homologous chromosomes); with the only exception being most of the X chromosome in males, who are haploid for this region.

locus control region (LCR) A DNA segment located upstream of the β-globin gene cluster and required for its high-level expression in erythroid cells. LCRs may exist for other cell-specific genes.

mutation A particular change in the sequence of genomic DNA.

nonsense codon *See* termination codon.

northern blotting A technique for transferring RNA from an agarose gel to a nitrocellulose filter on which it can be recognized by a suitable probe. Widely used to identify expression of an individual gene.

open reading frame A series of triplets coding for amino acids and thus potentially translatable into protein.

phage (bacteriophage) A bacterial virus.

phenotype The appearance of an individual person. In relation to a particular genetic character, the phenotype reflects the genotype conferring that character, plus the possible effects of the environment. In addition, the phenotype (what appears) depends on what we analyse (the way we look at it). Thus, while genotype is an absolute concept, phenotype is a relative concept.

plasmid An autonomously replicating extrachromosomal circular supercoiled DNA.

polymerase chain reaction (PCR) A technique for amplifying *in vitro* by a very large factor (10^5 or more) an individual DNA sequence. The reaction must be primed by using specific oligonucleotides, and therefore prior sequence information is necessary for the procedure to be carried out.

probe (gene probe) A nucleic acid sequence that can be used, by hybridization, to recognize a specific cellular DNA sequence or a specific RNA molecule (usually a gene, or its vicinity, or its cognate mRNA).

prokaryocyte Simple organism such as a bacteria.

promoter A DNA sequence located upstream of the transcribed portion of a gene, and essential for its transcription because it is the binding site for RNA polymerase.

recessive An allele which is obscured in the phenotype of a heterozygote by the dominant allele, often due to inactivity or absence of the product of the recessive allele.

recombinant DNA Any DNA molecule constructed artificially by bringing together DNA segments of different origin. The impact of the respective technology has been so great that the phrase 'recombinant DNA revolution' has been coined.

recombination An event whereby two non-allelic genes, located in tandem on a chromosome, are not transmitted together to the offspring because a cross-over with the homologous chromosome has taken place at meiosis. It is possible that a similar event may take place sometimes in somatic cells (mitotic recombination).

restriction enzymes Recognize specific short sequences (mostly four or six bases) of DNA and cleave the duplex wherever those sequences are found. These sequences are therefore called restriction sites.

reverse transcription Synthesis of DNA on a template of RNA; accomplished by the enzyme, reverse transcriptase.

RFLP (restriction fragment length polymorphism) Genetic variation in the size of a DNA fragment detectable, after digestion with a particular restriction enzyme, by a particular probe. RFLP results from a point mutation in a restriction site, or from a shift in its position due to a deletion or to a duplication.

Southern blotting The procedure for transferring denatured DNA from an agarose gel to a nitrocellulose filter, where it can be recognized by an appropriate probe.

splicing Describes the removal of introns from an RNA primary transcript and joining of the exons; thus introns are spliced out, while exons are spliced together.

termination codon This is one of three triplet sequences, UAG, UAA or UGA, that cause termination of protein synthesis; these are also called stop codons or nonsense codons.

trans Configuration of two sites is called *trans* when their location is on two different chromosomes.

transcription This is synthesis of RNA on a DNA template.

transcription unit *See* gene.

transfection This is the acquisition by eukaryotic cells of new genetic properties or markers by incorporation of added DNA.

transformation This refers to the conversion of eukaryotic cells to a state of unrestrained growth in culture, resembling or identical with neoplastic growth.

transgenic Animals produced by introducing new DNA sequences into the germ-line by microinjection into the egg or into the blastocyst.

translation Synthesis of protein on an mRNA template.

vector A DNA molecule capable of replication and specially engineered to facilitate cloning of another DNA molecule of interest. The vector is mostly a plasmid, a phage or a YAC (see below), but may also be an animal virus, such as a retrovirus.

yeast artificial chromosomes (YAC) Eukaryocyte vectors suitable for cloning large pieces of DNA (up to 2000 kb).

Index

Page numbers in *italic* refer to figures; in **bold** to tables.

ABO blood group system   *393*, **394**, *395*
acanthocytes   *29*
acquired immune deficiency syndrome
        (AIDS)   179−84
  aetiology   179, *180*
  clinical features   **181**, *182*, *183*
  diagnosis   183−4
  epidemiology   180
  haematological aspects   183−4
  myeloid growth factors in   147
  pathogenesis   180−1
  post-transfusional transmission   401−2
  treatment   184
  virus structure   179−80
activated partial thromboplastin time   **316**
  and circulating anticoagulant   **347**
  disseminated intravascular coagulation   **347**
  and heparin therapy   **347**
  liver disease   **347**
  massive transfusion   **347**
  and oral anticoagulant therapy   **347**
acute immune thrombocytopenia *see* immune
        thrombocytopenia purpura, acute
acute lymphoblastic leukaemia
  bone marrow transplantation   **226**
  cells of origin   193−4
  chromosome translocations in   *200*
  clinical features   211−13
  cytotoxic drug therapy   224, *225*, **226**
  differentiation from acute myeloid form   217,
        218
  drug resistance   227
  histology   *216*
  maintenance chemotherapy   227
  Philadelphia-positive   **238**
  prognosis   **225**
acute myeloid (myeloblastic) leukaemia
  clinical features   211−13, *214*
  bone marrow transplantation   **226**
  cells of origin   194
  chromosome translocations in   200
  cytotoxic drug therapy   **228**, **229**
  differentiation from acute lymphoblastic
        form   217, **218**
  drug resistance   227
  histology   *215*
  trans-retinoic acid therapy   228, 229−30
acute phase response   389−91
acylated plasminogen streptokinase activator
        complex (APSAC)   362

adhesion molecules   147−8
adhesion of platelets   *302*
adenocarcinoma, blood film   *370*
adult T-cell leukaemia/lymphoma   270
African lymphoma, *see* Burkitt's lymphoma
African trypanosomiasis, haematological effects of
        379
aggregation of platelets   303
  irreversible   304
AIDS, *see* acquired immune deficiency syndrome
Alder−Reilly anomaly   153, *154*
alkylating agents
  in acute leukaemia   **223**
  in chronic lymphocytic leukaemia   242
alloimmune haemolytic anaemias   90
alpha-interferon, use in treatment   235−6
amyloidosis   282−4
  classification of   **283**
  and monoclonal immunocyte proliferation
        283, *284*
  pathogenesis   **282**
  and protein deposition   284
  reactive systemic   283−4
anaemia   24−31
  aplastic, *see* aplastic anaemia
  blood film   *29*, *30*
  of chronic disorders   48−9, 366−7
    causes   **48**, **366**
  classification and laboratory findings   27−31
    blood film   *29*, *30*
    bone marrow examination   30, *31*, **32**
    red cell indices   27, **28**
    reticulocyte count   28, **29**
  clinical features   25−6
  congenital dyserythropoietic   129−30
  haemolytic, *see* haemolytic anaemias
  hypochromic
    differential diagnosis   50, **51**−2
    see also anaemia of chronic disorders; iron
        deficiency anaemia; sideroblastic anaemia
  immune haemolytic   **369**
  iron deficiency, *see* iron deficiency anaemia
  macrocytic, *see* megaloblastic anaemias
  malignant disease   367, *368*, **369**, *370*
  megaloblastic, *see* megaloblastic anaemias
  in renal failure   370−1, *372*−3
  sickle cell, *see* sickle cell anaemia
  sideroblastic, *see* sideroblastic anaemia
  signs   26, *27*
  symptoms   26

anaemia (*continued*)
  see also erythropoiesis
androgens, in treatment of aplastic anaemia   128
angioimmunoblastic lymphadenopathy   270
anisocytosis   *29*
antibody-mediated coagulation deficiency   346
anticoagulant drugs   356−64
  antiplatelet drugs   *363*−4
  direct thrombin inhibitors   358
  fibrinolytic agents   **361**, **362**
  heparin   *356*−7
    administration and laboratory control   357
    bleeding during therapy   357
    complications   357
    and haemostasis tests   **347**
    indications   357
    mode of action   *356*
    and platelet function disorders   329
  oral   357−61
    bleeding during warfarin therapy   **361**
    drug interactions   **360**−1
    and haemostasis tests   **347**
    laboratory control   *359*−60
    mode of action   *358*−9
    overdose   348
antiglobulin (Coombs) test
  direct   396, *397*
  indirect   397
antihaemophilic factor   **306**
antihuman globulin   396
  specificity of   397−8
anti-lymphocyte globulin, in treatment of aplastic
    anaemia   126, *127*
antimetabolites, in treatment of acute leukaemia
    222
anti-oncogenes   199
antiplatelet drugs   *363*−4
aplastic anaemia   121−8
  clinical features   124
  congenital   122, *123*
  diagnosis   124, **125**
  idiopathic acquired   123
  laboratory findings   124, *125*
  pathogenesis   **121**, *122*
  secondary   123−4
  treatment   125−6, *127*−8
    androgens   128
    anti-lymphocyte globulin   126, *127*
    bone marrow transplantation   128
    cyclosporin   127
    haemopoietic growth factors   128
    methylprednisolone   127
    myeloid growth factors   147
aplastic crises of sickle cell anaemia   112
apoptosis   8
aspirin   328−9, *330*, 362, *363*−4
autoimmune haemolytic anaemias   87−91
  cold type   **87**, 89−90
    clinical features   90
    laboratory findings   90
    treatment   90
  warm type   87−9
    blood film   *88*
    clinical features   87−8

  laboratory findings   *88*−9
autotransfusion   404

B cells   **163**, *164*
  maturation of   172, *173*−4
  see also lymphocytes
basophilia   155
basophilic stippling   *30*
basophils   *142*, 144
  normal blood count   **142**, **419**
benign monoclonal gammopathy   281, **282**
Bernard−Soulier syndrome   301, 328
'blanket' cells, *see* reticulum cells
bleeding time   315
blood cell formation, *see* haemopoiesis
blood coagulation   305−11
  coagulation factors, *see* coagulation factors
  disorders of, *see* coagulation disorders
  enzymes, receptors and cofactors   *309*
  extrinsic pathway   307
  final common pathway   *307*−8
  intrinsic pathway   306−7
  pathways of   *305*
  physiological limitation of   310, *311*
  screening tests of   **316**
  see also fibrinolysis; haemostasis; platelets
blood count   315
blood films   315
  adenocarcinoma   *370*
  alpha-thalassaemia   *101*
  anaemia   *29*, *30*
  beta-thalassaemia major   *103*
  essential thrombocythaemia   *294*
  G6PD deficiency   *85*
  haemolytic disease of newborn   *409*
  hereditary spherocytosis   *82*
  iron deficiency anaemia   *43*, *44*
  liver disease   *374*
  malaria   *378*
  megaloblastic anaemia   *65*
  microangiopathic haemolytic anaemia   *91*
  multiple myeloma   *275*
  myelodysplastic syndromes   247, *248*
  myelofibrosis   *296*
  renal failure   *372*
  sickle cell anaemia   *114*
  warm autoimmune haemolytic anaemia   *88*
blood groups   394−5
  ABO system   *393*, **394**, *395*
  antibodies   392−3
  Rh system   394, **395**
  serology   396−8
blood transfusion   392−415
  ABO system   **393**, **394**, *395*
  acute blood loss   407
  blood blank and blood products   402, *403*−6
    cyroprecipitate   406
    freeze-dried factor VIII concentrates   406
    freeze-dried factor IX−prothrombin complex
      concentrates   406−7
    granulocyte concentrates   405
    human albumin solution   406
    human plasma preparations   405−6

immunoglobulin 407
packed red cells 403−4
platelet concentrates 405
red cell substitutes 404
whole blood 403
blood group antibodies 392−3
blood group serology 396−8
cross-matching and pretransfusion tests **398**
direct antiglobulin test 396, *397*
indirect antiglobulin test 397
specificity of antihuman globulin 397−8
complications of 398, **399**−402
febrile/non-febrile non-haemolytic allergic
reactions 401
febrile reactions due to white cell
antibodies 401
haemolytic transfusion reaction 398−400
HIV virus transmission 401−2
post-transfusion circulatory overload 401
post-transfusion hepatitis 401
post-transfusion iron overload 402
DNA fingerprinting *414*, 415
haemolytic disease of the newborn 407−11
ABO type 411
Rh type 407−8, *409*, *410*−11
human leucocyte antigen (HLA) system 411,
412−13, **414**
red cell antigens 392, **393**
Rh system 394, **395**
body iron distribution 37, *38*, **39**
bone marrow
examination of 30, *31*, **32**
acute leukaemia 215
aplastic anaemia *122*
chronic lymphocytic leukaemia 241
chronic myeloid leukaemia 233
Gaucher's disease *384*
iron deficiency anaemia *44*
megaloblastic anaemia *66*
multiple myeloma *274*
myelodysplastic syndromes 247, *248*
haemopoietic stem cells in *2*−4
stroma *3*, *4*
bone marrow transplantation 130−40
acute leukaemia **226**, 230
allogeneic *133*
post-transplant course *134*
in aplastic anaemia 128
autologous *133*
chronic myeloid leukaemia *236*
complications **135**−40
graft failure 138
graft-vs-host disease **137**, *138*
haemorrhage 137
haemorrhagic cystitis 138−9
infections 135, *136*−7
interstitial pneumonitis 138, *139*
late 139−40
donor 134
HLA matching **130**−1, *132*
indications for **131**
myelodysplastic syndromes 249
myeloid growth factors and recovery *146*−7
post-transplant course *134*, 135

recipient 132, *133*
in thalassaemia major 108
bruising 318
Burkitt's lymphoma **191**, *269*
chromosome translocations in *200*
Burr cells *29*
busulphan, in treatment of chronic myeloid
leukaemia 234, *235*

CD molecules, see cluster differentiation
molecules
central nervous system, leukaemia prophylaxis
226
centroblasts *173*−4
centrocytes *173*, 174
Chédiak−Higashi syndrome 153, *154*
chemicals, and susceptibility to leukaemia/
lymphoma 205
chemotaxis 149
defects of 152
chemotherapy, see cytotoxic drug therapy
chondroitin **5**
Christmas disease 338−9
carrier detection and antenatal diagnosis 339
laboratory findings **336**, 338−9
treatment 339
Christmas factor **306**, 307
deficiency of, see Christmas disease
chromosomal translocations 190, **191**
and oncogene activation 199−203
ABL *200*, *201*
BCL-2 201
MYC 199−*200*
retinoic acid receptor 199
chromosome nomenclature 186, *187*
chronic granulocytic leukaemia 232
chronic immune thrombocytopenic purpura, *see*
immune thrombocytopenic purpura,
chronic
clinical features 322−3
diagnosis 323
pathogenesis *322*
in pregnancy 324
treatment 323, *324*
chronic lymphocytic (lymphatic) leukaemia
238−44
cells of origin 194
classification of **239**
clinical features 239, *240*
course and prognosis 241, **242**
laboratory findings 240, *241*
treatment 241−3
variants of 243−4
chronic myeloid leukaemia 232, *233*−8
cells of origin 194
chromosome translocations in *201*, *202*
classification of **233**
clinical features 232−3
course and prognosis 237
accelerated phase and metamorphosis 237
variants of 237−8
juvenile form 237−8
laboratory findings 233, *234*

chronic myeloid leukaemia (*continued*)
  treatment of 234, *235, 236*
    allopurinol 236
    alpha-interferon 235−6
    bone marrow transplantation *236*
    busulphan 234, *235*
    hydroxyurea 235
    splenic irradiation or splenectomy 236
cigarette smoking, and polycythaemia 292
cluster differentiation (CD) molecules, principle
      features of **417−18**
coagulation disorders 332−49
  acquired **341−8**
    antibody-mediated coagulation deficiency
      346
    anticoagulant overdose 348
    disseminated intravascular coagulation **344,**
      345−6
    liver disease 343−4
    massive transfusion syndrome **347,** 348
    vitamin K deficiency 341, *342−3*
  factor VIII, calculation 337
  factor IX deficiency 338−9
  haemophilia A 332, *333−8*
    clinical features 332, *334, 335−6*
    laboratory findings **336−7**
    treatment 337−8
  von Willebrand's disease 339, *340*
coagulation factors **306**
  freeze-dried for transfusion 406
  inhibitors of 310
  properties of **309**
  specific assays of 317
collagen **5**
complement 170, *171−2*
congenital dyserythropoietic anaemia 129−30
connective tissue disorders 319
  haematological effects of 369−70, *371*
Cooley's anaemia, *see* thalassaemias,
      betathalassaemia major
C-reactive protein **390−1**
cryoprecipitate 406
cyclosporin
  in prevention of GVHD 138
  in treatment of aplastic anaemia 127
cytoadhesins 148
cytogenetics 190
cytotoxic drug therapy
  acute leukaemia **222−6,** 225
    Hodgkin's disease 257
    multiple myeloma 277−8
  myelodysplastic syndromes 249
  non-Hodgkin's lymphomas 266−8
  polycythaemia rubra vera 291

deoxyhaemoglobin *19*
deoxyuridine suppression test 67, *68*
dipyridamole 364
disseminated intravascular coagulation 326, **344,**
      345−6
  causes of **344**
  laboratory findings 345−6, **347**
  pathogenesis 344, *345*

and systemic malignant disease **369**
  treatment 346
DNA binding drugs in treatment of acute
      leukaemia **223**
DNA diagnosis of genetic haemoglobin disorders
      116, *117−19*
  ARMS technique 118, *119*
  gene mapping 116, *117*
  oligonucleotide probes 117
  PCR gene amplification 118, *119*
  RFLP linkage analysis 116−17, *118*
DNA fingerprinting *414,* 415
DNA synthesis, defects of causing megaloblastic
      anaemia 71
drug-induced immune haemolytic anaemias 90,
      91
drug-induced immune thrombocytopenia 325−6
drug resistance in acute leukaemia 227
dyskeratosis congenita 122

Ehlers−Danlos syndrome 319
elliptocytes *29*
elliptocytosis, hereditary *82,* 83
Embden−Meyerhof pathway 21, *22*
  defects in 86
endothelial cells **5,** 311, *313*
endotoxin, in regulation of haemopoiesis *7*
eosinophilia 155, **156**
  pulmonary 380
  and systemic malignant disease **369**
eosinophils *142,* 143−4
  normal blood count **142, 419**
erythroblastosis foetalis, *see* haemolytic disease of
      newborn
erythroblasts *13*
erythrocyte sedimentation rate (ESR) 389, **390**
  in connective tissue disorders 370
erythropoiesis 12, *13, 14−35*
  erythropoietin 12−13, *15, 16*
    indications for therapy 15
  haemoglobin 17−20
    function of 17, *19, 20*
    methaemoglobinaemia 19−20
    synthesis of **17,** *18*
  ineffective 31−2
  qualitative aspects of 32−5
    red cell lifespan 35
    tests of effective erythropoiesis *34−5*
    tests of total erythropoiesis 32, *33*
  red cell 20, *21−4*
    membrane of 22, *23−4*
    metabolism 21, *22, 23*
erythropoietin 12−13, *15, 16*
  indications for therapy 15
  production of *15*
essential thrombocythaemia 293−5
  course 295
  laboratory findings *294−5*
  treatment 295
Evans' syndrome 88
extracellular growth factors 197

FAB classification of

acute leukaemias 209, **210**
  myelodysplastic syndromes 245
Fanconi's anaemia 122, *123*
fat cells **5**
Felty's syndrome 369
ferritin
  iron content **38**
  serum levels
    iron deficiency anaemia 45
    normal values **419**
fibrin
  formation and stabilization of *307*
  stabilization of haemostatic plug by 315
fibrin stabilizing factor **306**
fibrinogen **306**, *308*
  defects of 353
fibrinolysis 311–12
  fibrinolytic system *311*
  tests of 317
fibrinolytic agents **361**–2
  contraindications to **362**
fibroblasts **5**
fibronectin **5**
Fitzgerald factor **306**
Fletcher factor, *see* prekallikrein
foetus
  foetal haemoglobin 17
    switch to adult form 96
  prenatal diagnosis of genetic haemoglobin
      disorders 116
    blood sampling 116
    DNA diagnosis 116, *117–19*
  sites of haemopoiesis in 1, **2**
folate 57–60
  abnormal metabolism of 71
  absorption and transport 58
  biochemical functions *58*, 59
  deficiency 62, 65, **67**, **68**–9
  dietary intake **55**
  normal values **419**
  prophylaxis 71
  red cell, normal values **419**
  reduction 60
  structure *59*
folate deficiency 62
  causes **62**
  effects of **64**
  laboratory tests for **67**, *68*–9
  treatment **69**, *70*–1
free erythrocyte protoporphyrin in iron deficiency
    anaemia 45

Gaucher's disease, haematological effects of 382,
    383, 384–5
  genetic aspects 384
  treatment 385
gene rearrangements
  immunoglobulins 169, *170*, 189–90, 207–8
  and oncogene activation 199–202
    ABL 200, *201, 202*
    BCL-2 201
    MYC 199, *200*
    retinoic acid receptor 199

T-cell receptors 170, *171*, 189–90
gene therapy for genetic haemoglobin defects 120
glandular fever, *see* infectious mononucleosis
Glanzmann's disease 328
glucose-6-phosphate dehydrogenase (G6PD)
    deficiency 83, *84*–6
  blood film *85*
  causes **85**
  clinical features 84–5
  diagnosis *85*–6
  treatment 86
glucose-6-phosphate dehydrogenase (G6PD)
    isoenzyme analysis 187–8
glutathione deficiency 86
'golf ball' cells *101*
graft failure, as complication of bone marrow
    transplantation 138
graft-vs-host disease, as complication of bone
    marrow transplantation *137, 138*
granulocytes 141–9
  basophils *142*, 144
  concentrates 405
  control of granulopoiesis 145–7
  eosinophils *142*, 143–4
  formation and kinetics 144, *145*
  neutrophils 141, *142, 143*
  phagocytic surface receptors 147–9
    adhesion molecules 147–8
    Fc and C3b receptors 148
    leucocyte antigens 149
Grey platelet syndrome 301, 328
growth factors
  extracellular 197
  haemopoietic 5, **6**, *7–10*, 128
  myeloid 145, *146*–7
  receptors 8–9, **10**

haem, structure of *18*
haem enzymes, iron content **38**
haematocrit, normal values **419**
haemoglobin 17–20
  foetal
    hereditary persistence of 110
    switch to adult form 96
  function 17, *19, 20*
  genetic defects of 94–120
    gene therapy for 120
    prenatal diagnosis 116–19
    sickle cell anaemia 111–18
    thalassaemias 97–110
  iron content **38**
  methaemoglobinaemia 19–20
  normal values **419**
  synthesis **17**, *18*, 94, *95*–7
    molecular aspects of 94–5, *96*
haemoglobin C disease 115
  geographical distribution **98**
haemoglobin D disease 115
  geographical distribution **98**
haemoglobin E disease 115
  geographical distribution **98**
haemoglobin H disease *101*
haemoglobin Lepore 110

haemoglobin S
  combination of with other genetic defects of
      haemoglobin   115
  see also sickle cell anaemia
haemoglobinuria
  March   91
  paroxysmal nocturnal   92–3
haemolytic anaemias   74–93
  acquired   87–93
    alloimmune   90
    autoimmune   87, 88–90
    chemical/physical agents   92
    drug-induced immune   90, 91
    infections   92
    March haemoglobinuria   92
    red cell fragmentation syndromes   91–2
  classification of   77
  clinical features   75–6, 77, 78
  hereditary   79–86
    elliptocytosis   82, 83
    G6PD deficiency   83, 84, 85–6
    glutathione deficiency   86
    pyruvate kinase deficiency   86
    spherocytosis   79, 81, 82–3
  intravascular haemolysis   78, 79, 80
  laboratory findings   77–8
  normal red cell destruction   74, 75, 76
  paroxysmal nocturnal haemoglobinuria   92–3
  secondary   92
haemolytic crises of sickle cell anaemia   112
haemolytic disease of newborn   407–11
  ABO type   411
  blood film   409
  Rh type   408–11
    clinical features   408
    laboratory findings   408, 409
    management of pregnant women   409,
        410–11
    pathogenesis   408
    treatment   409
haemolytic transfusion reactions   398, 399–400
haemolytic uraemia syndrome   326
haemonectin   5
haemophilia A   332, 333–8
  clinical features   332, 334, 335–6
  laboratory findings   336–7
  treatment   337–8
haemophilia B, see Christmas disease
haemopoiesis   1–11, 65
  bone marrow stroma   4, 5
  extramedullary   1
  haemopoietic growth factors   5, 6, 7–10
  haemopoietic stem and progenitor cells   1, 2–4
  regulation of   7
  signal transduction   8, 9, 10–11
    growth factor receptors   8, 9, 10
    second messengers   10–11
  site of   1, 2
haemopoietic growth factors   5, 6, 7–10
  in treatment of
    AIDS   147
    aplastic anaemia   128
    myelodysplasia   147
haemopoietic stem and progenitor cells   1, 2–4

haemorrhage
  acute   407
  and anticoagulant therapy   357, 360, 361
  as complication of bone marrow transplantation
      137
  in thrombocytopenia   320
haemorrhagic cystitis, as complication of bone
      marrow transplantation   138–9
haemorrhagic disease of newborn   342–3
  diagnosis   343
  treatment   343
haemosiderin, iron content   38
haemostasis   313, 314–17
  hereditary disorders of   352–3
  platelet reactions and haemostatic plug
      formation   313–14
  stabilization of platelet plug   315
  tests of haemostatic function   315, 316–17, 347,
      348
    bleeding time   315
    blood coagulation   316
    blood count and blood film examination   315
    coagulation factors   317
    fibrinolysis   317
    vasoconstriction   313
  see also blood coagulation; fibrinolysis; platelets
haemostatic plug
  formation of   313–14
  stabilization of by fibrin   315
Hageman factor   306
hairy cell leukaemia   244
hand–foot syndrome   112
heavy chain disease   281
Heinz bodies   30
Henoch–Schönlein syndrome   319
heparan   5
heparin, see anticoagulant drugs
heparin cofactor II   310
hereditary haemorrhagic telangiectasia   318, 319
hereditary susceptibility to leukaemia/lymphoma
      204–5
Hermansky–Pudlak syndrome   301, 328
hexose monophosphate pathway   21–2, 23
histiocytic tumours   271
HIV, see acquired immune deficiency syndrome
Hodgkin's disease   251–9
  biochemical findings   253
  clinical features   252
  clinical staging   255, 256, 257, 258
  diagnosis and histological classification   253,
      254, 255
  haematological findings   253
  immunological findings   253
  pathogenesis   251–2
  prognosis   259
  treatment
    chemotherapy   257
    radiotherapy   256–7
    relapse   257–8
Howell–Jolly bodies   30, 386, 387
human albumin solution
  4.5%   406
  20%   406
human leucocyte antigen (HLA) system   411,

412−14
  and blood transfusion   401, 413
  and disease   413, **414**
  recognized HLA specificities   **416**
  and transplantation   413
human plasma preparations   405−6
hydrops foetalis   *100*
hydroxyurea, in treatment of chronic myeloid
      leukaemia   235
hyperglobulinaemia   329
hyperviscosity syndrome   284−5
  see also Waldenström's macroglobulinaemia
hypoplastic anaemia, *see* aplastic anaemia
hypothyroidism, haematological effects of   375

immune deficiencies   **178**−85
  acquired immune deficiency syndrome
      179−85
immune response   164−5, *166−7*
immune thrombocytopenic purpura
  acute   324−5
  chronic   320, 322−4
    clinical features   322−3
    diagnosis   323
    pathogenesis   322
    in pregnancy   324
    treatment   323, 324
immunoblasts   *173*
immunoglobulin gene superfamily   148
immunoglobulins   165−6, *167*, **168**−9
  gene rearrangements   169, *170, 171*, 189−90,
      207−8
  pooled, for transfusion   407
infants, sites of haemopoiesis in   1, *2*
infection
  in acute leukaemia   220−2
    prophylaxis   220−1
    treatment   221−2
  as complication of bone marrow transplantation
      135, *136−7*
  haematological effects of   375, **376**−80
    bacterial   *375*, 377
    viral   377, *378−80*
  myeloid growth factors in   147
infectious mononucleosis   175−8
  clinical features   175−6
  course and development   178
  diagnosis   *176−7*
    differential   177
  treatment   178
integrins   148
interstitial pneumonitis, as complication of bone
      marrow transplantation   138, *139*
intracellular signal transducers   197−8
intravascular haemolysis   78, **79**, *80*
iron
  absorption   **38**, 39
  body distribution   36, *37*, **38**
  dietary   **38**−9
  requirements   **40**
  serum levels
    iron deficiency anaemia   45
    normal values   **419**

status, assessment   **106**
  transport   *37*, 39−40
iron deficiency anaemia   36−48
  blood film   *43, 44*
  causes   **42**−3
    investigation of   *46−7*
  clinical features   40, *41*
  diagnosis   **51**
  laboratory findings   43−5
    bone marrow iron   *44*
    free erythrocyte protoporphyrin   45
    red cell indices and blood film   *43, 44*
    serum ferritin   45
    serum iron and total ironbinding capacity   *45*
  nutritional and metabolic aspects of iron
      36−40
  and malignant disease   **369**
  treatment   **47, 48**
    oral iron   47
    parenteral iron   48
    prophylactic iron therapy   47
  see also iron

kala-azar, haematological effects of   *379*
Kaposi's sarcoma   *183*
killing, by neutrophils and monocytes   150−1
  defects of   153
koilonychia   *41*
Kostmann's syndrome   156

labile factor   **306**
laminin   **5**
'lazy leucocyte' syndrome   152
lead poisoning   50
Lepore syndrome   102
leucocyte cell adhesion molecules   148
leucocytes   141−60
  in anaemia   28
  antigens of   149
  benign disorders of   153−9
    basophilia   155
    eosinophilia   155, **156**
    leukaemoid reaction   155
    monocytosis   **156**
    neutropenia   156, **157**−9
    neutrophilia   154, **155**
    variations in neutrophil morphology   153,
      154
  effects of splenectomy   387−8
  normal blood count   **419**
  see also individual cell types
leukaemias
  acute   209−31
    bone marrow transplantation   230
    chromosome analysis   **218**
    clinical features   211, *212−16*
    CNS prophylaxis   226
    cytochemistry   217, **218**
    cytotoxic drug therapy   **222**−3
    differentiation of   217
    drug resistance   227
    hybrid form   219

leukaemias (*continued*)
    immunoglobulin and T-cell receptor gene
        rearrangements 218
    immunological classification 216, *217*
    immunological markers 218, **219**
    incidence 211
    lymphoblastic, *see* acute lymphoblastic
        leukaemia
    maintenance chemotherapy 227
    management 219–30
    myeloid, *see* acute myeloid leukaemia
    myeloid growth factors in 147
    pathogenesis 209–11
    patients over 60 years of age 230
    prognosis 231
    prophylaxis and treatment of infection
        220–2
    testicular disease 227
    treatment of relapse 227
    cells of origin 191, *192*, **193**–5
    chronic 232–45
        lymphocytic, *see* chronic lymphocytic
            leukaemia
        myeloid, *see* chronic myeloid leukaemia
        neutrophilic 238
        T-cell 244
        see also myelodysplastic syndromes
    classification of 209, **210**
    eosinophilic 238
    hairy cell *244*
    inherited/acquired predisposition to 203–4,
        205, 205–7
    plasma cell 281
    prolymphocytic 243
leukaemoid reaction 155
    and systemic disease 367, **369**
light chain restriction 189
liver disease
    blood film *374*
    and coagulation disorders 343–4, **347**
    haematological effects of **373**, *374*
loa-loa, haematological effects of *380*
lupus anticoagulant 354–5
lymphadenopathy 184, **185**
lymphoblasts 174
lymphocytes 161–85
    benign disorders of 175–8
        infectious mononucleosis 175, *176*–8
        lymphocytosis **175**
        lymphopenia 178
    circulation of 174
    complement 170, *171*–2
    functional aspects of **163**, *164*
    germinal follicle 172, *173*–4
    immune deficiencies 178–85
        acquired immune deficiency syndrome 179,
            180, **181**–2, *183*–4
        classification of **178**
    immune response 164–5, *166*–7
    immunoglobulins 165–6, *167*, **168**–70
        gene rearrangements *169, 170*, 189–90,
            207–8
    lymphadenopathy 184, **185**
    natural killer and lymphocyte-activated killer

    cells 172
    normal blood count **142**, **419**
    primary lymphocyte formation *161, 162*
    T-cell receptor rearrangements 170, *171*,
        189–90
lymphocytosis **175**
lymphokine-activated killer cells 172
lymphoma/leukaemia syndromes 244–5
lymphomas, malignant
    adult T-cell leukaemia/lymphoma 270
    angioimmunoblastic lymphadenopathy 270
    Burkitt's lymphoma *269*
    cells of origin 191, *192*, **193**–5
    Hodgkin's disease, *see* Hodgkin's disease
    inherited/acquired predisposition to 203–4,
        205–6
    malignant histiocytic tumours 271
    mycosis fungoides 194, 269–70
    non-Hodgkin's, *see* non-Hodgkin's lymphomas
    Sézary's syndrome 194, 269–70
lymphopenia 178

macrocytes *29*
    megaloblastic anaemia *65*
macrocytic anaemias 72–3
macrophages **5**
malaria, haematological effects of 377, *378*
    blood film *378*
malignancies 186–206
    cell transformation 195–9
        oncogenes **195**, *196*–8, 199, *200*–2, 203,
            204–5, *206*
        tumour suppressor genes 198
    chromosome, gene rearrangement and oncogene
        studies in diagnosis and disease monitoring
        207–8
    chromosome nomenclature 186, *187*
    clonal progression 190, **191**
    establishment of clonality 187, *188*, **189**–90
        X-linked RFLP 188–9
        chromosomal translocation analysis by
            breakpoint probes 190
        cytogenetics 190
        G6PD isoenzyme analysis 187–8
        immunoglobulin and T-cell receptor
            rearrangements 189–90
        light chain restriction 189
        point mutations 190
    inherited and acquired predisposition to
        leukaemia and lymphoma 203–4, *205*–6
    originating cells 191, *192*, **193**–5
    systemic, haematological effects of 367, *368*,
        369, *370*
    see also leukaemias; lymphomas, malignant;
        multiple myeloma; myeloproliferative
        disorders
massive transfusion syndrome 327, 348
    laboratory findings **347**
May–Hegglin anomaly 153
mean corpuscular haemoglobin (MCH), normal
    values **419**
mean corpuscular haemoglobin concentration
    (MCHC), normal values **419**

mean corpuscular volume (MCV), normal values **419**
Mediterranean anaemia, *see* thalassaemias, beta-thalassaemia major
megakaryocytes, platelet production from *299, 300*
megaloblastic anaemias 53–73
  abnormal vitamin B$_{12}$/folate metabolism 71
  biochemical basis for 59–60
  blood film *65*
  causes of **53**
  clinical features 62, *63, 64*
  defects of DNA synthesis 71
  folate 57–9
    absorption and transport 58
    biochemical reactions *58*, 59
    deficiency 62, 65, **67, 68**–9
    dietary intake **55**
    reduction 60
    structure *57*
  laboratory findings 65–9
    blood film *65*
    bone marrow picture *66*
  macrocytic anaemias 72–3
    differential diagnosis 72–3
  pernicious anaemia **61**–2
  treatment **69**–71
    inadequate response 71
    response to therapy *70*–1
  vitamin B$_{12}$ 53–7
    absorption 54, *56*
    biochemical function 56, *57, 58*
    deficiency 60–2, 65, **67, 68**–9
    dietary intake 54, **55**
    structure *54*
    transport of 55–6
  vitamin B$_{12}$ neuropathy 63, *64*
methaemoglobinaemia 19–20
methylprednisolone, in treatment of aplastic anaemia 127
microangiopathic haemolytic anaemia *91*
  blood film *91*
  and malignant disease **369**
microcytes *29*
  iron deficiency anaemia *43*
mitotic inhibitors in treatment of acute leukaemia **223**
monocytes *142*, 143
  formation and kinetics 149, *150*
  functions of 149–50, *151, 152*
    chemotaxis 149, 152
    killing and digestion 150–1, 153
    phagocytosis 149, *150, 151*, 152
  normal blood count **142, 419**
monocytosis **156**
  and systemic disease **369**
multiple myeloma 272–8
  blood film *275*
  cells of origin 191, *192*, **193**–5
  clinical features 272–3
  diagnosis *273–6*, 277
  laboratory findings *275, 276*–7
  prognosis 278
  treatment 277–8

mycosis fungoides 194, 269–70
myelodysplasia, *see* myelodysplastic syndromes
myelodysplastic syndromes 245–50
  blood film 247, *248*
  chromosomal and oncogene abnormalities 247
  classification **245**–6
  clinical features *246*
  laboratory findings 246–7
  management 247
    high-risk 249–50
    low-grade 247, 249
  myeloid growth factors in 147
myelofibrosis 295–8
  blood film *296*
  cells of origin 194
  clinical features 295–6
  laboratory findings *296, 297*
  treatment 297–8
myeloid growth factors 145–7
  in AIDS 147
  clinical applications of *146*–7
myeloproliferative disorders 286, *287*–98
  cells of origin 191, *192*, **193**–5
  essential thrombocythaemia 293–5
    course 295
    laboratory findings **294**–5
    treatment 295
  myelofibrosis 295–8
    clinical features 295–6
    laboratory findings *296, 297*
    treatment 297–8
  and platelet function disorders 329
  polycythaemia 286–93
    cigarette smoking and 292
    differential diagnosis of 293
    polycythaemia vera 286–93
    relative polycythaemia 292
    secondary polycythaemia 292

natural killer (NK) cells 172
neutropenia 157–9
  autoimmune 158
  causes of **157**
  clinical features 159
  congenital 156
  cyclical 158
  diagnosis 159
  drug-induced 156–8
  idiopathic benign 158
  kinetic mechanisms of *157*
  management 159
  severe, myeloid growth factors in 147
neutrophilia 154, **155**
neutrophils 141, *142, 143*
  functions of 149–50, *151, 152*
    chemotaxis 149, 152
    killing and digestion 150–1, 153
    phagocytosis 149–50, *151, 152*, 152
    morphology, variations in 153, *154*
    normal blood count **142, 419**
    precursors 141–2, *143*
Niemann–Pick disease, haematological effects of 385

non-Hodgkin's lymphomas   159–68
  blood chemistry   264
  chromosome findings   263
  classification and histopathology   259, *260*,
    261–2
  clinical features   262–3
  diagnostic investigations and clinical staging
    264–7
  gene rearrangements   264
  haematological findings   263
  immunological markers   263, **264**
  predisposing diseases   262
  prognosis   268
  prognostic features   266
  treatment   266–8
    high-grade malignancy group   268
    intermediate-grade malignancy group   266–8
    low-grade malignancy group   266
    relapse   268
normoblast   *30*

oncogenes   **195**, *196*–8
  abnormalities of in myelodysplastic syndromes
    247
  activation in haematological malignancies
    199–205, *206*
    amplification   204–5, *206*
    inactivation   203
    point mutations   202–3
    promoter insertion   203, *204*
    translocations and rearrangements   199,
      200–2
  classification of   197
  diagnosis and disease monitoring   207–8
  function of protein products   197–8
    amplification   203
    extracellular growth factors   197
    inactivation   202–3
    intracellular signal transducers   197–8
    membrane-associated tyrosine kinases
      197–8
    nuclear oncogenes   198
    point mutations   202
    retroviral infection causing   203
  nuclear   198
  prevention of cell death   198
  recessive   199
osmotic fragility in hereditary spherocytosis   82,
    83
osteoporosis, and heparin therapy   357
oxyhaemoglobin   *19*

packed cell volume (PCV), normal values   **419**
pancytopenia   **123**
  and systemic malignant disease   **369**
Pappenheimer bodies   *30*, 386, *387*
Paterson–Kelly syndrome   *41*
Pel–Ebstein fever   252
Pelger–Huët anomaly   153, *154*
pentose phosphate pathway, *see* hexose
    monophosphate pathway
pernicious anaemia   **61**–2

  antibodies   61–2
Persantin   363–4
phagocytes   *143*
phagocytosis   149, *150*, *151*
  defects of   *152*
phosphorus-32 therapy in polycythaemia rubra
    vera   291
plasma cell tumours
  heavy chain disease   281
  plasma cell leukaemia   281
  soft-tissue plasmacytoma   280
  solitary plasmacytoma of bone   280
  see also multiple myeloma
plasma cells   *173*
plasma thromboplastin antecedent   **306**, 307
plasma viscosity   **390**
plasma volume, normal values   **419**
plasmacytomas
  soft-tissue   280
  solitary, of bone   280
plasmin   *311*, *312*
  inactivation of   *312*
plasminogen   311
  defects of   353
platelet count
  and circulating anticoagulant   **347**
  disseminated intravascular coagulation   **347**
  essential thrombocythaemia   **294**
  and heparin therapy   **347**
  liver disease   **347**
  massive transfusion   **347**
  normal   **419**
  and oral anticoagulants   **347**
platelet-derived growth factor   301, 304–5
platelet disorders   328–31
  acquired   328–9
  antiplatelet drugs   329
  diagnosis of   329, *330*–1
  hereditary   328
  renal failure   373
  and systemic malignant disease   367–8
  thrombocytopenia, *see* thrombocytopenia
platelets   299–304
  abnormal distribution of   **321**
  adhesion   *302*, 313–14
  aggregation   303
  antigens   302
  circulation of   300
  concentrates   405
  disorders of, *see* platelet disorders
  effects of splenectomy   388
  increased consumption of   *321*
  irreversible aggregation   *304*
  normal blood count, *see* platelet count
  procoagulant activity   303–4
  production   *299*, *300*
    failure of   **321**
  release reaction   303, *304*, 313–14
  structure   300, *301*–2
  transfusions, indications for   331, 405
  von Willebrand factor   303
  see also antiplatelet drugs
Plummer–Vinson syndrome   *41*
Pneumocystis carinii   *182*

poikilocytosis *29*
  iron deficiency anaemia *43*
point mutations 190
  and oncogene activation 202−3
polycythaemia 286−93
  cigarette smoking and 292
  differential diagnosis of 293
  and malignant systemic disease 367, **369**
  relative 292
  rubra vera 286−92
    cells of origin 194
    clinical features 287, **288**, *289, 290*
    course and prognosis 291−2
    laboratory findings **288**
    treatment 289, *291*
  secondary 292
polymorphs, *see* neutrophils
post-transfusion circulatory overload 401
post-transfusion hepatitis 401
post-transfusion purpura 325
pregnancy, and autoimmune thrombocytopenic
      purpura 324
prekallikrein **306, 309**
proconvertin **306**
prostacyclin 303, *304*
protein C 310, *311*
  deficiency 353
protein S deficiency 353
proteoglycans **5**
prothrombin **306, 309**
prothrombin time **316**
  and circulating anticoagulant **347**
  disseminated intravascular coagulation **347**
  and heparin therapy **347**
  liver disease **347**
  massive transfusion **347**
  and oral anticoagulant therapy **347**
pseudopolycythaemia 292
pseudoxanthoma elasticum 319
pyruvate kinase deficiency 86

radiation, and susceptibility to leukaemia/
      lymphoma 205−6
radiotherapy in
  bone marrow transplantation 132, *133*
  chronic lymphocytic leukaemia 243
  Hodgkin's disease 256−7
  multiple myeloma 277
  non-Hodgkin's lymphomas 266−8
red cell aplasia 128, **129**
red cell fragmentation syndromes *91−2*
red cells 20, *21−4*
  abnormal morphology *29*
  antigens 392, **393**
  defective metabolism 83−6
  effects of splenectomy 386, *387*
  ^{59}Fe incorporation into 34−5
  folate, normal blood count **419**
  fragments *29*
  haemoglobin synthesis in *18*
  inclusions *30*
  indices
    in anaemia 27, **28**, 43

  normal **24**−5
  lifespan 35
  membrane 22, *23−4*
  metabolic defects
    Embden−Meyerhof pathway 86
    G6PD deficiency 83, *84*, **85**−6
    glutathione deficiency 86
  metabolism 21−2, *23*
    Embden−Meyerhof pathway 21, *22*
    hexose monophosphate pathway 21−2, *23*
  normal blood count **419**
  normal destruction 74, *75, 76*
  packed 403−4
  substitutes for 404
relative polycythaemia 292
release reaction of platelets 303, *304*
renal failure, haematological effects of 370−1,
      372−3
  blood film *372*
restriction fragment length polymorphism 188−9
reticulocyte count 34
  in anaemia 29, **30**
reticulum cells **5**
trans-retinoic acid therapy for acute promyelocytic
      leukaemia 228, 229−30
retroviruses, and oncogene activation 203, *204*
Rh blood group system 394, **395**
rheumatoid arthritis, haematological effects of
      369−70, *371*
ring sideroblasts *49*, 50

scurvy 319
second messengers 10−11
secondary polycythaemia 292
selectins 148
senile purpura 318
serine protease, and blood coagulation *306−7*
Sézary's syndrome 194, 269−70
sickle cell anaemia 111−16
  blood film *114*
  homozygous form 111−15
    aplastic crises 112
    clinical features *111, 112, 113*
    haemolytic crises 112
    laboratory findings 113, *114*
    treatment 113−15
    vascular−occlusive crises 111−12
    visceral sequestration crises 112
  sickle cell trait 118
sickle cells *29, 114*
sideroblastic anaemia *49−52*
  classification of **50**
  differential diagnosis 50, **51**−2
  lead poisoning 50
  in myelodysplastic syndromes 247
siderotic granules, *see* Pappenheimer bodies
signal transduction 8, *9*, 10−11
  growth factor receptors 8−9, **10**
    second messengers 10−11
sinus histiocytosis 271
spherocytes *29*
spherocytosis, hereditary 79, 81−3
  blood film *82*

spherocytosis, hereditary (*continued*)
  clinical features 81
  haematological findings 81, *82*
  inheritance 81
  pathogenesis 79, **81**
  tests for 81, *82*–3
  treatment 83
splenectomy
  in autoimmune thrombocytopenic purpura
    323, *324*
  in chronic lymphocytic leukaemia 243
  in chronic myeloid leukaemia 236
  haematological effects **386**, *387*–8
  immunological effects 388
splenic atrophy
  causes of *387*, 388–9
  see also splenectomy
splenic irradiation, in treatment of chronic
    myeloid leukaemia 236
splenomegaly 381–2
  causes of **381**
  haematological effects of 382
steroid purpura 319
stomatitis in megaloblastic anaemia *64*
streptokinase *311, 312*, 361–2
stress polycythaemia 292
Stuart–Prower factor **306**
subacute combined degeneration of cord 63, *64*
sulphinpyrazone 364
systemic disease, haematological involvement in
    366–91
  acute phase response 389, **390**–1
    C-reactive protein 390–1
    erythrocyte sedimentation rate 389
    plasma viscosity 390
  anaemia of chronic disorders **366**–7
  Gaucher's disease 382, *383*, *384*–5
  hypothyroidism 375
  infections 375, **376**–80
    bacterial *375*, 377
    viral 377, *378*–80
  liver disease *373*, *374*
  malignant diseases 367, *368*, **369**, *370*
    anaemia 367, *368*
    leucocyte changes 367
    platelet and blood coagulation abnormalities
      367–8
    polycythaemia 367
  Niemann–Pick disease 385
  pulmonary eosinophilia 380
  renal failure 370–1, **372**–3
    anaemia 370–1, *372*
    platelet and coagulation abnormalities 373
  rheumatoid arthritis 369–70, *371*
  splenectomy, effects of **386**, *387*–9
  splenomegaly **381**–2
  systemic mast cell syndrome 386
  tropical splenomegaly syndrome 385–6
systemic lupus erythematosus 369–70
systemic mast cell syndrome 386

T cells **163**, *164*
  maturation of 172, *173*–4

  receptor rearrangements 170, *171*, 189–90
  see also lymphocytes
target cells *29*
Tay–Sachs disease, haematological effects of
    382, *383*
testicular involvement in leukaemia 227
thalassaemia intermedia 108, *109*
thalassaemia trait, laboratory diagnosis **51**
thalassaemias 97–110
  alpha-thalassaemia syndromes 97–*100*, *101*
    blood film *101*
    classification of **99**
    genetics of *100*
  beta-thalassaemia major 101–8
    blood film *105*
    clinical features *103*, *104*
    diagnosis, laboratory 104, *105*–6
    geographical distribution *101*
    molecular pathology of **102**
    treatment 106, *107*–8
  beta-thalassaemia trait 109
    association with other haemoglobinopathies
      110
  classification of **99**
  delta, beta-thalassaemia 110
  geographical distribution of *98*
  haemoglobin Lepore 110
  hereditary persistence of foetal haemoglobin
    110
thrombasthenia 328
thrombin 308, **309**, 310
  inhibitors of 358
thrombin time **316**
  and circulating anticoagulant **347**
  disseminated intravascular coagulation **347**
  and heparin therapy **347**
  liver disease **347**
  massive transfusion **347**
  and oral anticoagulant therapy **347**
thrombocythaemia
  blood film *294*
  cells of origin 194
thrombocytopenia *320*–7
  acute immune 324
  causes of **321**
    failure of platelet production 320, **321**
    increased platelet destruction 320, **321**–7
  chronic immune 320, 322–4
  drug-induced *320*, **321**
  drug-induced immune *325*–6
  post-transfusion purpura 325
thrombocytosis, and systemic malignant disease
    369
thrombosis
  arterial 350–1
    clinical risk factors **351**
    pathogenesis 350–1
  laboratory tests for increased risk 355–6
  treatment of, *see* anticoagulant drugs
  venous 351–5
    pathogenesis 351–2
    risk factors 352, **353**, **354**–5
thrombosthenia 301
thrombotic thrombocytopenic purpura 326

thromboxane A$_2$ 303, *304*, 314
tissue factor **306**
tissue plasminogen activator *311, 312*
  inhibition of 312
  recombinant 362
total iron-binding capacity
  chronic inflammation/malignancy **51**
  iron deficiency anaemia *45*
  normal values **419**
  sideroblastic anaemia **51**
  thalassaemia trait **51**
toxoplasmosis, haematological effects of 379
transcobalamins 55—6
transferrin-bound iron **38**
tropical splenomegaly syndrome 385—6
tumour suppressor genes 198
tyrosine kinases, membraneassociated 197—8

uraemia, and platelet function disorders 329
urokinase *311, 312*, 361—2

vascular bleeding disorders 318—19
  acquired 318—19
  hereditary haemorrhagic telangiectasia 318,
    319
vascular—occlusive crises of sickle cell
    anaemia 111—12
vasoconstriction 313
venesection, in polycythaemia 289
very late activation (VLA) antigens 148
visceral sequestration crises of sickle cell
    anaemia 112
vitamin B$_{12}$ 53—7
  abnormal metabolism of 71
  absorption 54, *56*

biochemical reactions 56, *57, 58*
deficiency, *see* vitamin B$_{12}$ deficiency
dietary intake 54, **55**
normal values **419**
structure *54*
transcobalamins 55—6
transport 55—6
vitamin B$_{12}$ deficiency 60—2, 65, **67**, **68**—9
  causes of **60**
  effects of **64**
  laboratory tests for **67**, *68*—9
  neuropathy 63—*4*
  pernicious anaemia **61**—2
  prophylaxis 71
  treatment **69**, *70*—1
vitamin K antagonists, *see* anticoagulant drugs,
    oral
vitamin K deficiency 341, *342*—3
  children and adults 343
  haemorrhagic disease of newborn 342—3
    diagnosis 343
    treatment 343
von Willebrand factor *301, 302*, 303
  deficiency of, *see* von Willebrand's disease
von Willebrand's disease 339—40
  laboratory findings **336**, 339—40
  treatment 340

Waldenström's macroglobulinaemia 278—80
  clinical features *279*
  diagnosis 280
  treatment 280
warfarin, *see* anticoagulant drugs, oral
white cells, *see* leucocytes
whole blood transfusion 403
Wuchereria bancrofti, haematological changes
    380